DATE DUE

DE 19 '97			
NO 21 '03			

DEMCO 38-296

R

Improving Outcomes in Public Health Practice

Strategy and Methods

G. E. Alan Dever, PhD, MT
Associate Dean for Primary Care
Grassmann Chair of Rural Medicine
Director and Professor, Community Science Program
Director, Office of Health Policy
Mercer University School of Medicine
Macon, Georgia

An Aspen Publication®
Aspen Publishers, Inc.
Gaithersburg, Maryland
1997

Riverside Community College
Library
'97 4800 Magnolia Avenue
AUG Riverside, California 92506

rary of Congress Cataloging-in-Publication Data

Dever, G. E. Alan.
outcomes in public health practice : strategy and
methods / G.E. Alan Dever.
p. cm.
Includes bibliographical references and index.
ISBN 0-8342-0637-4
1. Public health administration—Evaluation. 2. Public health
administration—Quality control. 3. Total quality management.
4. Public health administration—Research—Statistical methods.
I. Title.
[DNLM: 1. Public Health Administration—standards. 2. Quality
Assurance, Health Care—organizational & administration. 3. Program
Evaluation—methods. 4. Epidemiologic Methods. WA 525 D4911 1997]
RA427.D48 1997
362.1'068'5—DC21
DNLM/DLC
for Library of Congress
95-24231
CIP

About Aspen Publishers • For more than 35 years, Aspen has been a leading professional
publisher in a variety of disciplines. Aspen's vast information resources are available in both
print and electronic formats. We are committed to providing the highest quality information
available in the most appropriate format for our customers. Visit Aspen's Internet site for more
information resources, directories, articles, and a searchable version of Aspen's full catalog,
including the most recent publications: **http://www.aspenpub.com**
Aspen Publishers, Inc. • The hallmark of quality in publishing
Member of the worldwide Wolters Kluwer group.

Editorial Resources: Bill Fogle

Library of Congress Catalog Card Number: 96-45614
ISBN: 0-8342-0637-4

Printed in the United States of America

1   2   3   4   5

He who you shake and

is active

—Creates Life

He who you shake and

is still

—Creates Thought

To

Wallace Earl Dever

1935–1994

and

Donald Andrew Dever

1930–1996

Table of Contents

Introduction

Public health and community health have faced some difficult challenges in the past few years, especially since the Institute of Medicine reported that public health was in disarray and that the infrastructure was in need of improvement. The condemnations of this institution have been many. And certainly in many sections of this book, I point these out so we are able to focus on improvements and emerge out of this crisis to be successful in our mission. To build a healthy public health and promote healthy communities, the practice of public health must, however, move beyond the rhetoric of public health and begin to base programs, plans, evaluation, and outcomes on evidence. The practice of evidence–based public health, however, requires the knowledge and ability of public health professionals to use and understand the methods and tools of quality improvement. During the early 1990s, public health began to adopt the principles and concepts of continuous quality improvement (CQI) as a management philosophy. Unfortunately, most agencies adopted the "team–building" components of this management style—the more "touchy–feely" aspects—and did not focus on the methods and tools to bring about this change, monitor the change, assess the change, and hold the gains made as a result of this change and monitor this on a continuous basis. Many books have described these team–building efforts, how to gain support for CQI in an agency, and how to develop and build this philosophy within the agency. This book is not an attempt to deliver the principles and concepts of CQI management; it is, however, a book that illustrates and describes the tools and methods for quality improvement and outcome measurement in public health practice so that agencies can develop assessments, policies, and assurances based on evidence and not on rhetoric or anecdotal situations.

I believe this book is a blueprint for public health to reinforce its traditional role of health education, health promotion, and disease prevention by assessing the needs of populations in communities through the three core functions of public health assessment, policy development, and assurance. The public health role of providing services to individuals in clinics, although declining, will also benefit significantly from the use and application of the tools and methods of quality improvement measurement. The book is divided into two parts—Part 1, entitled "Quality Improvement in Public Health Practice," addresses the basic issues facing public health from a quality improvement and outcome measurement perspective; and Part 2, "Basic Methods," presents some familiar approaches to analyzing public health problems but also gives the public health practitioner a new set of tools to analyze problems from a quality improvement and outcome measurement perspective.

QUALITY IMPROVEMENT IN PUBLIC HEALTH PRACTICE

The first part of this book outlines in four chapters the concepts of quality improvement as applied to public health. Clearly, some of our current efforts in public health are directed toward a more meaningful analysis of our problems by indirectly embracing methods and concepts of continuous measurement and quality improvement. Chapter 1, "Toward a Healthy Public Health," deals with the heavy criticism that public health has endured. Specifically, public health has been attacked for being in disarray and not having the ability to effectively communicate results and accomplishments of funded programs (i.e., no evidence–based practices). However, to develop a healthy public health, we must develop a vision that strengthens and enhances public health as being the primary provider of health promotion/education and disease prevention activities. The suggestion is to embrace quality improvement methods; however, the dependence of use of these methods must understand the nature of building healthy communities—are they ready, how can they solve problems, and what is their overall focus on how to achieve health? It is proposed that improved community health may be facilitated by using the appropriate quality improvement tools. Chapter 2, "Public Health Practice: Assessment," is not a strange topic to the public health practitioner. In fact, to meet the demands of determining the needs for population-based services, an assessment is of major importance. There are several traditional tools to accomplish this task using the Year 2000 objectives as a guide. Such traditional tools detailed are Model Standards, Assessment Protocol for Excellence in Public Health and Planned Approach to Community Health. Typically, these are the tools used in conjunction with the Year 2000 objectives. This chapter proposes an extension of these typical assessment tools to include the quality improvement model based on the plan, do, check, act (PDCA) cycle in meeting the Year 2000 objectives. The parallels drawn between the PDCA cycle and the traditional tools present alternatives for assessing needs and improving decision making at the community level. Chapter 3 is the only chapter that illustrates the difference in CQI, quality control, and quality assurance and how public health may benefit from understanding the CQI process. The concepts presented in this chapter represent major shifts in thinking from conventional to CQI. For complete understanding and incorporation of the basic methods of quality improvement into the everyday practice of public health practitioners, shifts in thinking must occur that encompass divergent/convergent thinking, creative/empirical thinking, and critical thinking. A process improvement model using these thinking concepts and the CQI approach is applied to public health. The final chapter of Part 1 is "Evidence-Based Public Health Practice." Public health must meet the challenges of the health industry, notably, scarce resources, government down–sizing, improved performance, and improved health outcomes. For these challenges to be met, decisions based on evidence must become commonplace as opposed to the present process of supporting decisions based on intuition, opinions, or anecdotes. This chapter provides a comprehensive framework for developing evidence–based public health practices. Thus, a model for setting priorities, setting guidelines, measuring performance, and improving performance for evidence–based decisions is detailed. The success of this model is predicated on the philosophy of life-long learning, and it is suggested that public health grand rounds, the learning cube, and critical appraisal become the tools to move the evidence–based process of decision making to a reality. Part 1 clearly defines why quality improvement measurement is so critical to the future of public health practice. The primary purpose of this part is to illustrate this need for expanded models that embrace the CQI philosophy yet show how the traditional public health perspective may be blended to move toward quality outcome measurement using quality improvement methods.

BASIC METHODS

A major objective of this book is to provide public health managers—present and future, epidemiologists, health planners, statisticians, and policy makers—with the knowledge and information needed for the analytical study of public health program processes by using the basic methods of quality improvement. In fact, this part on basic methods is intended to provide the public health practitioners with the methods for identifying problems and analyzing problems. Specifically, the evaluation of the effectiveness of management practices, the ability of management to be knowledgeable about a process improvement, the understanding of establishing program/process control, and the maintenance of current levels of program performance are four major benefits to public health practitioners who apply these basic methods to their situation. If the basic methods presented are viewed only as a means of reporting on program operations and not on the management practices that establish the program guidelines for improvement, then the opportunity to improve program outcomes (i.e., plans, methods, practices, and even program materials) will likely go unnoticed. To ensure the effective use of these basic methods, management must lead and direct the change. Thus, whether evaluating program change, assessing program performance, or ensuring program improvements are maintained, the methods for completing these tasks are presented in the part on "Basic Methods." The material in Chapter 5 will be most familiar to the public health practitioner. The basics of epidemiology become the building blocks of quality measurement for program improvements. Typically, the quality improvement tools presented in later chapters require the knowledge of understanding rates, ratios, and proportions. Further, certain technical considerations, such as statistical instability, validity, and reliability, are discussed as important in the evaluation of rates when measuring quality improvement. Critical to the understanding and evaluation of control charts—discussed in Chapters 9 and 10—is the discussion of measures of central location and dispersion presented in Chapter 6. To some it may seem trivial to discuss the use, advantages, and disadvantages of the mean, median, mode, range, and standard deviation; however, having this knowledge in hand is essential to the critical appraisal of the methods for quality improvement.

Quality improvement tools and methods may be generally described as being used for problem identification or problem analysis. The methods for problem identification are detailed in Chapter 7. Thus, such methods as surveys, checksheets/logs, focus groups, brainstorming, nominal groups, and flowcharts are presented. Many of these methods are used in public health practice to elicit data and describe situations; but in the context of quality improvement, these methods are also used for measuring process change and process improvement. The quality improvement methods for problem identification are outlined in Chapter 8. They are histograms, Pareto charts, cause–and–effect diagrams, run charts, stratification, scatter diagrams, control charts, and force–field analysis. Most of these tools for quality improvement are used very little by public health practitioners. Knowledge and guidance are needed for process improvements and change in public health practice. A critical component of this improvement work for the public health practitioner is the management and technical knowledge brought to the team for determining where and how to use these quality improvement tools that focus heavily on understanding statistics. The essence of the previous statement is brought to bear in the understanding and use of control charts, which are discussed in Chapters 9 and 10. Chapter 9 outlines the various types of control charts to be used when your data are discrete (i.e., counts). Thus, attribute control charts (control charts for counts) such as the "p" chart, "np" chart, "c" chart, and "u" chart are illustrated. Each chart is applicable to a typical public health problem. The material in this chapter is definitely new information for most public health practitioners. In fact, this requires the understanding of basic probability models (binomial and Poisson distributions) and further, this chapter guides the reader as to which chart should be selected based on the problem to be analyzed. This definitely strengthens the skills of the new public health scientist as they become more involved in the "where" and "how" of using these tools for quality improvement and outcome assessment. Likewise, the control charts presented in Chapter 10 are used in situations in which the program data represent continuous measurement. These control charts for continuous measurement (variables control charts) are mean and range charts ($\overline{X}$ and R charts), mean and standard deviation charts ($\overline{X}$ and s charts), median and range charts ($\overline{X}$ and R charts), and individual and moving range charts (X and mR charts). Situations are presented for the public health practitioner that illustrate the charts use and application in public health programs. As one might expect, the application of these charts requires a bit more statistical sophistication because some of the control limits (upper and lower) to be determined require the use of constants. However, tables are supplied giving the constants; therefore they do not have to be derived, but the reader is instructed as to where to find material or the derivation of these constants. Control charts become the basis for quality improvement measurement in public health, so it is critical that the reader become familiar with their use, application, and importance to the improvement and outcome measurement process.

Chapter 11 takes a familiar topic, small area analysis, from a hospital use perspective and, less familiar, from a public health perspective and demonstrates how these methods are used for quality improvement measurement in public health. On occasion, the combination of geography and/or rates/numbers results in small values that are difficult to interpret or, in most instances, are accepted as presented even though they may be in error. Small numbers produce large error, so methods are presented within the context of quality improvement so that the reader will have the skills to deal with small numbers in the context of process improvement and outcome assessment.

The demands in public health practice to base decisions on evidence has been mounting and now requires the proper analysis and interpretation of methods to demonstrate improvements based on sound scientific evidence. To do this, there is also a demand for increased statistical skills for process investigation in public health. As a result, an effect on the content of public health courses will occur in all public and community–based evidence programs to further the professional education of public health practitioners in the area of quality improvement methods. Clearly, this book has been written to meet the need of the public health practitioner who will be faced with providing evidence-based decisions related to assessing outcomes using the appropriate quality improvement tools and methods for determining priorities, setting guidelines, measuring performance, improving performance, and holding the gains.

Acknowledgments

Many talents were instrumental in the completion of this endeavor. I especially would like to thank Douglas W. Skelton, MD, Dean of the Mercer University School of Medicine, who has always provided me with resources, encouragement, and support. He is a man of science who understands the "art of things" and possesses both vision and insight—a powerful mixture. His confidence in this project has been unfailing.

I would also like to thank Bunnie V. Stamps who waded through books, articles, and magazines to find resources and references, typed drafts, designed and created charts, and finally, performed a thorough review of the galley proofs. She worked long and painful hours and was thoroughly committed to keeping the project on schedule.

In addition, I thank all the professionals and students who were exposed to this material through various consultations and course offerings at the national level for their constructive criticism and viewpoints on several quality improvement/ outcome assessment issues. I thank the Community Science faculty and staff at Mercer University School of Medicine, and particularly Diana Wilson and Martha Davis for handling all the logistical issues. I would also like to thank Dee Hansen and Joy Miller, who gave me opportunities to express my views on many of the issues detailed in this book.

The constant and never ending support for my writing comes from my best friend and wife Georgie. I could quite possibly be one of the most fortunate men to ever have such a true companion for life. Georgie's laughter, compassion, and understanding of my needs is why I am able to do these things. Thank you, Georgie. Thanks to my son Jamie and his fiance Mickey, my daughter Tammy and my son-in-law Marc, and especially to my grandson Andrew, who always makes my life playful and lets me see the humor in madness.

Thanks also to the Aspen team for keeping this project on schedule and for having the insight to develop ideas for improving the product. Thank you Michael Brown, Bob Howard, Bill Fogle, and Loree Sichelstiel.

Part I

Quality Improvement in Public Health Practice

Chapter 1

Toward a Healthy Public Health

"If you always do what you always did, You'll always get what you always got."[1(p.142)]

Arthur R. Tenner and Irving J. DeToro

To achieve a healthy public health to develop healthy communities in America requires the monitoring and surveillance of populations in communities as opposed to individuals in clinics. The perception of improved outcomes as proposed by intuition, rhetoric, generalities, and anecdote must be replaced by the reality of rigorous measurement of outcomes using quality improvement methods. For far too long, many public health practice claims have been forged by using the prevailing social conditions to substantiate future funding. To clarify the role of public health, a vision must be developed that is representative of a system of measurement for designing improvement and not a system oriented toward the status quo or mediocrity for defining improvement.

Typically, the public health vision must demonstrate excellence, the best in class, and be responsive to the community needs by developing healthy strategies that build a healthy public health.

An example vision for a healthy public health is the following: "During the next decade, we want to become the best health care organization (public health, state department, community health center, etc.) in the United States and an excellent agency overall and be recognized as such." This vision statement is strong, but we must develop a better one. Thus, "We will be the preferred provider of disease prevention and health promotion activities, surveillance of health trends, assessment of health status, assurance activities, and health development policies that satisfy the health needs of all customers." This vision tells us what is important. It has the potential of moving public health agencies toward a healthy public health. What has activated this need for a new vision? What has happened to public health? What is the future for public health? How do we get public health on track? In the next several chapters, answers are provided to these questions by focusing on the topic of quality improvement methods. Quality improvement methods, which may be applied on a continuous basis, are used to aid in developing the vision of public health and, further and more important, to provide the opportunity to grasp the tools and techniques to develop public health practice measurement. The belief is that this approach of understanding and applying quality improvement methods to public health practice problems, although not a panacea, will create the environment for developing a healthy public health.

TRENDS SHAPING A QUALITY IMPROVEMENT FOCUS IN PUBLIC HEALTH PRACTICE

Most of the health care organizations today are focusing on quality and continuous improvement to an unprecedented degree. However, public health's acceptance of ongoing and continuous measurement of progress using quality improvement methods is poor. To meet the demands of government regulations, to develop ongoing evaluation/monitoring systems, and to satisfy the public health customer, public health must develop and sustain a reputation for quality and continuous improvement by using the appropriate methods in public health practice. These types of changes suggest a new environment for health care.[2]

- Challenge, choice, and change threaten quality at a time when the general public is demanding higher levels of quality and service from government than ever before. If government health programs do not focus on quality improvement, the result is the dissatisfaction of customers, communities, employees, and public health clients;
- The trend toward quality measurement for aiding communities in assessing health outcomes and monitoring indicators for showing improvement in clinical services;
- "A commitment to quality reduces expenditures. Research on the cost of quality repeatedly shows that 20 to 30 percent of a typical organization's expenses are the result of redundancy of effort, rework, error, inefficiency, recurrent problems, untrained personnel, and cumbersome systems;"[3(p.3)]
- Attention to quality helps public health practitioners feel proud to be associated with their organization. Further, most public health care professionals want to ensure their organization supports excellence in service—few want to be taken for granted by saying that this is "the way we've always done things here."
- The public health organization that is focused on quality and has developed effective strategies and measurements for ensuring quality improvement will clearly be more effective in meeting the public evaluation and scrutiny.

Further, a report by the Pew Health Professions Commission notes that the health care system will face drastic changes that will have an effect on all aspects of medicine and public health. Specifically, by the end of this century, the health care system will, in general, be:

- more managed with better integration of services and financing
- more accountable to those who purchase and use health services
- more aware of and responsive to the needs of enrolled populations
- able to use fewer resources more effectively
- more innovative and diverse in how it provides for health
- more inclusive in how it defines health
- less focused on treatment and more concerned with education, prevention, and care management
- more oriented to improving the health of the entire population
- more reliant on outcomes data and evidence[4]

These changes in our health care system have significant implications for public health practice. Notably, the focus of public health practice on assessment, policy development, and assurance will most assuredly require public health officials to use fewer resources more effectively, be innovative and decisive in the provision (assurance) of health, adopt an epidemiologic model of health policy (lifestyle, environment, biology, and health care delivery system) (i.e., a broader definition of health),[5] be less focused on treatment and more focused on education and prevention, be oriented to improving the health of the entire population (assessment), and finally base decisions on outcomes and evidence-based parameters. To meet these challenges, the Pew Commission makes some specific recommendations for public health.

- Create new public health education programs that bring together the traditional public health disciplines with the clinical professions. These programs should be created in conjunction with state government, local government, managed care organizations, and other nonacademic institutions.
- Develop partnerships to apply population-based health management skills to the problems that are now faced by highly managed and integrated systems of care. These partnerships should include research, service, and training components.
- Create programs at the federal, state, and managed care organization levels to continue and enlarge the support base for a broad range of psycho-social-behavioral research and training.

- Reframe public health as a basic science in the personal and clinical health sciences and incorporate the new knowledge, skills, and competencies related to the analysis of health care as a system and the redesign of work for continuous quality improvement and innovation of care.
- Recognize the obligation at the state and federal level to adequately fund public health education and practice, particularly in an era of market-driven health care.[6]

QUALITY IMPROVEMENT IN PUBLIC HEALTH

As in other industries that have implemented quality improvement using the appropriate methods, quality improvement and measurement in public health also mean *doing the right things right* and *making continuous improvements.* Leebov and Ersoz have suggested that an organization can do right or wrong things and do them in a right or wrong way (Figure 1–1).

For example, *processes* that would meet the expectations of the public health customer in a streamlined, cost-effective manner are the right things. The processing and registering of vital events in a state vital records division would represent a streamlined cost-effective process. The *performance* by the employees and departments that conforms to these processes of registering vital events is things done right. Fortunately, processes and performance interact. When you clarify and improve processes, performance improves as a result.[7]

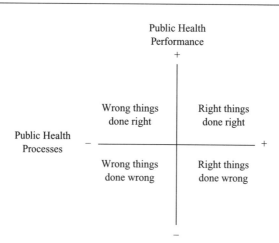

Figure 1–1 A Process/Performance Quality Improvement Scale. *Source:* Adapted with permission from *The Health Care Manager's Guide to Continuous Quality Improvement,* by Wendy Leebov, EdD, and Clara Jean Ersoz, MD, published by American Hospital Publishing, Inc., copyright 1991.

As suggested in Figure 1–1, there are four possibilities to consider when examining public health practice process and performance (i.e., assessment, policy development, and assurance). They are[8]

1. *Doing the right things wrong.* Your regional or district public health laboratory has a piece of equipment that is capable of producing very accurate and important test results, but the technicians do not use the equipment correctly; or your public health clinic providing family planning services has designed a very easy chart retrieval system, but the nurses using it do not return the clinic charts as appropriate.
2. *Doing the wrong things wrong.* You have an inefficient system for scheduling patients for block appointments, and the administrative people using this system make many mistakes when they give numbers and enter people's names on a check-in log sheet.
3. *Doing the wrong things right.* Always using the wrong definition of low birth weight but consistently using it the same way every time. Internationally, various countries define a low birth weight quite differently, resulting in making comparisons among countries almost impossible.
4. *Doing the right things right.* You have an excellent assessment model for health status evaluation, and you always apply it correctly in all situations. For example, Planned Approach to Community Health (PATCH),[9] Assessment Protocol for Excellence in Public Health (APEX*PH*),[10] model standards,[11] and the Plan Do Check Act (PDCA)[12] cycle.

These four scenarios may be viewed a little differently if one considers differences between traditional quality assurance and continuous quality improvement; "the right things done right" crossroads of public health performance and public health processes.[13] Leebov and Ersoz note that

> the emphasis in traditional quality assurance has been on monitoring whether the appropriate things are being done correctly. If they are not, actions are taken to correct *individual performance* to ensure better results in the future. In continuous quality improvement, the emphasis is also on doing the right things right, but in the face of problems, attention is directed first and foremost to [understanding and measuring] the *process.* Improvement efforts focus on identifying the root causes of problems (causes stemming from the process rather than individual performance) and intervening to reduce or eliminate these causes, taking steps to correct the process.[14(pp.4–5)]

In public health, doing the right things right and making continuous quality improvements make it possible for the organization to achieve the following: (1) establish appropriate prevention programs for communities, (2) achieve improvements in the health status of a population, (3) satisfy *all* customers (communities and patients [i.e., populations and individuals]), (4) recruit and retain professional personnel in the new sciences of population-based medicine and public health practice, and (5) be accountable to the customers, including the funding agencies.

Although communities cannot always judge the appropriateness and/or the types of public health prevention programs, professionals in your organization can. In the public health arena, doing the right things right is analogous to *doing appropriate things effectively.* The question to be asked by public health practitioners is, Is this action (i.e., a program, an analysis, or a management decision) relevant and necessary (appropriate), and if so, how can we be sure it will be done right (effectively)?

To answer this question, Leebov and Ersoz have suggested an Appropriate/ Effectiveness Quality Improvement Scale[15] (Figure 1–2). As with the Process/ Performance Scale (Figure 1–1), there are four possibilities for public health practitioners to consider when measuring and evaluating the appropriateness and effectiveness of public health programs.

1. *Appropriate things done ineffectively.* A family planning program with an objective to reduce or eliminate teenage pregnancy, but the teenage pregnancy rates do not change. Typically, the motive or reason for the family planning program is appropriate, but the effectiveness of the delivery of the program to reduce teenage pregnancy is questionable. There is significant "gut reaction" support or feeling that the program is appropriate to continue; however, we get ineffective results. This may be true or not true, but because

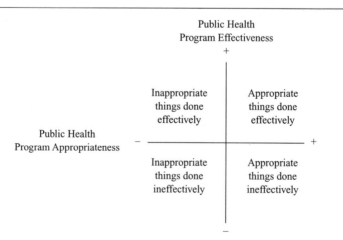

Figure 1–2 An Appropriate/Effectiveness Quality Improvement Scale. *Source:* Adapted with permission from *The Health Care Manager's Guide to Continuous Quality Improvement,* by Wendy Leebov, EdD, and Clara Jean Ersoz, MD, published by American Hospital Publishing, Inc., copyright 1991.

we do not have any evidence-based evaluation of the effectiveness of this program, it appears that it is done ineffectively or we just do not know.

2. *Appropriate things done effectively.* In public health practice, the immunization program is an excellent example of doing the appropriate things effectively. This is quite possibly the most successful prevention program with which public health is identified. There is clear evidence that increased immunization levels result in the effective reduction of childhood infectious diseases.

3. *Inappropriate things done effectively.* Quite possibly, the development of an integrated clinical management information system in public health is an effective tool, but given the changing nature of public health (i.e., moving away from providing clinic services and moving toward prevention), it is very likely that it may be most inappropriate. As noted earlier, public health is also being affected by managed care networks; in fact, the impact is such that many, if not all, clinical activities will be the domain of the managed care systems. Thus, a clinical management information system in public health would be most inappropriate.

4. *Inappropriate things done ineffectively.* From a public health clinical point of view and more recently from the medical profession point of view (costs considered), the Early and Periodic Screening, Diagnosis, and Treatment (EPSDT) program is done ineffectively, and it is certainly not appropriate for public health clinics to provide this service. Obviously, there is considerable debate over this issue. A main reason for this position is that in many states the current reimbursement for this service is at such a level that private physicians are now providing the care that was once traditionally only provided by public health clinics. In any event, this "loss leader" public health program appears to be inappropriate due to costs and ineffective due to time constraints needed to deliver the programs. A major debate about this EPSDT program is, Who gives the best quality of service? Again, without evidence-based evaluation about the outcomes and quality of the program, the program is at risk of being considered inappropriate and ineffective from a public health perspective. Of course, this debate may be moot with the current trend to managed care services.

Public health practice is faced with measuring and evaluating performance, process, effectiveness, and appropriateness. The key is to do what is appropriate effectively and do the right things right. The nature of continuous quality improvement and measurement as practiced from a public health perspective is to ensure that the core functions of assessment, policy development, and assurance are performed effectively and appropriately and that the right things are being done right. The vision of developing a healthy public health to produce healthy communities, including satisfying the customer, must adopt these strategies, which clearly indicates the need for quality improvement methods.

HEALTHY COMMUNITIES

The National Association of County and City Health Officials, in its July 1994 release of "Blueprint for a Healthy Community," summarized the following 10 essential activities that are required to be performed by health systems if communities are to be healthy. The essential required activities are as follows:[16]

1. conducting community diagnosis: collecting, managing, and analyzing health-related data for the purpose of information-based and evidence-based decision making
2. preventing and controlling epidemics: investigating and containing diseases and injuries
3. providing a safe and healthy environment: maintaining clean and safe air, water, food, and facilities
4. measuring performance/process, effectiveness/appropriateness, and outcomes of health services: monitoring health care providers and the health care system
5. promoting healthy lifestyles: providing health education to individuals and communities
6. providing laboratory testing: identifying disease agents
7. providing targeted outreach and forming partnerships: ensuring access to services for all vulnerable populations and ensuring the development of culturally appropriate care
8. providing personal health care services: treating illness, injury, disabling conditions, and dysfunction (ranging from primary and preventive care to specialty and tertiary treatment); probably an inappropriate activity for public health as managed care becomes more evident
9. conducting research and innovative programs: discovering and applying improved health care delivery mechanisms and clinical interventions
10. mobilizing the community for action: providing leadership and initiating collaboration

Public health at the federal, state, or local levels will not necessarily perform all these activities directly. But the structure and capacities of public health must ensure that each citizen lives in a community that is served effectively by these activities.[17]

The ways in which these activities are to be accomplished and the most appropriate and effective ways to ensure that communities can be healthy are significant challenges. However, by using quality improvement methods, principles, concepts, and tools, public health practitioners will be positioned to respond effectively to this challenge.

Meeting these recommendations and managing populations in communities as opposed to individuals in clinics will require the skills and competencies found only in the public health disciplines such as epidemiology, health policy and administration, biostatistics, health services research skills, health education, evaluation, and other parts of the intellectual core of the public health disciplines. These are the basic tools for assessing the health needs of populations, developing programs of intervention, and evaluating their costs and efficacy.[18] This will require "new links among schools of public health, the profession of public health and the emerging integrated delivery systems [of managed care]."[19(p.37)]

The Pew report states specifically that

> the needs of the integrated systems will not be met simply by hiring public health professionals. As care is managed throughout organizations, so clinicians throughout the system will need to develop the requisite skills to manage the health of and improve[ing] the value of care for the enrolled populations. This will require substantial and ongoing retraining of [public health professionals,] nurses, physicians, allied health personnel and managers. *Epidemiologists, biostatisticians, health educators and others will be essential to this undertaking, but they will be required to apply their skills in contexts. For example, large numbers of health professionals will require retraining in disease prevention, clinical epidemiology, process and systems analysis and managerial epidemiology [i.e., a new Public Health Practice]* (emphasis added).[20(p.37)]

Thus, all these activities and developments point to a renaissance for the public health professions, practice, and evaluation.

However, to create healthy communities also requires solving community problems, and this presents another challenge for public health practitioners.

Solving Community Problems

Solving community problems necessitates satisfying the customer—the community. In fact, according to a 1994 survey conducted by The Daniel Yankelovich Group for the Healthcare Forum, most Americans place their greatest confidence in others like themselves for solving community problems (Figure 1–3).[21] Most interesting about this survey is that local, state, and federal governments are ranked very low by Americans for solving community problems. Public health programs and the practice of public health are local or state efforts. Clearly, public health must turn to the communities, to friends, and to others if healthy communities are to be created. The notion of doing the most appropriate and effective thing must be tied to the appropriate activity to emphasize whether community

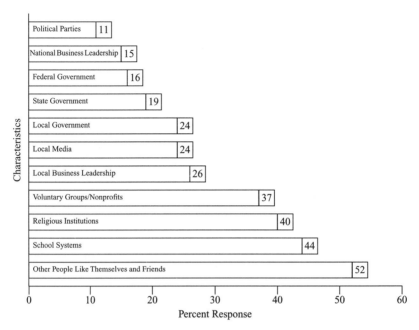

Figure 1–3 Where Americans Place Their Confidence for Solving Community Problems. *Source:* Adapted from *What Creates Health? Individuals and Communities Respond,* April 1994, by The Healthcare Forum.

problems are to be solved, thereby creating a healthy community. According to a Chinese proverb, *"Tell me, I forget. Show me, I remember. Involve me, I understand."* The message for solving community problems is to involve *me.* Thus, to solve is to involve.

Traditionally, citizens have had little opportunity to influence the decisions about the health of their communities, as well as other needs, priorities, and services. Citizen involvement has long been recognized as an important ingredient in developing appropriate and effective sustainable community development. Too often, however, involving citizens in the decision-making process consists of allowing them a few moments to state their view at public hearings held near the end of the process, when a decision has, for all intents and purposes, already been made. This amounts to extremely limited citizen *input* rather than meaningful citizen *involvement.* Citizens often leave these forums believing that their input will not be considered.[22] Our customers, in public health the citizens (community), become quite dissatisfied. In promoting quality improvement, it is imperative we give more attention to our community-based customers and measure (using appropriate improvement methods) their levels of satisfaction because this will certainly enhance the vision of creating healthy communities.

If community participation takes the form of more formal mechanisms, such as citizen advisory committees, task forces, commissions, or panels, research suggests that such forums are "generally ritualistic endeavors designed to shroud an elitist policy-making process in the cloak of democracy... the essence of decision making remains the triumph of conservative, business interests. Strategies designed specifically to facilitate direct involvement by certain groups (e.g., the poor) frequently do not work to their benefit."[23] Thus, it has been concluded that these deliberately designed mechanisms are rarely effective.[24] Certainly, as these authors note, the success rate is diminished when only "lip service" is given. This is certainly an example of doing the wrong things right or appropriate things ineffectively. Our goal in public health practice is to get on the right track and make a difference by enhancing community involvement and promote customer satisfaction—the number one tenet to be measured in a quality improvement endeavor for public health practice.

If public participation is to be meaningful, citizens must be heard not only before a final decision is made but from the beginning to the end of the decision-making process. Citizens must be able to influence the entire process, from defining the problem to developing alternative solutions and evaluating the alternatives to making the final decision (i.e., doing the right things right).[25]

In the healthy communities process, citizen participation involves a broad diversity of community representation *meaningfully* involved in addressing community health problems. Communities that have successfully implemented the healthy communities process recognize the importance of[26]

- including the citizens most affected at all stages of the process
- expanding ownership of the solutions so that a few individuals do not "burn out"
- creating a basis for communitywide priority setting and decision making
- using open-ended questions to identify health issues and to ensure that the agenda really comes from the residents
- connecting with the school system to gain more youth input
- finding other ways to reach vulnerable individuals in the community
- acknowledging the need to go where citizens feel comfortable
- using personal networking as one of the most important ways to bring more citizens into the healthy communities process.[27]

In a recent newsletter, a synopsis of McKnight's input on building communities is described:

> McKnight observed that community problems tend to be addressed using one of two major strategies. The first and most prevalent strategy identifies a community's needs and addresses them through problem-

oriented policies and programs. McKnight stated this approach leads to a view of the neighborhood and its residents as needy and deficient. Over time, residents view themselves as powerless to improve their neighborhoods and dependent on outside resources. McKnight believes this approach inherently breaks down a community's problem-solving skills and fosters dependence on outside agencies.

By contrast, the second approach identifies and builds on a community's skills and assets. McKnight's groundbreaking work shows this approach fosters community self-reliance, encourages independence, and succeeds even in the most destitute of urban neighborhoods. Yet, McKnight stated this approach is not widely used because funding agencies reinforce needs-based approaches, even though financial constraints demand approaches fostering self-reliance.

McKnight concluded that professionals successful in community-based programs tend to:

- have a deep respect for citizens and their communities, seeing themselves not as "the experts," but as *equal partners* in community efforts
- *share information* not easily known by the community in *usable, understandable* forms
- use their skills, contacts and resources to *magnify and empower* community commitment and efforts, rather than to gain credit or resources for themselves
- focus not on needs, but on *building community strengths by increasing social problem-solving skills.*[28(p.2)]

Thus, involving the individuals who are most affected by an issue from the very beginning is essential to developing sustainable efforts to improve health. They understand the underlying factors and know best what will make a difference. By participating in developing and sustaining their own solutions, they also gain a greater sense of control over their lives, which is the basis of improved health.[29]

McKnight's tenets have been embellished by Lundy, who developed 10 strategies to describe meaningful citizen participation. They are

1. power to make decisions and affect outcomes
2. citizen driven; from the community up, not top down
3. proactive, not reactive
4. encourages and facilitates broad community involvement
5. inclusive, not exclusive; accessible to all
6. balanced representation in the participation process; not just major "stakeholders"
7. consensus-oriented decision making
8. continuum of participation; support for entering at *your* level of participation

9. compromise; give and take
10. opportunities for involvement in *all* levels of activity, which include creating a vision, planning, prioritizing, deciding, evaluating[30]

To facilitate these strategies identified by McKnight and Lundy, the National Civic League has developed a "Civic Index," a checklist to evaluate a community's readiness for solving community problems.

Civic Index

The National Civic League (NCL) developed the "Civic Index"[*] to help communities evaluate and improve their civic infrastructure for building "healthy communities."[31] NCL defines the Civic Index as a description of the types of skills and processes that must be present for a community to deal effectively with its unique concerns.[32] The 10 components of the Index (i.e., the checklist) are presented in Table 1–1.

The 10 components of the Index represent a description of the types of skills and processes that must be present for a community to deal effectively with its unique concerns.[33] As the report notes, "The Civic Index assists communities in developing their problem-solving capacity by providing a method and a process for first identifying and recognizing their strengths and weaknesses, and then structuring collaborative approaches to solving shared problems. The Index provides a framework within which communities can undertake a self-evaluation of their civic infrastructure."[34(p.1)]

This community self-evaluation is a major step toward developing and building a healthy community. The outcome of this evaluation demonstrates the actions a community must take—the types of skills and processes it must develop or improve—to build its own capacity to deal with health-related critical issues.[35] Indicative of the need for this Civic Index checklist has been the trend away from analyzing individuals in clinics (or communities) and the trend toward analyzing populations in communities.

COMMUNITY FOCUS

Individual to Community Focus

The use and application of quality improvement methods within public health organizations have been very limited. In fact, the focus on the experience of the

---

[*]Civic Index is a perceptual tool, i.e., it measures how well citizens think their community is doing on the 10 dimensions, as opposed to a "hard data" analysis.

Table 1–1 Building Healthy Communities—A Civic Index Checklist

Index Components	Index Questions
1. Citizen participation	1. Do citizens volunteer to serve on local boards?
	2. How visible and active are local civic groups?
	3. Do citizens know how local government works?
	4. Is participation proactive or reactive?
	5. Are citizens actively involved in major projects?
2. Community leadership	1. Is there active leadership from all three sectors (public, private, nonprofit)?
	2. Is government willing to share leadership turf?
	3. Are there training programs to nurture new leaders?
	4. Is leadership results-oriented?
	5. Is leadership risk-taking?
	6. Do leaders take the long-term view?
	7. Do leaders from the three sectors work well together?
3. Government performance	1. Is government free of corruption?
	2. Does government address qualitative concerns about services?
	3. Is government professional and entrepreneurial?
	4. Is government responsive and accountable?
	5. Are services provided equitably?
	6. Does government consider and use alternative methods of service delivery?
	7. Is government a positive force in addressing community needs?
4. Volunteerism and philanthropy	1. Is there an active community foundation?
	2. Do local corporations have active giving programs?
	3. Does the community have long-term philanthropic goals?
	4. Do local programs encourage and honor volunteers and philanthropists?
	5. Do government and business work closely with the nonprofit sector?
5. Intergroup relations	1. Is the community dealing with ethnic and racial diversity?
	2. Does the community promote communication among diverse populations?
	3. Do all groups have the skills to become involved in the community?
	4. Do groups cooperate in resolving broad disputes?
	5. Do small, specific conflicts escalate into larger issues?
	6. Is the community dominated by narrow special-interest groups?

Table 1–1 continued

Index Components	Index Questions
6. Civic education	1. Do schools promote or require community involvement? 2. Do schools, churches, and youth agencies offer civic education? 3. Do civic education efforts involve the entire community? 4. Do youth have ample opportunity to engage in community service? 5. Are schools teaching citizenship and civic responsibility?
7. Community information sharing	1. Do citizens have information they need to make good decisions? 2. What role does government play in making information available? 3. Do schools and libraries play a role in informing the public? 4. Are there civic organizations designed for this purpose? 5. Do the media cover community issues fairly? 6. Do the media play an active and supportive role in the community?
8. Capacity for cooperation and consensus building	1. Are there neutral forums and processes in which all opinions are heard? 2. Are there informal dispute resolution processes? 3. Do community leaders have regular opportunities to share ideas? 4. Are all major interests represented in collaborative processes? 5. Do all three sectors work together to set common goals? 6. Do leaders reach collective decisions and implement them?
9. Community vision and pride	1. Is there a shared sense of a desired future for the community? 2. Has the community completed a broad strategic plan? 3. Does the community have a positive self-image? 4. Does the community preserve and enhance what is special and unique? 5. Does the community proactively monitor critical issues? 6. Does the community deal with problems before they become crises?
10. Intercommunity cooperation	1. How do local governments relate to each other? 2. How do regionwide policy challenges get resolved? 3. Is economic development addressed on a regionwide basis? 4. Do leaders in the region have a common forum to discuss issues? 5. Are any services provided on a regional basis? 6. Are any planning activities carried out on a regional basis?

individual patient in public health clinics has virtually gone unnoticed in a quality improvement sense. The application of quality improvement concepts and methods must go beyond the individual focus and focus on the population or community and reflect an epidemiologic or ecologic approach.[36]

Mettee has demonstrated, using a Community-Oriented Primary Care (COPC) model, the relationship of the individual focus to the community focus using the *s*ubjective, *o*bjective, *a*ssessment, *p*lanning (SOAP) format.[37] Mettee clearly acknowledged the importance of the community as a patient to have an effect on the health of the population to build healthy communities. A more recent study has elaborated on Mettee's approach by establishing a continuum to guide the clinical and public health practice from the individual to the community[38] (Table 1–2). This continuum using the SOAP format progresses from the individual, family, and institution to the community. As described in the matrix, each category of individual, family, institution, and community suggests variables to measure for the corresponding levels of measurement of the subjective, objective, assessment, prognosis, and plan process for building healthier communities. This shift in public health practices from an individual focus to a community focus must emphasize measurement and measures that use a quality improvement approach. Kaluzny has noted, "Given that groups starting to work on health care issues tend to revisit learned positions and old grievances, the community effort will probably do well to focus first on community health status indicators and community satisfaction measures to develop a common experience base and definition of the problem before trying to change specific organizational activities. Once these have been studied, leaders should be able to identify which limited sets of quality-of-care measures should be collected and monitored first."[39] (p.178)

The speed with which quality improvement methods can proceed and be applied will probably depend very much on the character of the community. As suggested previously, to build healthy communities a community must evaluate its readiness to implement and improve its health status by using the Civic Index checklist. Further, public health practitioners must be poised to identify a community's readiness and begin to establish a process whereby quality improvement outcome measurement can begin.

Illness (Disease) to Wellness (Prevention) Focus

Along with the shift in focus from the individual to the community is the shift from illness to wellness, which challenges the very nature of "the core business" of many participating institutions, specifically hospitals.[40] Historically, the hospital has been the leading major institution focusing on acute care; however, as the communitywide emphasis shifts to wellness and primary care from illness, the result is that acute care is no longer the core business of health care.

Table 1-2 Guide to Clinical and Public Health Practice

	Individual	Family	Institution	Community
Subjective				
Qualitative data	Medical history Interviewing	Medical history Family genogram Family interview	Institutional history Institutional charts Interviews with management/staff	Written and oral history of community Interviews with citizens
Profile of symptoms	Patient symptoms	Family symptoms	Institutional symptoms	Community symptoms
Explanation of problem(s)	Patient's explanation(s) of problems	Family's explanation(s) of problem(s)	Institution's explanation(s) of problems	Community's explanation(s) of problem(s)
Perception of resources	Patient's perception of personal resources	Family perception of family resources	Institution's perception of institutional resources	Community's perception of community resources
Objective				
Direct and indirect observations	Physical exam findings (signs)	Family observations Home visits Household assessment	Institutional observations and assessment of —human resources —financial resources —capital resources —building and space Site visits	Community's observations of —social conditions —housing characteristics —geology and geography —natural and man-made resources, barriers, and hazards —institutional resources —the county infrastructure
Quantitative data	Results of laboratory tests, imaging studies, and other ancillary investigations	Tests for familial diseases (hereditary) Family demographics and epidemiologic data list	Institutional documents, reports, files, and records Administrative data sets	Findings from —geographic information —photographs and maps —mortality/morbidity studies —demographic, epidemiologic, economic, and sociologic data sets
Assessment				
Diagnostic process	Individual problem and resource list—compared with normal values	Family problems and resource list—compared with accepted standards	Institutional problem and resource list—rating of institutions and physicians (profiling)	Community problem and resource list—compared with a standard (Year 2000 objective)
Prognosis				
Knowledge of the natural history	—of individuals in health and disease ("individual life cycle")	—of families that are functional or dysfunctional ("family life cycle")	—of institutions that are thriving or failing ("institutional life cycle")	—of communities and cultures in adaptive or maladaptive states ("community life cycle")
Plan				
Disease prevention Health promotion (primary prevention) Treatment (secondary prevention) Rehabilitation (tertiary prevention) Supportive care	Advice Patient education Medication Counseling	Advice Family education Family counseling Family therapy	Advice Institutional education Innovations and change strategies Total quality management	Advice Community education Community-based programs and social services Jobs Advocacy

Source: Adapted from "Family Health Science and the New Generalist Practitioner" by R.C. Like, *Family Systems Medicine* 11, no. 2 (1993):161.

Kaluzny noted that "this shift has upset the natural leadership pattern within communities. Hospitals as the historical 'center' of the system once had the managerial leverage to drive the system, but with acute care no longer the 'core business,' there exists a leadership vacuum within many communities."[41(p.180)] How this is resolved will vary by the state of community readiness—and will perhaps be resolved in the communitywide improvement process.[42] One thing is certain: The shift from inpatient care to outpatient has hospitals re-creating themselves to focus on disease prevention and health promotion. Such a shift leads to the establishment of wellness programs.

Wellness Focus

Travis makes a distinction between holism and wellness: "The primary orientation of holistic health is still towards healing conditions of illness. In contrast, the primary orientation of wellness is on increasing conditions of wellness."[43(p.102)] Specifically, the wellness model focuses on four dimensions: (1) physical activity, (2) nutritional awareness, (3) stress management, and (4) self-responsibility.

Travis developed the concept of an illness–wellness continuum[44] (Figure 1–4). The neutral point indicates no illness or wellness. Movement to the left shows poorer conditions of illness; movement to the right shows better levels of wellness. For instance, it is possible to be not quite physically ill, yet to experience depression, anxiety, frustration, and an overall dissatisfaction with life. Although traditional medicine may eliminate discernible physical illness, wellness goes beyond this point and deals with aliveness and enlightenment. The Year 2000 objectives have been more directed to wellness and community and support the tenets of Travis.[45]

Achieving Health for All—2000

Thinking about the components of health care and ways to achieve health for all has shifted from the "self-centered" activities of the holistic models in the

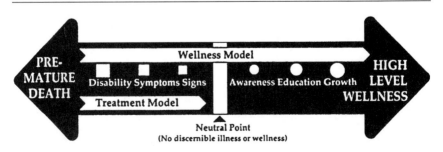

Figure 1–4 Illness–Wellness Continuum. *Source:* Reprinted from J.W. Travis, *Wellness Workbook,* p. 10, © 1988, Ten Speed Press.

1980s to an approach that embraces communities yet supports the tenets of individual participation in achieving health. This new vision of health requires an understanding of the changing nature of society as portrayed in the social transformation disease model.[46] Many countries, as well as the World Health Organization (WHO), have embraced this shift in focus to a more balanced policy that promotes health by supporting communities and fostering individual participation.[47–51]

In the United States, efforts have been directed toward establishing health objectives for the year 2000[52,53] (e.g., reducing tobacco use and improving surveillance and data systems)[54] and studying the future of public health.[55] Despite these efforts, public health in the United States is in a state of disarray. Although there is a focus on issues, such as preventive services, health protection, health promotion, objectives for vulnerable groups, expansion of access, social and physical correlates of disease, data collection needs, the objective process, and funds for health promotion and disease prevention,[56,57] there is not a framework for action—no overall strategy or policy. Similarly, there is no strategy for dealing with the health care priorities: human immunodeficiency virus (HIV) infection, drug abuse, health problems of the poor and minorities, the high cost of health care, long-term care, and health care for the uninsured and underinsured.[58]

Given the fragmented situation in the United States, the Canadian experience is to be evaluated. Epp outlined a model with components that are not topical or issue-based but are concepts, challenges, and strategies for achieving health for all Canadians by the year 2000 (Figure 1–5).[59]

The health *challenges* identified in Epp's model are (1) reducing inequities in the health of low- versus high-income groups in Canada, (2) increasing the prevention effort to find new and more effective ways of preventing the major cripplers and killers (e.g., estimated 45 percent reduction in mortality through lifestyle changes alone),[60] and (3) enhancing one's capacity to cope with chronic problems, disabilities, and mental health problems. The latter requires a capacity-building strategy at the individual level in contrast to traditional services-building policies that can be incapacitating or can foster dependency.[61,62] This point is critical to health care in the twenty-first century as the baby boom becomes the senior boom.

These critical challenges of the twenty-first century can be met through a broadened application of health promotion and disease prevention efforts. In the process of enabling individuals to increase control over and to improve their health, self-care, mutual aid, and healthy environments are the mechanisms to be promoted. Self-care comprises the decisions and actions that *individuals* take in the interest of their own health or simply healthy choices. Mutual aid, however, involves groups such as families, neighborhoods, communities, voluntary organizations, and self-help groups, in which individuals work together; support each other emotionally; and share ideas, information, and experiences. Thus, informal

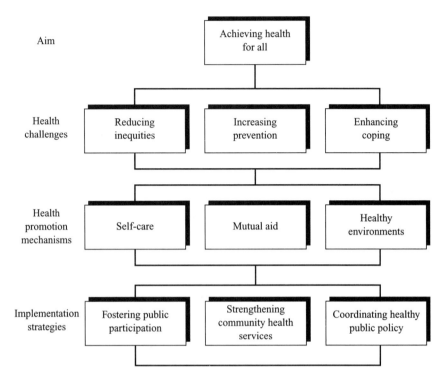

Figure 1–5 Framework for Health Promotion. *Source:* Reprinted with permission from *Canadian Journal of Public Health* 77, No. 6, p. 402, © 1986, Canadian Public Health Association.

networking is a basic resource in the promotion of health. The value of such mutual aid is that it enables individuals to live interdependently within a community while maintaining their independence. Ironically, the third health promotion mechanism, the healthy environment, was all but discarded during the transition from infectious diseases to chronic diseases. Now, in the 1990s and in the twenty-first century, the environment is seen as a major and critical component of health and well-being. This perspective must broaden to include social and economic, not just physical, elements. Education, labor, transportation, and health agencies must come together to promote legislation that will achieve a healthy environment.

To meet these health challenges and ensure that the health promotion mechanisms are implemented, Epp identified a set of strategies: (1) fostering public participation, (2) strengthening community health services, and (3) coordinating healthy public policy.[63] Health is a function of participation, and a strategy that is directed toward public participation is of paramount importance to the improvement in disease patterns. Individuals must participate not only to improve their own health but also to deal with such societal problems as drug abuse, homelessness, illiteracy, acquired immune deficiency syndrome (AIDS), social injustice, inequity, and ecologic threats.

Community health services must be strengthened in two ways. First, public health professionals must strengthen and expand their services to promote health. Second, communities must build their capacity to resolve their own health problems. This concept of capacity building versus service assistance in communities has emerged in the 1990s as a major policy shift that will be essential to our aim of ensuring conditions in which individuals and communities can be healthy.

The third strategy—coordinating healthy public policy—will be the most critical in ensuring health for all in the 1990s and well into the twenty-first century. It will require changes in thinking about ways to improve and promote health in the next 10 to 20 years. This change in direction will result in our directing change.[64] In the 1980s, health was recognized as a function of lifestyle, environment, biology, and health care delivery system. This model, which is still useful, was initially adopted in the United States in the public health arena. Yet, outside this arena, it has seldom been recognized. This lack of recognition cannot continue in the 1990s and into the 2000s. It is essential to coordinate policies among various sectors, which obviously do not share the same priorities. For example, a chemical company that dumps toxic waste into a river may argue that it would have to release employees if forced to clean up the pollution. This creates a dilemma, as a community needs both clean water and jobs. This type of ethical conflict will dominate the 1990s and will require health-promoting policy in such fields as energy, transportation, food, agriculture, economics, environment, education, and technology—not just in the health care sector. Thus, the challenge will be to advocate and coordinate healthy public policy.

The health promotion framework outlined by Epp may be of value to the United States in formulating a health policy. Epp stated, "Use it to visualize the kinds of mechanisms and strategies that are needed to support and encourage *Americans* as they strive to live healthy full lives. The framework links together a set of concepts, providing us with a particular way of thinking about and taking action toward achieving our aim of health for everyone in this country."[65(p.393)]

WHAT IS PUBLIC HEALTH PRACTICE?

Public health practice is composed of the core functions of public health—assessment, policy development, and assurance. These three core functions of public health represent 10 organizational practices as outlined by the Centers for Disease Control and Prevention (CDC) in their working draft report of August 1991.[66] Table 1–3 summarizes the three core functions and the 10 organizational practices

Table 1–3 Public Health Organization Practices

Core Function	Organizational Practices	Definition	Application of Practice
A. Assessment practices	1. Assess the health needs of the community by establishing a systematic needs assessment process that periodically provides information on the health status and health needs of the community	*Assessing health needs* is the process of systematically describing the prevailing health status and needs of a community	The organizational application of this practice provides the systematic collection and organization of health data in a usable format for analysis to determine health problems of a population. It provides the coordination and structure required to collect, transmit, organize, and make available information, from both internal and external data sources, to users in the public health system. The data collected should provide information on morbidity, mortality, disability, environmental health hazards, available heath services, and other health needs. Through this practice, information is provided to analyze health needs, establish health policy, develop health plans, and target health service delivery
	2. Investigate the occurrence of adverse health effects and health hazards in the community by conducting timely investigations that identify the magnitude of health problems, duration, trends, location, and populations at risk	*Investigation* is to initiate a systematic response to obtain information regarding health *effects*, acute and chronic diseases, premature death, disability, and environmental health hazards	The organizational application of this practice provides for the initiation of investigations and the appropriate response to protocols to control and prevent disease, injury, and exposure to biologic, chemical, or environmental health hazards that may result in death or disability
	3. Analyze the determinants of identified health needs to identify etiologic and contributing factors that place certain segments of the population at risk for adverse health outcomes	*Public health analysis* is the process of examining data to establish the *determinants* of community health needs	This organizational practice provides for the systematic study of health data to determine health problems and their magnitude, temporal trends, location, affected population, and causes. Within the organization, the practice must provide an operational framework for the synthesis of data to determine the community health status and identify determinants and contributing factors of health problems. Through this practice, interpretation and presentation of findings are made so appropriate health policy, plans, and programs can be developed

B. Policy development practices			
	1. Advocate for public health, build constituencies, and identify resources in the community by generating supportive and collaborative relationships with public and private agencies and constituent groups for the effective planning, implementation, and management of public health activities	To *advocate for public health* is the process of generating support among constituent groups that address community health needs and issues. *Community resources identification* and *constituency building* are the processes of establishing collaborative relationships between a public health agency and the public it serves, the government body it represents, and other health-related organizations in the community	This organizational practice coordinates and directs agency actions to identify issues where constituent support will be solicited, to identify where support and opposition coexist within the community, to design methods to promote community support and resource development, to establish and use networks and communication channels, and to facilitate and empower the community to act in its own behalf. Constituent support is critical to agency operation and performance of all organizational practices such as management of system resources, plan and policy development, and implementation of public health programs
	2. Set priorities among health needs based on the size and seriousness of the problems and the acceptability, economic feasibility, and effectiveness of interventions	*Priority setting* is the process of listing, ordering, and classifying community health problems based on the size and seriousness of the problem and the acceptability, economic feasibility, and effectiveness of interventions	This organizational practice provides structure for ordering health needs according to their importance, determined on the basis of qualitative, quantitative, social, economic, and political analyses, and to the availability of scientifically effective intervention methods. Through it, a decision-making structure is provided to direct and select methods and participants who will implement the priority-setting process and establish rank order of the health needs. Through the use of this practice, the agency arrives at decisions that direct its efforts in the practice of plan and policy development and resource management
	3. Develop plans and policies to address priority health needs by establishing goals and objectives to be achieved through a systematic course of action that focuses on local community needs and equitable distribution of resources and involves the participation of constituents and other related governmental agencies	The development of public health *plans and policies* is the process in which health agencies, working together with their constituents and other groups, formulate *goals and objectives* to meet the priority health needs of the community, and identify a *course of action* to achieve those goals and objectives	The organizational application of this practice provides the establishment of strategic, managerial, and programmatic direction in response to an analysis of existing and potential health problems in the community. It links the administrative direction provided from these three different levels to one another in accomplishment of the agency's mission. It provides coordination and control of preparation, review, approval, integration, and implementation of strategic, managerial, and programmatic direction for a public health agency. Plan and policy development provides direction to the practices of constituency development, managed resources, and implementation of public health programs

continues

Table 1–3 continued

Core Function		Organizational Practices	Definition	Application of Practice
C. Assurance practices	1.	Manage resources and develop organizational structure through the acquisition, allocation, and control of human, physical, and fiscal resources; and maximize the operational functions of the local public health system through coordination of community agencies' efforts and avoidance of duplication of services	To *manage resources and develop organizational structure* is the process of acquiring, allocating, and controlling resources, both human and fiscal, that will enable a public health agency to improve its leadership, work force, and operational systems that respond to both current and future community health needs	The organizational application of this practice links agency direction, as established in Plan and Policy Development to Program Implementation I, and ties the decision-making activities of resource acquisition utilization and delegation of organizational responsibility to the accomplishment of public health objectives. It uses the principles of financial management, organizational management, human resources development, and organizational development
	2.	Implement programs and other arrangements ensuring or providing direct services for priority health needs identified in the community by taking actions that translate plans and policies into services	To *implement programs* refers to the process of taking action on plans and policies to accomplish the community's public health objectives	The organizational application of this practice is demonstrated through the delivery of services and practices to accomplish a community's public health objectives. It uses internal and external support and resources to translate policy and plans into services. It provides for operating control and methods for outcome evaluation and the use of that evaluation data to revise programs.
	3.	Evaluate programs and provide quality assurance in accordance with applicable professional and regulatory standards to ensure that programs are consistent with plans and policies and provide feedback on inadequacies and changes needed to redirect programs and resources	*Evaluate programs and provide quality assurance* are the *process of continuous inquiry* to determine the efficiency and effectiveness of organizational management and program services for the purpose of providing feedback to the organization so that corrections can be made to improve activities and outcomes	The organizational application of this practice provides the coordination and direction within the agency to examine, monitor, and improve management and system services, the quality of patient/client and community service, and the impact and outcome of services provided. It directs the establishment of standards for operation and service performance, selects evaluation and monitoring methods, and uses those methods in analysis and interpretation of findings and recommendations for improvement of system performance

4. Inform and educate the public on public health issues of concern in the community, promoting an awareness about public health services availability, and health education initiatives that contribute to individual and collective changes in health knowledge, attitudes, and practices toward a healthier community	*Inform and educate* is the process of influencing behaviors by increasing knowledge, shaping attitudes, and developing skills and health practices through informed individual and collective choice and support systems within the community	This organizational practice provides coordination and direction in identifying the role of information and education in addressing community health risks, problems, or issues, directing communications to constituent groups, managing information and education interventions, and using community resources to support information and education of the public. It uses community outreach, public relations, information dissemination, and community and patient education principles to increase awareness, shape attitudes, and develop skills and health practices. Through this practice, constituency development and program implementation are supported

Source: Data from by B.J. Turnock et al., Implementing and Assessing Organizational Practices in Local Health Departments, *Public Health Reports,* Vol. 109, No. 4, pp. 478–484, 1994 and W.W. Dyal, *Public Health Practice Program Office: Organizational Practice Definitions,* 1991, Centers for Disease Control and Prevention.

that local public health departments must focus on and energize their resources to ensure their practice application and strengthen the public health system.

All this activity to define the breadth and depth of public health was created by the Institute of Medicine (IOM) Report of 1988. This report was a scathing attack on public health, suggesting public health was in a state of disarray and that the future of public health was in serious jeopardy and was considered a threat to the health of the public. Such a broad condemnation of the system engendered responses locally and globally in the U.S. health care reform debate. For the first time, public health was being singled out as a failing component of the delivery of health care. Public health lost its mission and followed misguided goals and objectives of providing client direct personal services and dismissed the basic tenets of health promotion and disease prevention. In essence, public health became largely invisible, except for specific services (e.g., immunizations) and was strongly identified as delivering health care services only to the poor. Population-based advocacy was limited, yet the public health system was based primarily on delivering population-based services. Simply stated, it did not deliver health to the public. Further, the system did not focus on health promotion and disease prevention. In a 1986 report by the Public Health Foundation, an analysis of agency spending by public health prevention foundations for 1984 reveals an interesting pattern.[67] Ninety-six percent of all monies were spent on assurance functions, 0.08 percent on policy, and 3.96 percent on assessment. Health spending for health education was only 0.2 percent of all expenditures. A 1992–1993 report on expenditures for core population-based public health functions shows that to provide essential services of public health to communities it cost approximately $11.4 billion in 1993—up from the $7.5 billion in 1984.[68,69] The *Morbidity and Mortality Weekly Report* (MMWR) reports further indicate the following:

> In addition, during this period, PHS spent an estimated $3.0 billion on core public health functions. Therefore, during fiscal year 1993, the combined estimated state, local, and PHS expenditures on core public health functions were $14.4 billion (range: $11 billion–$17 billion). Based on an estimate by the Health Care Financing Administration (HCFA), total health-care–related expenditures for the United States in 1993 were $903 billion. Thus, core public health functions accounted for approximately 1.6% (range: 1.2%–2.0%) of national health-care expenditures in 1993. If expenditures by environmental agencies and PHS are not considered, only 0.9% was spent on core public health functions. In comparison, HCFA estimated that, in 1993, expenditures for federal, state, and local public health activities were $24.2 billion— or 2.7% of national health expenditures. In addition, a previous report indicated that, in 1988, prevention-related activities accounted for 3.4% of national health expenditures.[70(p.427)]

Clearly, with minimal funding of planning and assessment activities, the maps for policy and, therefore, assurance become misguided. As a result of these recent failures, the public health community is picking up the pieces and moving the public health system forward.[71] Specifically, they agreed that to put public health on the map again (it was surely derailed during the recent health care reform debate, especially with the evolving emphasis on managed care programs), there must be a combined approach. They recommended four strategies:[72]

1. Boost awareness of public health as a *system.*
2. Build understanding of *essential services.*
3. Develop community partnership.
4. Aid elected officials to understand and appreciate public health.

These strategies, among others, were put to use by the Essential Public Health Services Work Group by adopting the Public Health in America vision and mission statements. These statements reflecting the enhancement of public health and support of the essential public health services are outlined in Exhibit 1–1 (Public Health in America—Vision). Given these efforts, there are still others who believe that "public health practices" will be influenced dramatically by managed care and universal coverage[73] (Exhibit 1–2). However, these events will primarily have an effect on personal care services—specifically, no matter the level of managed care (i.e., capitation) associated with universal coverage, the public health practices related to primary care will decrease. However, while under managed care if universal coverage does not become a reality, personal health care will potentially increase for those not covered by insurance. As to the impact on the specific core functions—assessment, policy development, and assurance—these public health practices will increase in importance. The extent of increase in the importance of these core functions must be tied to the measurement and demonstrated improvement in the health status of the population. This requires the development and use of quality improvement methods to measure the ongoing public health practices of assessment, policy development, and assurance.

TOWARD A HEALTHY PUBLIC HEALTH

A review of the literature on the status of public health and its role in the future suggests public health is under siege and is in drastic need of "rebound"—a rejuvenation. The terms that are echoed all convey a singular purpose of moving toward and creating a "healthy public health." Table 1–4 is derived from the recent barrage of articles that are directed toward this issue of re-creating the ministry of public health. Notably, the viewpoints are similar and the message is quite clear—public health has a role to fill in the rapidly changing health care environment. It is evident from the selective list that there are several strategies

Exhibit 1–1 Public Health in America

PUBLIC HEALTH IN AMERICA
Vision:
Healthy People in Healthy Communities

Mission:
*Promote Physical and Mental Health and
Prevent Disease, Injury, and Disability*

Public Health

- Prevents epidemics and the spread of disease
- Protects against environmental hazards
- Prevents injuries
- Promotes and encourages healthy behaviors
- Responds to disasters and assists communities in recovery
- Assures the quality and accessibility of health services

Essential Public Health Services

- Monitor health status to identify community health problems
- Diagnose and investigate health problems and health hazards in the community
- Inform, educate, and empower people about health issues
- Mobilize community partnerships to identify and solve health problems
- Develop policies and plans that support individual and community health efforts
- Enforce laws and regulations that protect health and ensure safety
- Link people to unneeded personal health services and assure the provision of health care when otherwise unavailable
- Assure a competent public health and personal health care workforce
- Evaluate effectiveness, accessibility, and quality of personal and population-based health services
- Research for new insights and innovative solutions to health problems

Source: Courtesy of Essential Public Health Services Work Group of the Core Public Health Functions Steering Committee, Fall 1994.

suggested that presumably will rescue public health, which once more will resume its role of preventing illness and death and promoting health. Table 1–5 outlines the evolution of public health from 1700 to 2010. It is evident that public health was at the pinnacle of protecting the health of population and communities during the 1700s and 1800s. The role of public health strayed, and in the early 1900s, personal care became commonplace. This expanded role continued well into the 1980s. In addition, during this time public health neglected to measure or

Exhibit 1–2 Predictions for Public Health under Differing Conditions of Universal Coverage and the Penetration of Capitation

		Universal Coverage	
		Present	*Absent*
Penetration of Capitation	High	⇑ Population focus ⇑ Preventive focus ⇑ Health promotion ⇑ Assessment ⇑ Policy development ⇑ Assurance ⇓ Public health agencies providing personal care services—if so, only to very select/vulnerable populations	⇑ Population focus ⇑ Preventive focus ⇑ Health promotion ? Assessment ? Policy development ? Assurance ⇑ Public health agencies providing personal care services to those not covered
	Low	? Population focus ? Preventive focus ? Health promotion ⇑ Assessment ⇑ Policy development ⇑ Assurance ⇓ Public health agencies providing personal care services—if so, only to very select/vulnerable populations	? Population focus ? Preventive focus ? Health promotion ? Assessment ? Policy development ? Assurance ⇑ Public health agencies providing personal care services to those not covered

Note: ⇑, increase; ⇓, decrease; ?, unclear.

Source: Adapted from C.A. Williams, Beyond the Institute of Medicine Report: A Critical Analysis and Public Health Forecast, *Family and Community Health*, Vol. 18, No. 1, p. 20, © 1995, Aspen Publishers, Inc.

evaluate the success or failures of programs. Nowhere was there information to tell government leaders the outcomes of the programs based on the dollars that were allocated to improve the health of the public. Thus, in the late 1980s, when the crisis in financing, the growth of government, and the growth of government spending on health care took center stage, public health was not able to respond. These events shook, shattered, and devalued the public health system. As noted in Table 1–4, there are several viewpoints as to how public health should move forward and fit with the current health care reform movement. In addition to those noted (e.g., building the infrastructure, training, partnerships, and reinventing the system), the single most important role public health must create is to put public health into practice by providing measurement and improvement methods that focus on the core public health practice functions of assessment, policy development, and assurance.

Table 1–4 Toward a Healthy Public Health—A Selective List of Recent Viewpoints on Creating a New Public Health

Year	Author	Viewpoint
1989	A. Scott-Samuel	Building the New Public Health[74]
September 1992	C.W. Keck	Creating a Healthy Public[75]
November–December 1992	W.L. Roper et al.	Strengthening the Public Health System[76]
February 1993	V.W. Sidel	Public Health vs. Health Care Debate Goes On[77]
July 1993	W.H. Foege	Preventive Medicine and Public Health[78]
Autumn 1993	L. Gordon	Public Health Is More Important than Health Care[79]
December 1993	P.R. Lee	Reinventing Public Health[80]
April 1994	R. Crawshaw	Grass Roots Participation in Health Care Reform[81]
May–June 1994	S. Dandoy	Filling the Gaps[82]
December 1994–January 1995	U.S. Public Health Service	A Time for Partnership[83]
Fall 1995	S.S. Addiss	Communicating the Public Health Message[84]
Fall 1995	N. Milio	Beyond Informatics: Electronic Community Infrastructure for Public Health[85]
Fall 1995	T.B. Richards et al.	Evaluating Local Public Health Performance at a Community Level on a Statewide Basis[86]
Fall 1995	L. Rowitz	A New Approach to Public Health Practice Experiences[87]
Fall 1995	P.J. Wiesner et al.	Taking Training Seriously[88]

CONCLUSION

Public health must be re-created by reinventing itself and focusing on populations in communities versus individuals in clinics. It has been attacked for being in disarray and not having the ability to effectively communicate results and accomplishments of funded programs. The movement toward a healthy public health must develop a vision that strengthens and enhances public health as being the premier provider of health promotion and disease prevention activities. This vision requires that the practitioner of public health practice must be familiar with and have the ability to use quality improvement methods. However, the use of quality improvement methods is dependent on understanding the nature of communities—how they solve problems, community readiness, and their focus on achieving health for all. The building of a healthy public health and healthy communities must focus on the core functions of assessment, assurance, and policy. It is the ability to use quality improvement methods for measuring outcomes and improvement in these core functions that is the foundation for developing healthy communities.

Table 1–5 Evolution of Public Health 1700–2010

Time	Disease Cycle	Major Conditions	Epidemiologic Risk	Role of Public Health
Pre-1700	Infectious	Plague Cholera Smallpox Tuberculosis	• Sign of poor moral and spiritual condition	• Attempt to isolate the ill and quarantine travelers • Authorities adopted and enforced isolation and quarantine measures and the reporting and recording of deaths
1700–1800	Infectious	Cholera Smallpox Tuberculosis	• New ideas about the cure and prevention of disease were seen as natural effects of the human condition	• Laws for isolation of smallpox patients and quarantine. Councils to enforce laws • Control through public action • 1st volunteer hospitals • 1st public mental hospital
1800–1900	Infectious	Diphtheria Cholera Typhoid Tuberculosis Smallpox	• The identification of filth as both a cause of disease and a vehicle of transmission • Illness—an indicator of poor social and environmental conditions • Cleanliness was embraced	• "The great sanitary awakening" • Disease control continued to focus on epidemics, but control turned from isolation and quarantine of the individual to cleaning and improving the common environment • Public boards, agencies, and institutions were formed • Sanitary/social reform provided the basis for the formation of public health organizations at local/state levels • Federal activities limited to Marine Hospital • State boards of health, state health departments, and local health departments were established
1875–1900	Infectious	Anthrax Tuberculosis Diphtheria Typhoid Yellow fever Smallpox	• Bacteria • Discovery of bacteriologic agents that produced diseases • Interventions: Immunization and water purification controlled	• "Germ theory" of disease provided a scientific basis for public health • Expansion into laboratory service and epidemiology
1890s	Infectious	Anthrax Tuberculosis Diphtheria Typhoid Yellow fever Smallpox	• Science revealed that both environment and individuals could be agents of disease	• State/local health departments established laboratories (the 1st in Massachusetts) • 1st major success of the public health system—bacteriology • 10 glorious years "Before 1880 we knew nothing; after 1890 we knew it all"

continued

Table 1–5 continued

Time	Disease Cycle	Major Conditions	Epidemiologic Risk	Role of Public Health
Boundary of Public Health Shifts: A Major Shift from Population- to Individual-Based Health Care				
1900–1925	Infectious	Tuberculosis Infant mortality High childhood mortality Syphilis Polio Influenza	• It became clear people were often the source of disease transmission rather than things	• Move toward personal care—tuberculosis and infant mortality • Expanded role of state/local public health departments • Clinical care and health education was the focus • Shift from disease prevention to health promotion • Epidemiology provided scientific justification for health program • Disease registries required reporting—required reporting implied obligation to treat
1912–1922	Infectious	Infant mortality Parasitic diseases Nutritional	• Environment • Hygiene • Public health cleanliness	• Major investment of federal health activities—Children's Bureau formed in 1912 • 1st White House Conference on Child Health—1919 • 1922—Funds to state to establish programs in maternal/child health
1930–1970	Infection/chronic	Heart disease Cancer Stroke Motor vehicle accidents Diabetes Syphilis Polio	• Lifestyle • Environment • Biology • Health care delivery system	• Major expansion of "personal care" as a role for the government • NIH—1937, by the 1970s several institutions were formed • Medicaid/Medicare (1966) • Parallel changes at the state/local levels • Growth of maternal/child health, family planning, immunizations, venereal disease control, tuberculosis control • Major statistical and surveillance efforts
1970–1990	Chronic/social transformation	AIDS Homeless Drugs Crime Environmental waste Alcoholism	• Lifestyle • Environment	• Crisis in care and financing • Block grants (1981) • New problems identified that conflict with concerns about the growth of government and government spending in health

Table 1–5 continued

Time	Disease Cycle	Major Conditions	Epidemiologic Risk	Role of Public Health
Boundary of Public Health Shifts: A Major Shift from Individual- to Population-Based Health Care				
1990–2010	Social transformation	AIDS Aging Crime Environmental problems Genetics Education	• Lifestyle • Environment	• Universal coverage/ managed care for special populations • Public health turns back to its intended purpose— population-based medicine • Epidemiology takes center stage—assessment, policy development, assurance • Public health is based on monitoring, surveillance, research, and evaluation • Movement toward quality improvement and outcome measurement

Source: Data from *The Future of Public Health,* pp. 56–71, © 1988, The Institute of Medicine.

NOTES

1. A.R. Tenner and I.J. DeToro, *TQM: Three Steps to Continuous Improvement* (Reading, MA: Addison-Wesley Publishing Co., 1992), 142.

2. Pew Health Professions Commission, *Critical Challenges: Revitalizing the Health Professions for the Twenty-First Century* (San Francisco: UCSF Center for the Health Professions, 1995), v.

3. W. Leebov and C.J. Ersoz, *The Health Care Manager's Guide to Continuous Quality Improvement* (Chicago: American Hospital Publishing, 1991), 3–4.

4. Pew Health Professions Commission, *Critical Challenges,* v.

5. G.E.A. Dever, *Community Health Analysis: Global Awareness at the Local Level,* 2d ed. (Gaithersburg, MD: Aspen Publishers, 1991), 21.

6. Pew Health Professions Commission, *Critical Challenges,* xi.

7. Leebov and Ersoz, *Health Care Manager's Guide,* 4.

8. Ibid.

9. American Public Health Association (APHA) and the Centers for Disease Control and Prevention (CDC), *The Guide to Implementing Model Standards: Eleven Steps toward a Healthy Community* (Washington, DC: American Public Health Association, 1993), 14–15.

10. Ibid., 12–13.

11. American Public Health Association, *Healthy Communities 2000: Model Standards,* 3d ed. (Washington, DC: Government Printing Office, 1991).

12. M. Brassard, *The Memory Jogger Plus+* (Metheun, MA: GOAL/QPC, 1989), 1–3.

13. Leebov and Ersoz, *Health Care Manager's Guide,* 4.

14. Ibid., 4–5.

15. Ibid., 5.

16. National Association of County and City Health Officials et al., *Blueprint for a Healthy Community: A Guide for Local Health Departments* (Washington, DC: 1994), 5–6.

17. Ibid.

18. Pew Health Professions Commission, *Critical Challenges,* 36.

19. Ibid., 37.

20. Ibid., 37.

21. Office of Planning and Policy Development of South Carolina, DHEC, "Citizen Participation," *Blueprint* 2, no. 1 (1995).

22. Ibid., 1.

23. G.A. Persons, "Defining the Public Interest: Citizen Participation in Metropolitan and State Policy Making," *National Civic Review* 79, no. 2 (1990): 118–131.

24. "Citizen Participation," *Blueprint,* 1.

25. Ibid.

26. Ibid., 1–2.

27. British Columbia Ministry of Health, *Healthy Communities Yearbook* (Vancouver, BC: 1992).

28. V. Look, ed. "McKnight Describes Building Communities from the Inside Out," *Connections: California Healthy Cities Project* 7, no. 1 (1995): 2.

29. "Citizen Participation," *Blueprint,* 2.

30. T. Lundy, *Community Health Councils, Strategies for Increasing Community Participation* (Vancouver, BC: British Columbia Ministry of Health; 1993).

31. Office of Planning and Policy Development, South Carolina Department of Health and Environmental Concerns, "Civic Infrastructure Affects Community Problem-Solving Capacity," *Blueprint* 2, no. 3 (1995): 1.

32. Ibid.

33. Ibid.

34. Ibid.

35. Ibid.

36. A.D. Kaluzny et al., "Quality Improvement: Beyond the Institution," *Hospital & Health Services Administration* 40, no. 1 (1995): 177–178.

37. T.M. Mettee, "Community Diagnosis: A Tool for COPC," in *Community-Oriented Primary Care,* ed. P.A. Nutting (Albuquerque: University of New Mexico Press, 1990), 52–59.

38. R.C. Like et al., "Family Health Science and the New Generalist Practitioner," *Family Systems Medicine* 11 (1993): 161.

39. Kaluzny et al., "Quality Improvement," 178.

40. S.M. Shortell et al., "Creating Organized Delivery Systems: The Barriers and Facilitators," *Hospital & Health Services Administration* 38 (1993): 447–466.

41. Kaluzny et al., "Quality Improvement," 180.

42. Ibid., 178, 180.

43. J.W. Travis, *Wellness Workbook* (Mill Valley, CA: Ten Speed Press, 1988), 102.

44. Ibid.

45. U.S. Department of Health and Human Services, *Healthy People 2000: National Health Promotion and Disease Prevention Objectives,* DHHS Pub. (PHS) 91-50212 (Washington, DC: Government Printing Office, 1991), GPO Stock No. 017-001-0474-0.

46. G.E.A. Dever, *Community Health Analysis,* 25.

47. J. Epp, "Achieving Health for All: A Framework for Health Promotion," *Canadian Journal of Public Health* 77 (1986): 393–407.

48. Swedish Ministry of Health and Social Affairs, *Health in Sweden, The Swedish, The Swedish Health Services in the 1990's* (Stockholm: Swedish Ministry of Health and Social Affairs, 1982).

49. Department of Health and Environmental Welfare, *Healthy People—The Surgeon General's Report on Health Promotion and Disease Prevention* (Washington, DC: 1979) (PHS) Publ. 79550712.

50. World Health Organization, *Global Strategy for Health for All by the Year 2000* (Geneva: 1981).

51. "Promoting Health/Preventing Disease. Public Health Service I Implementation Plans for Attaining the Objectives for the Nation," *Public Health Reports* suppl. (September–October 1983).

52. M.A. Stoto, "Memorandum to Members of the Year 2000 Health Objectives Consortium. Update on the Year 2000 Objectives." National Academy of Sciences, June 14, 1988, 10.

53. U.S. Department of Health and Human Services, *Healthy People 2000: Midcourse Review and 1995 Revisions* (Washington, DC: Government Printing Office, 1995.)

54. Stoto, "Memorandum," 10.

55. Institute of Medicine, Committee for the Study of the Future of Public Health, The Future of Public Health (Washington, DC: National Academy of Sciences, 1988), 225.

56. Stoto, "Memorandum," 10.

57. U.S. Department of Health and Human Services, *Healthy People 2000.*

58. U.S. Department of Health and Human Services, *The 1990 Health Objectives for the Nation* (Washington, DC: 1990).

59. Epp, "Achieving Health for All," 393–407.

60. G.E.A. Dever, "An Epidemiological Model for Health Policy Analysis," *Social Indicators Research* 2 (1976): 456–461.

61. J. Stewart and M. Clarke, "The Public Service Orientation: Issues and Dilemmas," *Public Administration* 65 (Summer 1987): 161–177.

62. J. McKnight, "Why 'Servanthood' Is Bad," *The Other Side* (January–February 1989): 38–41.

63. Epp, "Achieving Health for All," 393–407.

64. G.L. Siler-Wells, *Directing Change and Changing Direction—A New Health Policy Agenda for Canada* (Ottawa: Canadian Public Health Association, 1988), 131.

65. Epp, "Achieving Health for All," 393–407.

66. W.W. Dyal, *Public Health Practice Program Office: Organizational Practice Definitions* (Atlanta, GA: Centers for Disease Control, Public Health Practice Program Office, Division of Public Health Systems, 1991), 1.

67. Institute of Medicine, *The Future of Public Health* (Washington, DC: National Academy Press, 1988), 182.

68. S. Addiss et al., "Estimated Expenditures for Core Public Health Functions—Selected States, October 1992–September 1993," *Morbidity and Mortality Weekly Report (MMWR)* 44, no. 22 (1995): 421–429.

69. Institute of Medicine, *Future of Public Health,* 182.

70. Addiss, "Estimated Expenditures for Core Public Health Functions," 427.

71. "Essential Public Health Services' Document Offers Tools for Marketing Public Health," *The Nation's Health* December (1994): 1,3.

72. Ibid.

73. C.A. Williams, "Beyond the Institute of Medicine Report: A Critical Analysis and Public Health Forecast," *Family and Community Health* 18, no. 1 (1995): 20.

74. A. Scott-Samuel, "Building the New Public Health: A Public Health Alliance and a New Social Epidemiology," in *Reading for a New Public Health,* eds. C.J. Martin and D.V. McQueen (Edinburgh: Edinburgh University Press, 1989), 29–44.

75. C.W. Keck, "Creating a Healthy Public," *American Journal of Public Health* 82 (1992): 1206–1209.

76. W.L. Roper et al., "Strengthening the Public Health System," *Public Health Reports* 107, no. 6 (1992): 609–615.

77. V.W. Sidel et al., "Letters to the Editor: Public Health vs. Health Care Debate Goes On," *The Nation's Health* February (1993): 1,3.

78. W.H. Foege, "Preventive Medicine and Public Health," *JAMA* 270, no. 2 (1993): 251–252.

79. L. Gordon, "Public Health Is More Important Than Health Care," *Journal of Public Health Policy* Autumn (1993): 261–264.

80. P.R. Lee, "From the Assistant Secretary for Health, US Public Health Service," *JAMA* 270, no. 22 (1993): 2670.

81. R. Crawshaw, "Grass Roots Participation in Health Care Reform," *Annals of Internal Medicine* 120 (1994): 677–681.

82. S. Dandoy, "Filling the Gaps: The Role of Public Health Departments under Health Care Reform," *Journal of American Health Policy* 4, no. 3 (1994): 6–13.

83. U.S. Public Health Service, "A Time for Partnership: Report of State Consultations on the Role of Public Health," *Prevention Report* December–January (1994–1995): 1–12.

84. S.S. Addiss, "Communicating the Public Health Message," *Journal of Public Health Management and Practice* 1, no. 4 (1995): 105–106.

85. N. Milio, "Beyond Informatics: An Electronic Community Infrastructure for Public Health," *Journal of Public Health Management and Practice* 1, no. 4 (1995): 84–94.

86. T.B. Richards et al., "Evaluating Local Public Health Performance at a Community Level on a Statewide Basis," *Journal of Public Health Management and Practice* 1, no. 4 (1995): 70–83.

87. L. Rowitz, "A New Approach to Public Health Practice Experiences," *Journal of Public Health Management and Practice* 1, no. 4 (1995): 102–104.

88. P.J. Wiesner et al., "Taking Training Seriously: A Policy Statement on Public Health Training by the Joint Council of Governmental Public Health Agencies," *Journal of Public Health Management and Practice* 1, no. 4 (1995): 60–69.

Chapter 2

Public Health Practice: Assessment

The discussion in Chapter 1 outlined the issues of why public health was at a crossroads. The shift from clinical medicine (evaluating individuals in clinics) to population-based medicine (understanding populations in communities) produced the need to focus on the practice of public health and the three core functions of assessment, policy development, and assurance. A major factor contributing to this shift was the managed care movement and the greater acceptance of Medicaid and Medicare by physicians. This change resulted in a major decline in the delivery of public health clinical services. This decline was so extreme that major revenues coming from Medicaid programs declined dramatically. Elaine Conley has offered a very succinct view of this demise of how public health lost touch with its population-based practice that once was a significant component of its foundation. Conley states,

> The answer is multifaceted and complicated, but at the heart of it is lack of funding. As a means of survival, public health...was seduced into believing that Medicaid, fee-for-service (FFS), and programmatic funding were the answer to all of its ills and with each step public health...moved further away from its origins. *The problem with Medicaid dollars, FFS, and programmatic funding is that they do not fund population-based services. These dollars fund a specific service for an individual or family but do not pay for assessment or assurance activities that are not individual or family oriented. Thus, public health...lost the capacity to provide services to the larger communities it was originally dedicated to serving.* Compounding this problem, public health...moved from a generalist to a specialist practice in order

to effectively carry out programmatic services, which resulted in fewer [professionals] serving the larger community. (emphasis added)[1(p.1)]

Conley further explains that the public-private competition for individual and family services has diminished the role of public health. This has led to confusion and uncertainty about public health's role and how it will fit in with managed care and health care reform.[2] This overall decline in the role of public health was more apparent in urban areas where managed care programs became more prevalent. The rural impact of these programs has yet to be determined. There may be opportunity in rural areas to actually become the managed care provider. In fact, even in urban areas the opportunity exists for public health and community health centers to contract with managed care programs for services delivered to the Medicaid population. No matter the status of clinical services delivered by public health clinics, the future of public health practice must address the three core functions. The methods and tools proposed in this book may be equally applied to the clinical assessment of programs and patients as well as to the community assessment of populations. To meet these parallel needs of clinical and community assessment, the public health practitioner must develop new skills, understand basic methods, and be prepared to respond to the new challenges of public health practice.

ASSESSMENT

To meet the demands of determining the need for population-based services, a health status assessment is of paramount importance. A health status needs assessment is not an end product in itself but is part of a process that provides information that is continuously monitored. The continuous monitoring of information from programs and/or communities is a major and critical component of continuous quality improvement (CQI). In strengthening public health, the CQI process is crucial. For too long now public health programs have not monitored their outcomes, and in many instances programs do not even have any outcome measures. The intent of assessment—a core public health function—is to determine the health needs of a community from a population-based perspective. Assessment is one of the major phases of public health problem solving (i.e., identification of problems). The other core public health functions of policy development and assurance correspond to the phases of the "mobilization of necessary effort and resources" and "*assurance* that vital conditions are in place and that crucial services are received."[3(p.43)] Assessment is defined as the systematic collection, analysis, and sharing of information about health conditions, risks, and resources in a community. Included in these actions are the concepts of community diagnosis such as surveillance, identifying needs, analyzing the causes and variations of problems, collecting and interpreting data (special cause versus common cause[*]) case finding, monitoring and forecasting trends, researching, and evaluating outcomes. The linkage of the assessment function to a regular and systematic analysis by using quality improvement methods that continuously monitor outcomes is essential. The statistical methods for measuring quality improvement are presented in subsequent chapters. Thus, the foundation for public health activities is the assessment function that continuously monitors data (surveillance). Developing this assessment function provides the capacity to identify problems (assessment), provides data to assist in decisions about appropriate actions (policy development), and monitors progress of delivery service (assurance). The essential science of public health to carry out these actions (core functions) has been epidemiology. A strong assessment function and surveillance system (continuous monitoring—using quality improvement methods) based on sound epidemiologic principles is a fundamental part of a technically competent public health practice program.[4]

Conley has suggested that assessment activities may be categorized by community, family, and individual.[5] She further categorizes policy development and assurance activities by the same categories (Table 2–1). The assessment activities are clearly identified and reflect a public health nursing perspective. The significance of this approach being offered is the extension of the assessment activities to the family and the individual. This model, as Conley notes, is that intervention at both of these levels (family and individual) is critical to population-based public health services because they provide the linkage that effectively ensures an interaction with the community. In Chapter 1, the community diagnosis functions were similarly categorized by these three levels with an additional institutional component. This public health practice guide to community assessment used the *S*ubjective, *O*bjective, *A*ssessment, *P*lanning (SOAP) format for developing a clinical and population-based diagnosis. It is evident the assessment function is the cornerstone of public health practice. In fact, it will behoove the public health practitioner to acquire and master the skills for diagnosing a community to ensure that public health programs are evaluated on the basis of outcome and not based on rhetoric, generalities, or anecdotes.

ASSESSMENT—A NEW CONTEXT

Health care reform has created a flurry of assessment activity by insurance groups, managed care networks, hospitals, primary care settings, and federal, state, and local agencies. Most of this activity has been directed toward the indus-

---

[*]This is defined and discussed in subsequent chapters on quality improvement methods.

Table 2–1 Public Health Practice: Core Functions of Assessment, Policy Development, and Assurance Categorized by Community, Family, and Individual

Assessment Functions		
Community	*Family*	*Individual*
Analyze data on needs of specific populations or geographic areas	Evaluate a specific family's strengths and areas of concern	Identify individuals within the family who are in need of services
Identify and interact with key community leaders both formally and informally	Evaluate the family's living environment, looking specifically at support, relationships, and other factors that might have a significant impact on family health outcomes	Evaluate the functional capacity of the individual through the use of specific assessment measures
Identify target populations that may be at risk and participate in data collection on these populations	Assess the larger environment in which the family lives for safety, access, and other related issues	Develop a diagnosis for the individual that describes a problem or potential problem, etiology, and contributing factors
Conduct surveys or observe targeted populations to gain a better understanding of needs		Develop a nursing plan or critical care map for the individual
Participate in formal community assessment process		
Policy Development Functions		
Provide leadership in convening and facilitating community groups to evaluate health concerns and develop a plan to address the concerns	Recommend new or increased services or programs to meet specific family needs within a geographic area	Recommend or assist in the development of standards for individual client care
Recommend specific training and programs to meet identified health needs	Facilitate networking of families with similar needs. Make recommendations to policy makers about specific issues affecting clusters of families	Recommend or adopt risk classification systems to assist with prioritizing individual client care
Raise awareness of key policy makers about health regulations, budget decisions, and other factors that may negatively affect the health of the community	Request additional data and analyze information to identify trends in a group or cluster of families	Participate in establishing criteria for opening, closing, or referring individual cases
Act as an advocate for target populations that are not willing or able to speak to policy makers about issues of concern	Identify key families in a community and develop appropriate and effective intervention strategies to use with these families	Participate in the development of job descriptions to establish roles for various team members who will provide service to individuals

Table 2–1 continued

Assurance Functions		
Community	*Family*	*Individual*
Ensure that prevention and intervention efforts for communicable diseases or other public health candidates are being appropriately implemented	Ensure that families are linked with health services	Provide generalist public health nursing services to individuals across the age continuum based on identified need
Collaborate with the community including various health care providers to reduce barriers to accessing health care	Provide public health nursing services to a cluster of families within a geographic setting	Consult regularly with other health care providers and team members regarding individuals' care
Assist the community in implementation of its intervention plan		

Source: Adapted from E. Conley, "Public Health Nursing within Core Public Health Functions," *Journal of Public Health Management and Practice,* Vol. 1, No. 3, pp. 4–6, © 1995, Aspen Publishers, Inc.

try of the above groups' representative communities (i.e., policy holders, clients, patients, and community populations). Further, each of the agencies is in someway focusing its assessments on the Year 2000 objectives. As important as these assessment efforts are and as critical as they are in this era of health care reform, it is not a new endeavor for public health agencies.

Lloyd F. Novick has noted that: "Assessment is not new in public health... [such] activities were the major force spurring the inception of organized public health in England at the end of the Elizabethan period and later in the United States."[6(p.v)] He further states that the newness may be the result of an increased recognition of assessment as a fundamental and basic tool of public health practice. A further point made is that the change is less likely due to the assessment–policy development–assurance categories outlined by the Institute of Medicine report, but a more reasonable explanation is the change in public health during the past 15 years and, as noted earlier, the high profile of the health care reform debate.[7] This new recognition has been demonstrated by several authors, and their contributions were noted in Table 1–4 in Chapter 1. The most recent example of these trends is the Spring issue of the *Journal of Public Health Management and Practice.*[8] Significant to this trend of a renewed interest in assessment is that assessments must not be initiated without a framework, model, or purpose. Community health assessments in the past have been major data collection activities with the purpose of providing a compendium of information that many times is of little use to the community. A usable database assessment that was developed for the purpose of improving the health status of the community makes more sense and would be extremely valuable to the community planning effort. A database-driven assessment as sanctioned by a specific protocol developed by a community must be supported by a system or network that allows for an ongoing monitoring of the programs and priorities as determined by the community. Philip C. Nasca has specifically stated that "the future of databased assessment, planning, and evaluation of public health programs will most certainly be tied not only to the maintenance of existing systems, but also to the development of more sophisticated approaches to information gathering, analysis, and dissemination."[9(p. vii)] To accomplish this approach as part of the public health practice function of assessment, there must be widespread interest in developing networks of public health data systems. Such systems if designed and implemented properly will provide rapid access to health data (defined in a holistic sense) for providing an integrated and comprehensive approach to public health assessment.[10]

ASSESSMENT—PROCESS TOOLS

Although there are as many ways to develop the assessment process as there are communities, it would be most prudent to use established protocols. The degree to which standard protocols are used is a function of community size and available expertise to that community. Most state agencies are able to develop unique approaches to the community assessment process but are unable to implement sound approaches at the community level. In this event, the state may recommend to the community that standard protocols be used to perform their public health practice function of assessment. Many times, local communities are on "fast forward," and the state agencies may be taking their cues from the community. For a community to become active in the community needs assessment process, it must develop an awareness of the national objectives and how these established Year 2000 objectives may become part of community planning efforts within a quality improvement process.

Year 2000 Objectives

The Year 2000 objectives are detailed in the report *Healthy People 2000: National Health Promotion and Disease Prevention Objectives.*[11] The context of this report began taking shape in 1987 when a collaborative effort between the Public Health Service and state and local organizations, health professionals, and interested citizens identified broad goals and priority areas for action. This product became the guiding vision for states and communities to do health planning for the year 2000. The primary purpose of the *Healthy People 2000* document was to commit the United States to three broad health goals: (1) increase the span of healthy life for Americans; (2) reduce health disparities among Americans; and (3) achieve access to preventive services for all Americans.[12(p.6)]

An outgrowth of these specified goals was a set of measurable objectives to be achieved by the year 2000. The selection of these objectives was based on a specified set of criteria (Exhibit 2–1). These criteria should be used by communities to aid in identifying problems and establishing priorities. The adaption of such criteria for setting the year 2000 objectives will facilitate the planning process and further will ensure a standardized process. However, the objectives and the levels to be attained were not based on evidence nor were public health practice guidelines established to ensure appropriate and standard guidelines for assessment. These objectives were organized into 22 priority areas, including specific age-related categories (Table 2–2). As shown, the 22 priority areas were organized into four groups: health promotion, health protection, preventive services, and surveillance and data systems. This latter category, although the most significant to the success of an ongoing CQI movement process, has received the least attention. This certainly relates to the discussion earlier that public health lost sight of

---

Exhibit 2–1 Healthy People 2000 Criteria

CRITERIA FOR SETTING HEALTHY PEOPLE 2000 HEALTH OBJECTIVES

1. *Credibility:* Objectives should be realistic and address the issues of greatest priority.
2. *Public comprehension:* Objectives should be understandable and relevant to a broad audience, including those who plan, manage, deliver, use, and pay for health services.
3. *Balance:* Objectives should be a mixture of outcome and process measures, recommending methods for achieving changes, and setting standards for evaluating progress.
4. *Measurability:* Objectives should be quantified.
5. *Continuity:* Current objectives should be linked to previous objectives where possible but reflect the lessons learned in implementing them.
6. *Compatibility:* Objectives should be compatible, where possible, with goals already adopted by the community as a whole and by major groups within the community, such as the public health department and/or major health care providers.
7. *Freedom from data constraints:* The availability or form of data should not be the principal determinant of the nature of the objectives. Alternate and proxy data should be used when necessary.
8. *Responsibility:* The objectives should reflect the concerns and engage the participation of professionals, advocates and consumers, as well as state and local health departments.

Source: Reprinted from *Healthy People 2000: National Health Promotion and Disease Prevention Objectives,* DHHS Pub. No. (PHS) 91-50212, p. 90, 1991, U.S. Department of Health and Human Services, Washington, DC.

Table 2–2 *Healthy People 2000* Priority Areas

Health Promotion	Health Protection	Preventive Services	Surveillance and Data Systems
1. Physical Activity and Fitness 2. Nutrition 3. Tobacco 4. Alcohol and Other Drugs 5. Family Planning 6. Mental Health and Mental Disorders 7. Violent and Abusive Behavior 8. Educational and Community-Based Programs	9. Unintentional Injuries 10. Occupational Safety and Health 11. Environmental Health 12. Food and Drug Safety 13. Oral Health	14. Maternal and Infant Health 15. Heart Disease and Stroke 16. Cancer 17. Diabetes and Chronic Disabling Conditions 18. HIV Infection 19. Sexually Transmitted Diseases 20. Immunization and Infectious Diseases 21. Clinical Preventive Services	22. Surveillance and Data Systems

Age-Related Objectives
Children Adolescents and Young Adults Adults Older Adults

Source: Reprinted from *Healthy People 2000: National Health Promotion and Disease Prevention Objectives,* DHHS Pub. No. (PHS) 91-50212, p. 7, 1991, U.S. Department of Health and Human Services, Washington, DC.

its population-based perspective and became more concerned and consumed by the provision of clinical services.

Health promotion strategies for community health improvement include activities related to individual lifestyles that can exert powerful influences on one's health. Health protection strategies are environmental or regulatory measures that confer protection on large community-based population groups (i.e., populations in communities). Preventive services include counseling, screening, immunization, and chemoprophylactic intervention for individuals in clinics. Clearly, the categorization of these activities represents an epidemiologic model for assessing community health status, specifically lifestyle, environment, health care delivery system, and biology (i.e., genetics) as part of the preventive services category.[13]

From a public health practice perspective, it is evident that the assessment function includes individuals in clinics and populations in communities. Thus, the quality improvement concepts and methods discussed in this book may be used in either setting.

In addition to the *Healthy People 2000* priority areas, the Centers for Disease Control and Prevention/National Center for Health Statistics developed a set of indicators by consensus to monitor, evaluate, and assess the improvement in the health status of a population or county. Table 2–3 lists the consensus indicators by

---

Table 2–3 CDC/NCHS Consensus Indicators

Health Status	Mortality Rates (per 100,000)	Reported Incidence (per 100,000)	Indicators of Risk Factors
1. Race/ethnicity-specific infant mortality, as measured by the rate (per 1,000 live births) of deaths among infants less than age one	2. Motor vehicle crashes 3. Work-related injury 4. Suicide 5. Lung cancer 6. Breast cancer 7. Cardiovascular disease 8. Homicide 9. All causes	10. AIDS 11. Measles 12. Tuberculosis 13. Primary and secondary syphilis	14. Incidence of low birth weight, as measured by percentage of total number of infants weighing less than 2,500 grams at birth 15. Births to adolescents (females age 10 to 17 years) as a percentage of total live births 16. Prenatal care, as measured by the percentage of mothers delivering live infants who did not receive prenatal care during the first trimester 17. Childhood poverty, as measured by the proportion of children less than age 15 living in families at or below the poverty level 18. Proportion of persons living in counties exceeding U.S. Environmental Protection Agency standards for quality during the previous year

Source: Data from Centers for Disease Control and Prevention and the National Center for Health Statistics.

---

health status, mortality rates, incidence, and indicators of risk factors. As is seen later, some of these indicators are selected to illustrate the quality improvement process in public health practice. This set of standard indicators in essence becomes practice guidelines for the assessment function in public health practice. However, the indicators were developed by the consensus method and not based on evidence. This theme of improving public health performance by basing decisions on evidence is developed in a later chapter.

Model Standards

Model Standards is a guidebook and tool for community health planning.[14] This document serves as a link between the Year 2000 objectives and the efforts communities can make in meeting the national objectives. The flexibility of the model standards is a major advantage to its implementation of establishing objectives and developing strategies that are responsive to their own situation, specifically setting local priorities and using local resources. The *Model Standards* suggests, in addition to the principle of flexibility for adaption of specific objectives, other principles that guide the application of these standards. The other principles are

- emphasis on health outcomes
- focus on the entire community
- government presence at the local level
- accessibility of services
- emphasis on programs
- importance of negotiation[15]

To assist in implementing these guiding principles as outlined in the guidebook, a series of 11 steps is recommended. The 11 steps are listed in Table 2–4. It is suggested that the implementation of these 11 steps may vary depending on the community needs and the needs of the local health agency. Examples of these model standards as linked to the Year 2000 objectives are shown in Figure 2–1.[16] As shown, it is quite easy for a community to adopt its local priorities and set its own measurable objectives based on the standard recommended. The use of this process may be quite effective in monitoring the progress toward improvement. Although the nature of CQI is to continually show advances toward a high level, it does necessarily set objectives. However, for health programs, objectives are critical to success, and the monitoring of these objectives to show improvement is the function of quality improvement measurement for public health practice

Table 2–4 Model Standards for Healthy Communities: Steps for Attaining the Year 2000 Health Objectives

Steps	Task	Description
1	Assess and determine the role of one's health agency	The local public health department develops a mission statement and agrees on a long-range vision that provides the community with a clear description of the agency's role
2	Assess the lead health agency's organizational capacity	The director and the staff of the agency should assess the organization's readiness to exercise leadership. Such an assessment can be accomplished by conducting a review of a department's structure and capacity to determine if it has the skills, community support, and staff capacity to lead the community
3	Develop an agency plan to build the necessary organizational capacity	Once a department has conducted an assessment of its organizational capacity, an agency should develop a plan to build on its internal strengths, overcome its weaknesses, and enhance its organizational effectiveness for carrying out communitywide efforts
4	Assess the community's organizational and power structures	Each local health department should work in partnership with key community agencies, community leaders, interest groups, and community members. Identifying key people and organizations to involve in this effort is fundamental to its success and is an essential part of community leadership. The agency should conduct an assessment of the community's organizational and power structures either on a formal or informal basis as part of its strategy to develop such partnerships
5	Organize the community to build a stronger constituency for public health and establish a partnership for public health	The local health agency should convene community groups to assess health needs, to address health problems, and to assist in the coordination of responsibilities. *Model Standards* can be used internally with agency staff to develop a focus on health outcomes and strategies
6	Assess health needs and available community resources	A community assessment provides the information needed to identify a community's most critical health problems. Community assessment should include both formal and informal information collection. It should identify the perceptions and values of community leaders, groups, agencies, individuals, and health department staff about health priorities for the community. The effort should also examine pertinent health data and/or survey information to identify and verify the extent of major health problems and the level of risk for subpopulations. An inventory of available community resources should be developed
7	Determine local priorities	Establishing local priorities should involve major health agencies, community organizations, and key interest groups and individuals. Information gathered from a community assessment is intended to aid in determining local priorities
8	Select outcome and process objectives that are compatible with local priorities and the *Healthy People 2000* objectives	*Model Standards* can be used to establish local priorities for health achievements, and to negotiate and select appropriate goals and outcome and process objectives for resolving community health problems. *Healthy Communities 2000: Model Standards* provides an array of goals and objectives to establish these objectives; a community coalition can develop process objectives for achieving them.
9	Develop communitywide intervention strategies	Developing communitywide interventions provides the means to achieve selected community goals and objectives. Once interventions have been selected, responsibilities should be assigned so that activities can be distributed and coordinated among agencies and organizations
10	Develop and implement a plan of action	Establishing goals, objectives, and communitywide intervention strategies is an important step, but success depends on developing and executing a plan of action that implements intervention activities and services. Establishing timelines and the assignment of responsibilities for activities and services is an essential part of this process
11	Monitor and evaluate the effort on a continuing basis	The achievement of improved health status will attest to the effectiveness of community efforts. In the short term, achievement of local process objectives will show movement toward improved health status if effective interventions have been selected

Source: Adapted with permission from *The Guide to Implementing Model Standards: Eleven Steps toward a Healthy Community*, pp. 8–9, © 1993, American Public Health Association and Centers for Disease Control and Prevention, Washington, D.C.

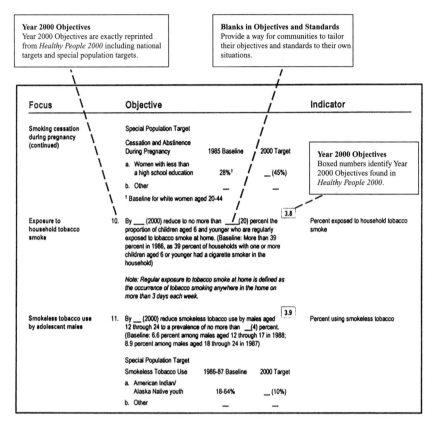

Figure 2–1 Quick Reference Guide to Model Standards. *Source:* From *Healthy Communities 2000: Model Standards,* 3rd edition. Copyright 1991 by the American Public Health Association. Adapted with permission.

application. To effectively build a successful public health practice, there also must be an established link between quality improvement and the Year 2000 objectives, which in turn is linked to the model standards. In summary, the *Model Standards* document suggests the following ways communities can use the information to enhance the planning process:

- Translate national objectives into community action plans tailored to meet community needs.
- Establish community-specific measurable objectives.
- Encourage communication and coordination of public health efforts.
- Foster opportunities for shared responsibilities among groups.

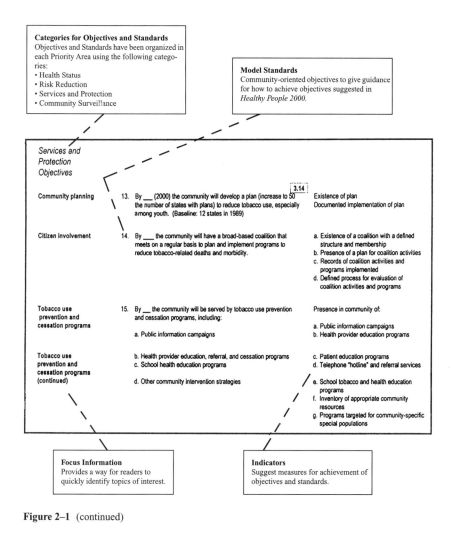

Figure 2–1 (continued)

- Determine service priorities based on existing patterns, needs, and resources.
- Support program and budget justification to legislative bodies.[17]

Probably, the most basic theme that is proposed in the *Model Standards* document is that the standards be used not only to link with the 2000 objectives but also be tied to the use of assessment tools. The health planning tools for assessment such as Assessment Protocol for Excellence in Public Health (APEX*PH*) and Planned Approach to Community Health (PATCH) are highly recommended. These are described in subsequent sections.

APEX*PH*

To assist the community in the implementation of the 11 steps put forth by the *Model Standards* document, two assessment and planning tools have been developed. These tools, APEX*PH* and PATCH, were designed to facilitate the community health planning process. These tools are quite similar but are distinguishable by *what* they are designed to accomplish and *how* they are used. Table 2–5 indicates a description of each of these tools and outlines their basic differences. The significance of these assessment tools to the quality improvement process and the linkage to the measurement issues is that they are very much a part of an ongoing monitoring process of the APEX*PH* and PATCH models. Specifically, the last phases of APEX*PH* and PATCH recommend a continuous monitoring and/or evaluation of the process that refines the assessment and planning functions. Although not discussed as of yet, the PDCA cycle attributed to CQI establishes a process of *p*lanning, *d*oing, *c*hecking, and *a*cting in a cyclical fashion, which moves the process toward continuous improvement each time the cycle is complete. The result is the assessment tools: the PDCA cycle, APEX*PH*, and PATCH will move a community forward toward achieving better outcomes health status, which is continuously monitored to ensure quality improvement.

The APEX*PH* model for assessment and planning is organized into three parts:

1. organizational capacity assessment
2. community process
3. completing the cycle[18]

There are eight steps to accomplish parts 1 and 2, whereas for part 3, it is a discussion of the policy development and assurance functions that results from the steps accomplished during the assessment function. Further, the monitoring and evaluation functions to carry out the organizational action plan and the community health plan are described. Thus carrying out this final part of the APEX*PH* assessment tool completes the core functions of public health assessment, policy development, and assurance and thereby becomes an ongoing part of management (i.e., CQI). The APEX*PH* model for parts 1 and 2 is outlined in Figure 2–2. Although the model is staged (i.e., parts 1, 2, and 3), it is not always going to be implemented in sequence; sometimes the community assessment may precede or may be conducted concurrently with the assessment of the organizational capacity of the community.

PATCH

PATCH is similar to APEX*PH* in that certain steps are suggested to improve the health status of the population. However, PATCH focuses on mobilizing the com-

Table 2–5 APEX*PH* and PATCH Assessment Tools: What They Are and How They Are Used

	APEX*PH*	PATCH
Description (what they are)	APEX*PH* improves the system of public health in a community by enhancing its capacity to perform the core functions of assessment, policy development, and assurance. APEX*PH* enables the agency to assess and improve its internal organizational structure by involving the local public health director and management team. The APEX*PH* process encourages and strengthens the ability of the local public health agency to provide leadership in the development and implementation of a community health plan	PATCH can be used as a generic planning/implementation process, but it is primarily geared toward chronic disease prevention and health promotion programs. PATCH is typically managed by a health agency's education/promotion program or through an outside community organization. It is often used to affect and change public policy and environmental factors as well as individual decisions regarding lifestyles and behavior in the community. PATCH materials provided in a series of workshops guide participants through the steps required for a planned approach to community health
Tasks (how they are used)	• Offers self-assessment to meet user needs • Produces a practical plan of action to address the community's priority problems • Focuses on administrative capacity, basic structure, and the role of the agency in the community • Encourages assessment of community, state, and federal agency relations and how to obtain support • Easily adapts to fit local situations and resources • Is cyclical; by instituting the process, it allows for continued adaptation as changes occur	• Mobilizes the community • Collects and organizes data • Chooses priorities and target groups • Chooses and conducts interventions • Evaluates itself • Maintains and refines the PATCH process

Source: Adapted with permission from *The Guide to Implementing Model Standards: Eleven Steps toward a Healthy Community,* p. 16, © 1993, American Public Health Association and Centers for Disease Control and Prevention, Washington, D.C.

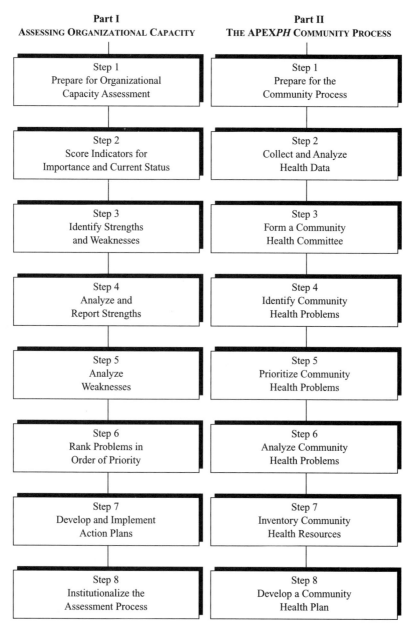

Figure 2–2 Flowchart of Steps To Assess the Organizational Capacity and To Assess the Community Needs Process within the APEX*PH* Model. *Source:* Adapted with permission from American Public Health Association et al., APEX*PH: Assessment Protocol for Excellence in Public Health,* pp. 10–78, March 1991, National Association of County Health Officials, Washington, DC.

munity to have an effect on chronic disease prevention and health prevention strategies. The model offers a good fit for analyzing many of the health promotion/disease prevention Year 2000 objectives. The primary mission of PATCH is to reduce the major causes of mortality and morbidity by addressing risk factors related to lifestyle, environment, biology, and health care delivery system areas. An added dimension to this analysis is to focus on the levels of prevention: primary, secondary, and tertiary. To achieve this mission, the PATCH model analyzes the community through the development of community profiles to find the specific causes of death and illness and the contributing factors significant to the community of interest. Further, this planning and implementing of various interventions is paramount to the success of improving health status in the community.

The PATCH model outlines five phases to carry out the community mission:

1. mobilizing the community
2. collecting and organizing data
3. choosing health priorities and target groups
4. choosing and conducting interviews
5. evaluating [19]

Table 2–6 outlines the phases, the description of the phases, and the tasks to be completed during each phase. An application of this approach has been developed by the Hospital Association of Pennsylvania (HAP) and has been outlined in five phases much like the PATCH model.[20] Their guide for assessing and improving the health status of Pennsylvania communities was developed to supplement the *County Health Profile* that they produced as well as to mobilize communities into action.[21] The report suggests five actions that are interrelated with the five phases of their community planning process:

1. Learn and understand from the *County Health Profile* what makes communities unique in terms of their demographic characteristics, available health care resources, health status and risk, and historical patterns of use of specific clinical services.
2. Recognize that information characterizing the health behavior of a community, a comprehensive inventory of human services agencies, and an appreciation for the economic impact of health care in a community provide an invaluable insight into the pervasive nature of health care.
3. Work together, using community-organized focus groups drawing on the perceptions, expertise, and support of local resources, to identify and establish a list of needs, priorities, and targets for attention.
4. Rally the local community to develop an aggressive action plan to address identified needs, combining the efforts of preventive measures and health promotion with programs to encourage early detection and treatment.

Table 2–6 Planned Approach to Community Health (PATCH) Key Concepts and Tasks

Phase	Description	Tasks
1. Mobilizing the community	Community mobilization is an ongoing component. A community group is formed to define the community, increase members' knowledge and skills for addressing health issues, and create working groups to carry out the PATCH process	✔ Define the PATCH community ✔ Complete community profile ✔ Publicize PATCH to the community ✔ Organize the community group ✔ Organize the steering committee ✔ Conduct first community group meeting ✔ Form working groups

2. Collecting and organizing data	Mortality, morbidity, community opinion, and behavioral and other community data are gathered and analyzed. Data are presented to the community group and form the basis for determining health priorities and for program planning and evaluation	✔ Gather data
		  ✓ Mortality and morbidity data
		  ✓ Community opinion data
		  ✓ Behavioral data
		✔ Analyze data
		✔ Present mortality, morbidity, and community opinion data to community group
		✔ Identify health priorities
		✔ Identify additional data needs
		✔ Identify ways to share data with community

3. Choosing health priorities and target groups	Health priorities are identified; factors that contribute to the health priorities are analyzed; existing community resources, policies, and programs are identified; potential target groups are selected; and community objectives are set in relationship to *Healthy People 2000* objectives	✔ Present behavioral and additional data ✔ Choose health priorities ✔ Set community objectives ✔ Determine contributing factors ✔ Select target groups ✔ Determine existing policies and programs ✔ Complete community resource inventory ✔ Develop community health promotional strategy ✔ Set behavioral objectives for intervention
4. Choosing and conducting interventions	A comprehensive community health promotion strategy is developed and the target groups are involved in the design and implementation of health intervention activities. Intervention and evaluation plans are developed. Volunteers are trained and recruited, and interventions are conducted and evaluated.	✔ Select interventions ✔ Involve target groups ✔ Develop intervention and evaluation plan ✔ Prepare activity and master timetables for interventions ✔ Recruit and train volunteers ✔ Publicize interventions ✔ Conduct interventions ✔ Provide intervention feedback

Table 2–6 continued

Phase	Description	Tasks
5. Evaluating PATCH process and interventions	Like phase 1, mobilizing the community, phase 5 is an ongoing component of the PATCH process. The evaluation should include monitoring the impact of the PATCH process on the community and assessing the impact of intervention activities.	✔ Review behavioral objectives ✔ Set criteria for success ✔ Determine evaluation questions ✔ Determine data sources ✔ Collect and analyze data ✔ Use results to enhance interventions ✔ Determine progress in completing phases ✔ Monitor participation ✔ Determine community impact ✔ Use results to improve process

Source: Adapted with permission from *The Guide to Implementing Model Standards: Eleven Steps toward a Healthy Community,* pp. 14–15, © 1993, American Public Health Association and Centers for Disease Control and Prevention, Washington, DC; and *Planned Approach to Community Health,* pp. 7–15, 1991, Centers for Disease Control and Prevention.

5. Measure and assess the impact that community action has on the health status of their population and continually strive to improve its effectiveness.[22]

These five actions are suggestions to help communities improve their health status. The actual five-phase process is shown in Figure 2–3. Notably, there is a strong parallel to the PATCH model discussed previously. Clearly the HAP has adapted its model to its own specific situation. Certainly, there is a message to be gained from this discussion (i.e., the core functions of public health practice [assessment, policy development, and assurance] may be implemented and assessed in various ways and that in any one community the approach must be population sensitive). A major theme in the HAP document is the use and application of quality improvement tools; however, the actual monitoring of the trends and the use of statistical measurement as reflected by run charts, control charts, and the like is not evident. These options and examples of using quality improvement tools are illustrated with applications in subsequent sections.

Continuous Quality Improvement Model

The public health practice core functions of assessment, policy development, and assurance may be viewed within the context of CQI. CQI is a process that incorporates the PDCA cycle, which begins and ends with an assessment of per-

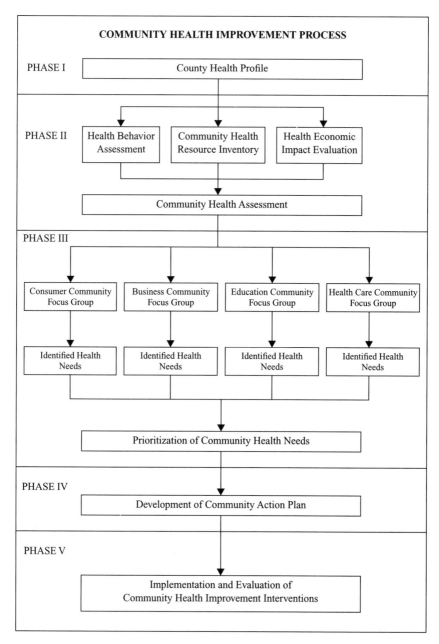

Figure 2–3 The Five Phases of the Community Health Improvement Process. *Source:* Reprinted with permission from *A Guide for Assessing and Improving Health Status: Community...Planting the Seeds for Good Health,* p. 3, © 1993, The Hospital Association of Pennsylvania.

formance. In public health practice, the community health needs assessment—an assessment of performance—should be viewed as a dynamic and ongoing process that may be considered as a quality improvement process, reflecting a community system as opposed to specific institutions. Of course, the public health agency responsible for the community needs assessment certainly can be viewed as the institution. The PDCA cycle may be viewed as an ongoing uphill action cycle that moves the process of assessing community need to a cycle of never-ending improvement. The illustration in Figure 2–4 suggests a 3- to 5-year cycle of addressing the community concerns by updating and completing the needs assessment. Each cycle produces a continuous advancement whereby the quality of the health status of the residents is continually improved. The goal of public health agencies in this country and as underscored by the Year 2000 objectives is to improve the health status of all Americans by increasing life span, reducing health disparities, and providing access to preventive services. The continuous application of the PDCA cycle to have an effect on these efforts will result in an ongoing monitoring, surveillance, and evaluation of the needs assessment process that moves an agency toward continuous improvement of the community health status.

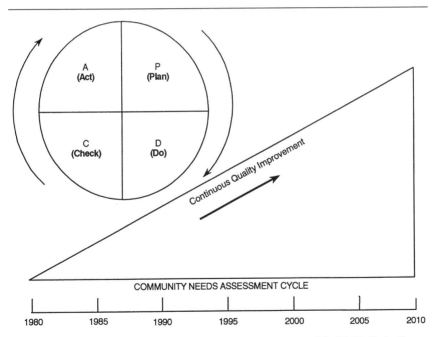

Figure 2–4 Public Health Practice—Community Needs Assessment and the PDCA Cycle. *Source:* Adapted with permission from H. Gitlow et al., *Quality Management: Tools and Methods for Improvement,* 2nd Edition, p. 108, © 1995, Richard D. Irwin, Inc.

The quality improvement model incorporating the PDCA cycle involves a 12-step process. Figure 2–5 illustrates the specific components of the 12-step process as it relates to the PDCA cycle.[23] It is this cycle and the specific steps related to quality improvement as applied to public health protocols that will become the focus of the remainder of this book. The application of the quality improvement methods to public health practice has been limited. However, it will become clear that many of the activities carried out in public health are actually using some of the concepts and principles that are peculiar to quality improvement. A comparison of the assessment tools (model standards, APEX*PH*, and PATCH) to the PDCA cycle and CQI illustrates that there are common aspects and approaches to assessing the performance of a process (Exhibit 2–2). Of specific interest is that the issues of monitoring, surveillance, and evaluation on a continuous basis are either directly indicated as in the *Model Standards* and APEX*PH* models or are

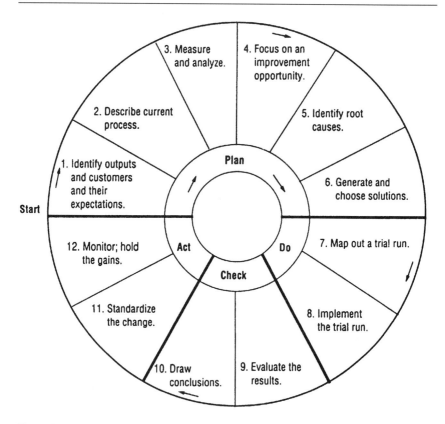

Figure 2–5 PDCA Model and Its 12 Substeps. *Source:* Courtesy of the Einstein Consulting Group, 1990, Philadelphia, Pennsylvania.

Exhibit 2–2 The Relationship of Assessment Tools to Continuous Quality Improvement

Steps	Model Standards	PDCA*	CQI Model	APEXPH	PATCH
1	Assess and determine the role of the public health agency within the community		Identify outputs and customers and their expectations	Introduction	
2	Assess the lead health agency's organizational capacity		Describe current process	Preparation, score indicators, identify strengths/weaknesses, rank problems/priorities, institutionalize assessment	
3	Develop an agency plan to build the necessary organizational capacity			Develop/implement action plan	
4	Assess the community's organizational and power structures		Measure and analyze	Form a community health committee, procedures for scoring indicators, role description	Identifies and organizes community committees, conducts community opinion survey and behavioral risk data collection
5	Organize the community to build a stronger constituency for public health and establish a partnership for public health	PLAN	Focus on an improvement opportunity	Form a community health committee	Identifies and trains community citizens
6	Assess the health needs and available resources		Identify root causes	Collect/analyze community health problems, inventory resources scoring indicators	Data collection, analysis of community opinion, behavioral and mortality data
7	Determine local priorities and available resources			Prioritize community health problems, method for setting priorities	Identify priorities and target groups; conduct inventory of resources
8	Select outcome and process objectives that are compatible with local priorities and the *Healthy People 2000* objectives		Generate and choose solutions	Develop a community health plan	Objective setting
9	Develop communitywide intervention strategies	DO			Develop a detailed work plan
10	Develop and implement a plan of action		Map out a trial run; implement the trial run	Implement a community health plan	Expansion of initial activities intervention planning, progress in overall implementation
11	Monitor and evaluate the effort on a continuing basis	CHECK/ACT	Evaluate the results; draw conclusions; standardize the change; monitor, hold the gains; continuous quality improvement	Basic monitoring and evaluation functions to progress toward policy development and assurance; continuous monitoring of data	Process, outcome, and impact evaluation

*Plan Do Check Act Cycle
Source: Adapted with permission from *The Guide to Implementing Model Standards: Eleven Steps toward a Healthy Community,* p. 17, © 1993, American Public Health Association and Centers for Disease Control and Prevention, Washington, DC.

suggested as in the PATCH model. However, how this activity is implemented and measured by the different approaches varies widely. The next issue to be addressed is the practice of public health and the application of quality improvement methods.

CONCLUSION

To meet the demands of determining the need for population-based services, a health status assessment is of paramount importance. This chapter discusses the role of the Year 2000 objectives, model standards, APEX*PH*, PATCH, and the CQI model in meeting a major core function of public health—assessment. Each of these process assessment tools is compared based on the 11-step model standards approach. Typically, in public health practice APEX*PH* and PATCH have been used in conjunction with the Year 2000 objectives and the model standards. This chapter proposed an extension of these typical assessment tools to include the CQI model based on the PDCA cycle for meeting the Year 2000 objectives and beyond. The CQI model is adapted to show the parallels of this approach to the model standards, APEX*PH*, and PATCH. Eventually, it is the application and use of the quality improvement methods that become the basis for improving effective decision making and completing sound community assessments in public health practice.

NOTES

1. E. Conley, "Public Health Nursing within Core Public Health Functions," *Journal of Public Health Management and Practice* 1, no. 3 (1995): 1–8.
2. Ibid.
3. Institute of Medicine, *The Future of Public Health* (Washington, DC: National Academy Press, 1988), 43.
4. Ibid., 113.
5. Conley, "Public Health Nursing within Core Public Health Functions," 1–8.
6. L.F. Novick, "Editorial: Public Health Assessment in a New Context," *Journal of Public Health Management and Practice* 1, no. 3 (1995): v–vi.
7. Ibid.
8. L.F. Novick, ed., *Journal of Public Health Management and Practice* 1, no. 2 (1995).
9. P.C. Nasca, "Editorial: Public Health Assessment in the 1990s," *Journal of Public Health Management and Practice* 1, no. 2 (1995): vii–viii.
10. Ibid.
11. U.S. Department of Health and Human Services, *Healthy People 2000: National Health Promotion and Disease Prevention Objectives,* DHHS Pub. (PHS) 91-50212 (Washington, DC: Government Printing Office, 1991), GPO Stock No. 017-001-0474-0.
12. Ibid.

13. G.E.A. Dever, *Community Health Analysis: Global Awareness at the Local Level,* 2d ed. (Gaithersburg, MD: Aspen Publishers, 1991), 1–30.

14. American Public Health Association, *Healthy Communities 2000: Model Standards,* 3d ed. (Washington, DC: Government Printing Office, 1991).

15. Ibid., xvii–xix.

16. Ibid., xxx–xxxi.

17. Ibid., xxviii.

18. American Public Health Association and the Centers for Disease Control and Prevention, *The Guide to Implementing Model Standards: Eleven Steps toward a Healthy Community* (Washington, DC: 1993), 12–13.

19. Ibid., 14–15.

20. The Hospital Association of Pennsylvania, *A Guide for Assessing and Improving Health Status: Community...Planting the Seeds for Good Health* (Harrisburg, PA: 1993), 3.

21. The Hospital Association of Pennsylvania, "County Health Profile," in *A Guide for Assessing and Improving Health Status: Community...Planting the Seeds for Good Health* (Harrisburg, PA: 1993), 5–12.

22. HAP, *Guide for Assessing and Improving Health Status,* 2.

23. W. Leebov and C.J. Ersoz, *The Health Care Manager's Guide to Continuous Quality Improvement* (Chicago: American Hospital Publishing, 1991), 83.

Chapter 3

Public Health Practice and Continuous Quality Improvement

This book has been designed to focus on the quality improvement methods that are necessary to ensure that the results obtained from the implemented continuous quality improvement (CQI) process are being measured, reported, and evaluated. It is not about CQI as perceived by most readers. For instance, there is very little discussion about how to begin or implement CQI in an organization—there are many textbooks on this aspect of CQI,[1–6] and a few have been written on this approach as applied to public health.[7–12] However, it is important to outline some basic concepts of CQI and recognize that these concepts must be fully understood if the public health practitioner is to use effectively the methods presented in this book for quality improvement. Thus, a brief review of CQI implementation concepts is presented.

CQI has been defined by various authors in many different ways. It has been called total quality management, total quality measurement, and continuous quality improvement. CQI is defined as a very structured process that must involve agency employees in the planning and executing of improvements in the processes and/or systems to provide quality health care (assessment, policy development, and assurance) that meets the needs of the public health customer. This process is a continual ongoing improvement of the delivery of health services to the community and the patient and/or client (i.e., the customer). The process is usually focused on a problem or need that translates into a project (i.e., a problem needing a solution). A basic tenet of CQI is that improving processes will achieve far greater results than finding people who are causing the problems. Remember the process is cyclical and ongoing, always moving forward toward improved quality on a continuous basis (see Figure 2–5). Thus, CQI is a process that involves continuous evaluation and is always moving toward new levels with new standards.

Many times, however, confusion occurs as to the difference in quality improvement compared with quality control and quality assurance. The differences are subtle but are important to discuss because many individuals clearly think that CQI is a new fad and, in fact, is no different from other measurement models that have been proposed to evaluate and monitor health outcomes.

CQI, QUALITY CONTROL, QUALITY ASSURANCE

From a conceptual point of view, CQI and quality control are different, whereas quality assurance represents a paradigmatic shift when compared with CQI. Quality control is about problem solving that detects a change, makes efforts to identify the cause of the change, and finally returns the process to the status quo. CQI, however, has the goal of reaching a level of performance never before achieved. The identification of a project and/or problem changes the organization to perform via changes in attitude, knowledge, and skills (i.e., focus on results). To solve problems effectively, CQI requires the use of data and improvement methods within an organization that provides the opportunities for change. Thus, the focus is on continuous improvement as opposed to fixed goals, which are associated with quality assurance or quality control.

Most agencies, managers, and public health organizations are quite familiar with the traditional quality assurance approaches. In fact, many confuse quality assurance with CQI and believe CQI is not different from quality assurance—it only is a new term applied to a traditional concept. A very basic difference is that quality assurance is focusing on finding fault with a person, whereas CQI is focusing on the process to improve the quality. This basic distinction allows any agency to improve its quality by moving beyond the individual level of fault to the understanding of the process to determine the nature of the variation. Of course, there are several other differences between quality assurance and CQI, and they are detailed in Table 3–1. The comparisons noted in Table 3–1 do not necessarily apply to public health practice because public health agencies usually have not had a quality assurance program and only now, as the health care reform movement requires accountability in public health, are they taking on the challenge of embracing the principles, concepts, and tools of CQI. The traditional role of public health state and county health departments has undergone significant evolution. This evolution was outlined in Chapter 1. Changing government benefits, government programs, and the need for more accountability has left public health in disarray. The infrastructure was nonexistent. The Institute of Medicine report suggested a focus on assessment, policy development, and assurance (i.e., the public health core functions to build the infrastructure and move public health toward a community-based agency).[13] This shift reflects a gradual erosion of the traditional public health function of "patient–clinic" programs to

Table 3–1 Public Health Practice: Comparing Quality Assurance and CQI

Characteristic	Traditional Quality Assurance	Continuous Quality Improvement
Purpose	• Improve quality of patient care for patients and improve the health status of communities, government auditors, regulators	• Improve quality of all services and products for patients and other customers (communities), excel, compete effectively to satisfy customers
Scope	• Retrospective clinical processes and outcomes • Actions directed toward people studied • Selected departments and functions • Quality is a separate activity	• All prospective systems and processes—clinical and nonclinical • Actions directed toward process improvement • Organizationalwide and across functions • Quality is integrated activity
Leadership	• Managers and clinical leaders: planning committee • Reactive • Top down	• All clinical and nonclinical leaders in the agency • Proactive • Bottom up
Aims	• Problem solving • Identify individuals whose outcomes are outside specified thresholds—implies special causes	• Continuous improvement, even if no "problem" identified • Addresses both special and common causes—most attention toward common causes—community, clinics, population based
Focus	• Who focused (negative) • Peer review vertically focused by department or clinical process • Unacceptable few—education or elimination of those who do not meet standards • Inspection and repair • Focus on meeting clinical criteria • Focus on solving problems • Outcome oriented	• Why focused (positive) • Horizontally focused to improve all processes and people that affect outcomes • Improve performance of everyone, not just the unacceptable few • Prevention and design to improve the processes—then inspection to monitor process • Focus on all processes to improve • Focus on improving processes • Process and outcome oriented
Customers and requirements	• Customers are professionals and review organizations—patient is focus • Measures and standards established by health care professionals only • Year 2000 objectives	• Customers are patients, professionals, review organizations, and others—everyone • No long-term fixed standards— continuously improving standards established by customers and professionals • Monitor progress for improvement, establishing new standards

continues

Table 3–1 continued

Characteristic	Traditional Quality Assurance	Continuous Quality Improvement
Improvement methods/tools*	• Chart audits • Nominal group technique • Hypothesis testing • Indicator measurement	• Indicator monitoring and data use • Brainstorming • Nominal group technique • Force-field analysis • Coaching/mentoring • Flowcharting • Checklist • Histogram/Pareto chart • Cause–effect, fishbone diagram • Run/control charts • Stratification
People involved	• Actions decided by committees appointed for specific periods • Externally directed • Limited involvement • Required, defensive • Management focused (directing)	• Everyone involved with process • Actions decided by team of people familiar with process—no time period specified • Internally directed • Total institutional involvement • Chosen, proactive • Employee focused (involving)
Outcomes	• Includes measurement and monitoring • May improve performance of the few individuals addressed • Creates defensive posturing • Event based	• Includes measurement and monitoring • Improves performance of everyone involved in process • Focus on process improvement—reduces threat to individuals, promotes team spirit, and can break down organizational barriers • Process based
Continuing activities	• Monitor for deviations from thresholds/standards • Follow up when there are special cause deviations	• Monitor processes for deviations and continually improve standards (QI) • Follow up when there are special or common cause deviations

*Most of this book is about quality improvement methods and tools that are used to monitor and evaluate outcome, process, and change in CQI.
Source: Adapted with permission from R.J. Coffey, "Comparing TQM and Traditional QA: Considerations for Health Care Organizations," *Competitive Times,* No. 2, pp. 9–10, ©1991, GOAL/QPC.

more emphasis toward evaluating populations in communities. These communities (population-based) and the clinical-based activities represent the customers of public health. Whether the emphasis for public health in the future is on population-based health (i.e., evaluating populations in communities) or clinical-based services (i.e., evaluating individuals in clinics), the focus of CQI must certainly include satisfaction of the public health customers.

PUBLIC HEALTH PRACTICE AND CQI—SHIFTS IN THINKING

Conventional Thinking versus CQI Thinking

To use the concepts, principles, and tools of CQI applied to the core public health practices of assessment, policy development, and assurance requires a paradigm shift in thinking. Public health agencies must evolve to a form of CQI thinking and away from the typical conventional thinking that has dominated public health agencies for decades. The contrasts between these two modes of thinking are described in Table 3–2. Notably, some of the shifts that must occur in thinking are dramatic. For instance, thinking based on opinions that are based on subjectivity, rhetoric, or case reports (i.e., glittering generalities) must be replaced by data based on objective, empirical, and factual thinking. For other paradigm shifts in thinking to occur, we must focus on the concept of serving the customers (communities, patients, clients, business, etc.) as opposed to the thought that customers are not evident as part of delivering a service. The measure of this would be the "customer satisfaction index." Another example is quantity (process evaluation—counting how many are served) versus quality (outcome evaluation—determining/measuring improvements in health status). Public health thinking has been extremely successful in counting (quantity measurement [e.g., we served 1.2 million clients last year, we have family connection programs established in 23 counties]) but has been essentially unsuccessful in assessing improvements in programs that can be attributed to the public health program (quality measurement [e.g., improvement in infant mortality, teenage pregnancy]). These shifts in thinking are not necessarily drastic, but for CQI to be supported and implemented in a public health agency, they must be addressed. Although we have pointed out these differences in thinking and sometimes philosophy, there is no attempt in this book to focus on the management philosophy as embraced in public health agencies. However, to incorporate the content and context of the material expressed in this book, management must investigate and adopt the principles embraced by CQI.

Creating Critical Thinkers

As previously suggested, to implement CQI in a public health agency, a paradigm shift in thinking must occur. Assuming the leadership in an agency has agreed to implement CQI, then a policy must be adopted that allows agency personnel to develop critical thinking skills. The need to create critical thinkers is

Table 3–2 A Paradigm Shift—From Conventional to Quality Improvement Thinking[*]

Public Health Practice Management

Conventional Thinking	Quality Improvement Thinking
Control programs	Coaching change in programs
Quantity • As important as quality • Result of better inspection	Quality • Without quality, quantity is irrelevant • Is built in from the start
Opinion • Subjective, rhetoric, case reports	Data • Objective, empirical, factual
Resistance to change	Open to change
Customers are not evident as being served • Not part of continual thinking • Internal focus	Customers are an integral part of your organization • Communities, patients, clients, business, etc. • Internal/external focus
We/they mentality	Us mentality
Suspicion	Trust
Detection (diagnosis)	Prevention (assessment)
Objectives • 95% is great • Focus on fixed goals	Process • 100% is possible • Focus on improvement
Errors/mistakes (who is responsible)	Variation (statistical process control)
People as commodities • Do your job • Know your place • Individual • Do what I tell you	People as resources • Expand your job • Understand the big picture • Team • Do what is needed
Problems • Compliance • Need more and better people	Opportunities • Commitment • Can achieve with the people we have right now

[*]Public health requires a paradigm shift in which a new set of rules and regulations aids in defining boundaries that guide the agency on how to be successful. It is a shift from managing the public health agency to leading the public health agency (i.e., doing the right things right).

significant to the agency for following the Plan-Do-Check-Act (PDCA) cycle and the 12 steps for improving a process on a continuous basis (see Figure 2–5). Probably the most recognized critical thinker is Marilyn vos Savant. She has suggested, based on her book *Brain Building,* that in 12 weeks one will be able to acquire and learn the tools and techniques of critical thinking.[14] The learning and adoption of these skills and techniques will bear on every aspect of your daily working life, including problem solving (the heart of the CQI process), decision making, and personal relationships (intraorganizational people skills). The author has created a "public health learning series" for "creating critical thinkers" that was implemented in a six-county health district for all district and local health employees.[15] This training was designed to run for 12 months as opposed to 12 weeks and was embraced effectively. In any event, as indicated "once it becomes a habit, the technique...will be yours forever, your own permanent key to thinking better."[16(p.x)] The relationship of thinking critical to the PDCA cycle has been elaborated on by the Juran Institute.[17] Specifically, they suggest that two important thought (thinking) processes are critical to effective problem solving: (1) the divergent/convergent thinking cycle, and (2) the creative/empirical thinking cycle.

Divergent/Convergent Thinking

The cycle of divergent/convergent thinking refers to *expanding* the thinking in the CQI process by the individual and/or team members and thus narrowing it down to a focus. The relationship of the PDCA cycle and the 12 steps of process improvement to the divergent/convergent thinking cycle is shown in Table 3–3. Developing a "laundry list" of problems (divergent thinking) related to a particular process will result in selecting or focusing on one of these problems (convergent thinking). Thus, depending on the nature of the 12 steps in the CQI process, the cycle of divergent/convergent thinking will be altered. There is always the danger of too much convergent thinking too early in the process, which would focus too quickly and potentially be too specific—more brainstorming or divergent thinking would be in order. However, if quality improvement efforts were continually focused on divergent thinking, then the process could become bogged down and a specific project would never be identified. Obviously, as shown in the chart (Table 3–3), there must be balances between the cycle to process through the PDCA cycle.

Creative/Empirical Thinking

The cycle of creative/empirical thinking refers to solving problems by *opinion-driven* thinking in the CQI process by the individual and/or team members or

Table 3–3 Divergent/Convergent Thinking in Public Health Practice Problem Solving

PDCA Cycle	CQI Process Improvement Steps for Problem Solving in Public Health Practice	Divergent Thinking	Convergent Thinking
Plan	1. List and prioritize problems (identify outputs and customers and their expectations for public health)	■	
	2. Describe current process		■
	3. Measure and analyze	■	
	4. Focus on an improvement opportunity (formulate theories of causes; test theories)	■	
	5. Identify root causes		■
	6. Generate and consider alternative solutions	■	
Do	7. Design solution and controls (map out a trial run)		■
	8. Implement the trial run		■
Check	9. Evaluate the results	■	
	10. Implement solutions and controls (draw conclusions)		■
Act	11. Standardize the change (check performance)		■
	12. Monitor; hold the gains		■

Source: Adapted from *Quality Improvement Tools®: Problem Solving Glossary* by P.E. Plsek and A. Onnias, © 1989 Juran Institute, Inc., p. 23.

by relying on *data-driven* thinking. The relationship of the PDCA cycle and the 12 steps of process improvement to creative/empirical thinking cycle is shown in Table 3–4. As suggested by the cycle, there are times or points during the problem-solving process that the effort is based on theories, hunches, guesses, or opinions.[18] This creative (opinion-driven) thinking is most needed when deriving lists of problems, possible causes, potential solutions, or barriers to change. The data-driven (empirical) thinking is based on facts. The appropriate time for empirical thinking is when prioritizing problems, analyzing data, testing hypotheses about causes, constructing solutions, checking solutions, and monitoring (surveilling) the system. Obviously, for this creative/empirical cycle to be effective, there must be a balance between the two cycles just as indicated for divergent/convergent thinking cycles. The Juran Institute has summarized the issues that may need to be addressed to resolve the balance between the creative/empirical thinking strategies. Creative thinking may lead to the following:

Table 3–4 Creative/Empirical Thinking in Public Health Practice Problem Solving

PDCA Cycle	CQI Process Improvement Steps for Problem Solving in Public Health Practice	Creative Thinking	Empirical Thinking
Plan	1. List problems (identify outputs and customers and their expectations for public health)	■	
	2. Prioritize problems (describe current process)		■
	3. Measure and analyze symptoms		■
	4. Focus on an improvement opportunity (formulate theories of causes; test theories)	■	
	5. Identify root causes		■
	6. Generate and consider alternative solutions	■	
Do	7. Design solutions and controls (map out a trial run)		■
	8. Implement the trial run	■	
Check	9. Evaluate the results		■
	10. Implement solutions and controls (draw conclusions)		■
Act	11. Standardize the change (check performance)		■
	12. Monitor; hold the gains		■

Courtesy of the Juran Institute, 1989, Wilton, Connecticut.

Lack of empirical thinking is the major fallacy behind some so-called "creative problem-solving models." These approaches are typified by their reliance on voting among team members at key decision points. Proponents of these approaches argue that such voting techniques are data and fact based because the team members work in the process and observe it every day. There are two pitfalls in this argument. First, human memory is a notoriously biased data-collection tool. People tend to remember the problem or cause that happened recently, affected them most seriously, or came at a particularly memorable moment for them. The second pitfall lies at the heart of our discussion of breakthroughs in chronic problem areas. Substantial breakthroughs in performance require breakthroughs in knowledge. In many cases, chronic problems exist precisely because no one knows the *true* extent and cause of the problem. Team voting merely produces decisions; it cannot fill in the gaps in knowledge.[19(p.26)]

However, strategized thinking may inhibit the creative thoughts. As the Institute notes,

> There is also a danger in strict empirical thinking that does not allow for unique ideas, suggestions, and points of view. Contrary to the beliefs of some, the huge stores of data that currently exist in most organizations do not contain all the answers to improved performance. The reason for this is that no one has ever *asked the right questions* that would result in the right data being gathered. The situation that many organizations face regarding the costs of poor quality is a prime example of this. The practice of rework has never been questioned, and so, no one has ever collected the data to quantify it. "Question asking" is a creative-thinking process. Without good, creative questions, a problem-solving team will never cut the new windows into the process that are often needed in order to allow empirical thinking to drive breakthroughs in knowledge.[20(p.26)]

Public Health Practice and Thinking Cycles

The relationship of the two cycles of thinking (divergent/convergent and creative/empirical) to the public health practice core function of assessment, policy development, and assurance is illustrated in Table 3–5. The importance of this relationship to public health agencies is to avoid and prevent the public health agency from regressing into the conventional thinking model and promote the CQI thinking model. By following the paths of the various types of thinking to be adopted for analyzing the core public health functions, the agency will move into the CQI process-thinking model and realize the importance of using quality improvement methods.

THE PUBLIC HEALTH CUSTOMER

The very first step of the 12-step PDCA cycle is to identify outputs and customers and their expectations. In public health, we have stated that the public health customer is the community, the client, the citizenry of the state/county, and other business and industry. These various types of customers for public health are considered external customers from a CQI point of view. Internal customers are considered to be individual sections/units within the public health organization. I will not attempt to deal with the internal/external customer phenomenon of CQI because that decision may be made by each public health organization. The more important concern is how to meet the needs of the customers and their expectations and to identify the processes that must be addressed to inspire the customer-organization relationship. Figure 3–1 outlines a customer-driven CQI process model.[21,22] This eight-step improvement model should not be confused

Table 3–5 Relationship of Public Health Practice Core Functions and the Cycles of Thinking: Divergent/Convergent and Creative/Empirical

Public Health Practices Core Functions[*]		Cycles of Thinking			
		Divergent	Convergent	Creative	Empirical
Assessment practices	Assess health needs	■			■
	Investigate occurrences		■	■	
	Analyze determinants		■		■
Policy development practices	Advocate	■		■	
	Set priorities		■		■
	Develop plans and policies	■			■
Assurance practices	Manage resources	■		■	
	Implement programs		■		■
	Evaluate programs		■		■
	Inform and educate	■		■	

[*]Any one of the efforts of the core functions is to be part of the CQI process. Each of the 10 efforts would be analyzed using the PDCA cycle and the 12 steps of process improvement.

Courtesy of the Juran Institute, 1989, Wilton, Connecticut.

---

with the 12-step PDCA cycle, but this customer-driven model includes at step 8 the PDCA cycle, which is initiated to continually improve the process—in this instance, to improve the level of customer satisfaction. The eight-step customer-driven CQI process model may be separated into phases.[23] As presented by the Einstein Consulting Group, and as noted in Figure 3–1, phase 1 represents steps 1 through 4 and includes the following:

1. Identify customers.
2. Identify customer expectations and professional standards.
3. Translate both customer expectations and professional standards into process/operational requirements.
4. Decide on measures of both outcomes and process.

Although these steps begin the process, periodic updating and revision are important as departmental responsibilities, customer expectations, and professional

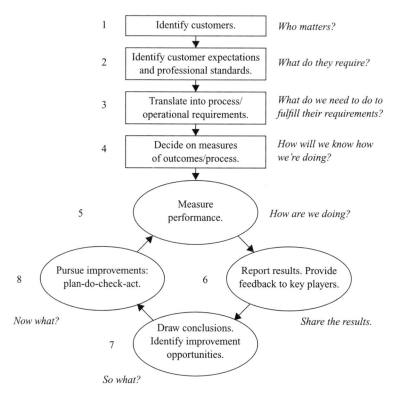

Figure 3–1 Customer-Driven CQI Management Model. Courtesy of The Einstein Consulting Group, 1990, Philadelphia, Pennsylvania.

standards change. Once start-up decisions are determined, implementation occurs. This is the second phase, a cyclical, closed-loop process for making improvements. The four steps in this phase, also noted in Figure 3–1, are as follows:

1. Measure performance using the indicators selected.
2. Report the results clearly and share the results with staff and leaders who are in influential positions.
3. Engage staff in drawing conclusions from the results and identifying and prioritizing opportunities for improvement.
4. Pursue specific improvement opportunities by using the PDCA process that was suggested previously and appropriate quality improvement tools to yield the desired outcomes.

The key to customer-driven management and CQI is to build this ongoing cycle of activities into the public health practice management routine.

THE PROCESS IMPROVEMENT MODEL FOR CQI

The customer-driven model, as we previously noted, has some of the steps that resemble the model for making specific quality process improvements (i.e., the PDCA cycle). In the process improvement model, the steps are applied to one process, not to overall departmental level management. Specifically, the process improvement model is applied at the micro level, whereas the customer-driven model is applied at the macro level.

The PDCA cycle represents four basic phases of plan, do, check, and act (Figure 3–2). The relationships of these four phases to the 12 steps for process improvement are shown in Figure 2–5. The use of the PDCA cycle may evolve in several ways. One does not have to follow exactly the 12 steps of the process model of the PDCA cycle. It is probably more critical to realize the importance of these steps and then apply them to your own specific situation by using the appropriate tools for dealing with the selected steps. In considering the elimination of steps, although possible, it is probably important to recall the pitfall of divergent/convergent and creative/empirical thinking models. Too much divergent thinking potentially eliminates some of the crucial steps and thereby could misguide the process.

Application of the PDCA Cycle

The use of the PDCA cycle and the 12 steps in the improvement process has been prevalent in the health care industry, mostly hospitals.[24] However, applications related to the patient care process by physicians and nurses have been detailed and are appropriate models for public health practice, especially focusing on the "individuals in clinics" component of the public health system. Two

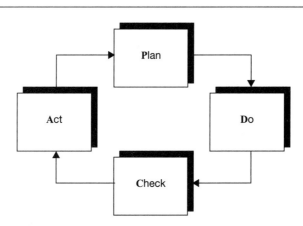

Figure 3–2 Generic PDCA Cycle for Quality Improvement

such approaches are shown in Figures 3–3 and 3–4. The Community Assessment Process model using the PDCA cycle illustrates the parallels between the approach of diagnosing and assessing communities' problems and the basic approach to problem solving. Further, for public health nursing the PDCA-CQI improvement process also parallels the clinical nursing aspect of public health programs. However, for the public health nurse who is more focused on community care (i.e., populations in communities), this quality improvement process would be modified to reflect a community assessment focusing on problems, priorities, interventions, and evaluations of the particular program.

The Public Health Practice—CQI Model

To implement the core public health functions of assessment, policy development, and assurance within a CQI framework—one that ensures an ongoing cycle

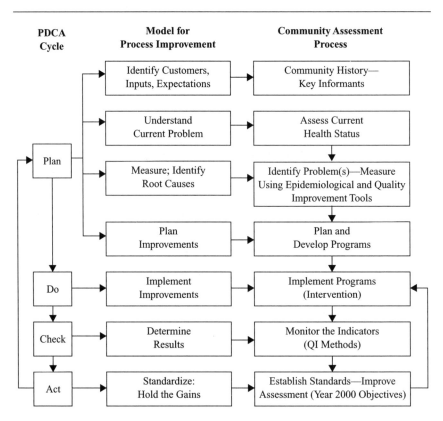

Figure 3–3 PDCA Cycle: A Community Assessment Model

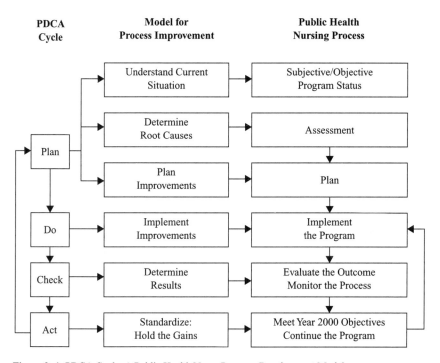

Figure 3–4 PDCA Cycle: A Public Health Nurse Program Development Model

moving toward continual improvement—a model is desirable. The *S*ubjective, *O*bjective, *A*ssessment, *P*lanning (SOAP) model originally developed for charting a patient's progress in a medical record has been expanded to show the parallels of this approach to analyzing community health problems.[25] Table 3–6 shows the CQI model and its relationship of the SOAP format to the PDCA cycle and its application to the clinical/community diagnosis and the CQI process in public health practice. In this instance, we have developed a SOAP-DCA model that illustrates the various steps to be completed for clinical, community, and clinical/ program public health practice improvement. There was an attempt to show parallel steps for each part of the SOAP-DCA cycle for continuity in analysis. However, there was no attempt to show, as has been illustrated previously, the cyclical nature of the SOAP-DCA model. Notably, as one reaches the act stage of the model, the steps point out revision, redirect, plan for the future, or more specifically, recycle to the beginning of the SOAP-DCA process. Certainly, a community health assessment will involve several cycles of learning, changing, and improving by continually following the SOAP-DCA model. Typically, the PDCA cycle must be viewed as an iterative process that is repeated over and over again with the primary goal of always improving the process and raising the standards.

Table 3–6 Relationship of Community Diagnosis and Clinical Diagnosis to Continuous Quality Improvement in Public Health Practice

SOAP-DCA Cycle	Diagnosis		CQI Process Model in Public Health Practice
	Clinical	*Community*	
Definition	*Individuals in clinics*	*Populations in communities*	*Clinics and programs in communities*
Subjective (S)	1. Patient's medical history 2. Symptoms 3. Explanations of illness 4. Resources	1. History of community 2. Community symptoms 3. Key community leaders' explanations of problems 4. Key community leaders' perception of resources	1. History of programs and clinics (recognize the process) 2. Program problems/symptoms 3. Leadership and customers' explanation of problems 4. Leadership and customers' perception of resources
Objective (O)	1. Physical findings (signs) 2. Lab work, test results, X-ray	1. Survey of community—a drive-through look for barriers/hazards 2. Use data (i.e., rates and numbers)	1. Understand the current programs—look for signs 2. Use data: rates, numbers 3. Measure, identify causes
Assessment (A)	1. Compare to standard—normal vs. abnormal 2. Develop problem list (i.e., differential diagnosis) 3. What is the problem?	1. Compare to standard—high risk vs. low risk 2. Develop problem list (i.e., establish priorities) 3. What is the problem?	1. Compare to previous measurement—look for improvement 2. Develop problem list (i.e., based on variation from the process)—look for root causes 3. What is the problem?
Plan (P)	1. Patient education and advice 2. Levels of prevention 3. Behavioral counseling 4. Degree of intervention (e.g., surgery, medication)	1. Community education and advice 2. Screening programs for disease problems 3. Levels of prevention 4. Working with community-based providers	1. Plan improvements based on identified causes 2. Continuous measurement for monitoring 3. Plan prevention to improve the process
Do (D)	1. Follow the appropriate protocol for implementing health improvement 2. Interventions	1. Implement improvements to the program 2. Develop new programs 3. Interventions	1. Implement changes to improve the process—determine options
Check (C)	1. Follow-up as determined by the condition or disease category 2. Evaluate	1. Follow up as appropriate for the program 2. Evaluate	1. Confirm changes and monitor for improvement 2. Measure changes
Act (A)	1. Continue protocol to determine outcome 2. Revise as appropriate	1. Analyze data to determine outcomes 2. Redirect resources and/or programs as warranted	1. Use quality improvement tools to determine progress of process 2. Plan for the future changes

Thus, a successful public health practice must be committed to a continuous and dynamic process directed toward improved assessment, policy, and assurance of health care.

CONCLUSION

Clearly, this book is not about the CQI management philosophy or the structure and organization that may be needed to implement CQI in a public health agency. However, a book that is focused primarily on quality improvement methods must at least highlight some of the CQI issues that are germane to the effective use of quality improvement methods in public health practice. To use these methods, an agency must realize CQI is not quality assurance or quality control revisited with a new name. There are differences, and these differences are important to the adoption and application of the quality improvement tools. Of specific importance is the nature of thinking: traditional or conventional versus quality improvement. To apply quality improvement methods effectively, the agency must create critical thinkers who understand the need for divergent/convergent and creative/empirical thinking. These concepts are applied to public health practice using the PDCA cycle of process improvement. The central issue for succeeding in these efforts must be the customer, the public health client. To ensure customer needs from a quality improvement perspective, the public health practitioner must clearly understand the relationship of applying the SOAP-DCA cycle to individuals in clinics, populations in communities, and programs and clinics in communities.

NOTES

1. W.C. Byham with J. Cox, *Zapp! The Lightning of Empowerment* (New York: Fawcett Columbine, 1988).
2. P.B. Crosby, *Quality without Tears: The Art of Hassle-Free Management* (New York: McGraw-Hill, 1984).
3. R. Fritz, *Think Like a Manager* (Shawnee Mission, KS: National Press Publications, 1991).
4. P.R. Scholtes, *The Team Handbook* (Madison, WI: Joiner Associates Inc., 1988).
5. A.R. Tenner and I.J. DeToro, *Total Quality Management: Three Steps to Continuous Improvement* (Reading, MA: Addison-Wesley Publishing Co., 1992).
6. M. Walton, *The Deming Management Model* (New York: Perigree Books, 1986).
7. A.F. Al-Assaf and J.A. Schmele, eds., *The Textbook of Total Quality in Healthcare* (Delray Beach, FL: St. Lucie Press, 1993).
8. E.J. Gaucher and R.J. Coffey, *Total Quality in Healthcare: From Theory to Practice* (San Francisco: Jossey-Bass, Publishers, 1993).
9. Juran Institute, Inc., *Quality in Healthcare.* Conference Proceedings: Day 2 of IMPRO91 Juran Institute's Ninth Annual Conference on Quality Management (Wilton, CT: 1991).

10. V.A. Kazandjian, ed., *The Epidemiology of Quality* (Gaithersburg, MD: Aspen Publishers, 1995).

11. C.P. McLaughlin and A.D. Kaluzny, eds., *Continuous Quality Improvement in Health Care: Theory, Implementation, and Applications* (Gaithersburg, MD: Aspen Publishers, 1994).

12. P.L. Splath, ed., *Innovations in Health Care Quality Measurement* (Chicago: American Hospital Publishing, 1989).

13. Institute of Medicine, *The Future of Public Health* (Washington, DC: National Academy Press, 1988), 87–98.

14. M. vos Savant, *Brain Building* (New York: Bantam Books, 1990), ix.

15. G.E.A. Dever, *Creating Critical Thinkers* (Atlanta, GA: Georgia Department of Human Resources, 1993).

16. vos Savant, *Brain Building*, x.

17. P.E. Plsek and A. Onnias, *Juran Institute Quality Improvement Tools: Problem Solving/Glossary* (Wilton, CT: Juran Institute, Inc., 1989), 23–27.

18. Ibid., 24.

19. Ibid., 26.

20. Ibid.

21. W. Leebov and C.J. Ersoz, *The Health Care Manager's Guide to Continuous Quality Improvement* (Chicago: American Hospital Publishing, 1991), 31.

22. Leebov and Ersoz, *The Health Care Manager's Guide,* 31.

23. Ibid., 32.

24. N. Goldfield et al., *Measuring and Managing Health Care Quality: Procedures, Techniques, and Protocols* (Gaithersburg, MD: Aspen Publishers, 1991).

25. T.M. Mettee, "Community Diagnosis: A Tool for COPC," in *Community-Oriented Primary Care,* ed. P.A. Nutting (Albuquerque: University of New Mexico Press, 1990), 52–59.

Chapter 4

Evidence-Based Public Health Practice

In the previous chapters, the focus was on public health practice. Specifically, efforts to create a healthy public health and models to perform public health practice assessments were outlined and presented. Further, a basic understanding of the quality improvement thought process was discussed based on concepts of convergent/divergent and creative/empirical thinking. A recurring message throughout this material was that public health must make sound scientific decisions based on evidence and not base decisions on anecdotal, rhetoric, or generalities that reflect unsound nonscientific thought or policies. Thus, this chapter furthers these concepts of promoting evidence-based public health and presents some very basic strategies for moving public health practice into the assessment, policy development, and assurance activities using evidence for making such decisions.

Public health must reframe, reconstruct its being, and quit believing the past will create the future. There have been recent accounts by individuals who still believe and espouse the ideas and thoughts that defend the tradition of public health.[1–3]

Thoughts such as "many of our services—WIC, prenatal, health education, for example—are seen as unnecessary and unproductive benefits for undeserving populations"[4(p. 8)] because Evans believes that "part of the problem we face is a hardened America, with a mean-spirited, begrudging attitude toward social justice, affirmative action, equity and compassion."[5(p. 8)] Koop has suggested that we must grumble, advocate for programs and offices, stand tall, articulate, and become confrontational.[6] These types of thoughts will not create a public health practice that emerges in the twenty-first century as a leader in providing population-based services to communities by implementing the core functions of public health—assessment, policy development, and assurance. Our public health services are not seen as unnecessary or unproductive because of a hardened attitude toward social justice, equity, etc., but because of our inability to provide evidence that these programs have been necessary or productive. Public health must shelve the rhetoric, reframe the system, and act on evidence-based policies. This chapter provides some approaches and directions to take public health into the twenty-first century by using evidence-based tools for the practice of public health.

ASSESSING PUBLIC HEALTH EVIDENCE

The Institute of Medicine (IOM) Report, as previously noted, suggested that public health lacks the infrastructure to successfully complete the core public health functions of assessment, policy development, and assurance. Further, in a recent edition of the *American Journal of Preventive Medicine,* the focus on research and measurement in public health practice is an indication of the need to provide the tools for effective measurement in public health practice. In fact, the main objective is this issue was how to best measure the effectiveness of public health practice.[7] Attempts for developing a strategy for measuring local public health practice and methods for assessing the public health core functions have been demonstrated by several authors.[8-11]

The attention to this topic indicates the need for public health practitioners to take notice and recognize that our abilities must be expanded to create a public health scientist, one with epidemiologic, behavioral, statistical, and quality improvement measurement skills.

Richards surveyed local health departments (370) to assess performance of the core functions by asking 26 questions related to assessment, policy development, and assurance (Table 4–1). The results clearly indicate public health is weakly positioned to implement evidence-based decisions because only 46 percent of the surveyed health departments are doing assessment functions. Within this function, the indicators on immunization (No. 7) received the highest response (79 percent) and the hospital indicator (No. 5) received the lowest (18 percent). Of further importance is that the functions of policy development recorded 53 percent and assurance was 68 percent. Within these functions, the indicators scoring the highest were meetings (95 percent), officials (91 percent), media (95 percent), and standards (87 percent). These results indicate that the practice of public health by local, state, and federal agencies must expand their capabilities beyond the levels that have been identified and promote population-based health (i.e., public health practice) from an evidenced-based perspective. Public health is failing with a grade of 56 percent. Note the indicators in Table 4–1 that receive a score of 90 percent or better (meetings, officials, and media). Our ability to promote the practice of public health is excellent, but it is not based on evidence because most evidence-based indicators all reflect values of less than 60 percent.

Table 4–1 Assessing Public Health Practices—Core Functions: Assessment, Policy Development, Assurance

Indicator	Question	% Yes*
Assessment		46
1. Needs	In the past three years in your jurisdiction, has there been a health needs assessment that included using morbidity, mortality, and vital statistics data?	51
2. Age-specific	In the past three years in your jurisdiction, have there been any age-specific surveys to assess participation in preventive and screening services?	32
3. Behavioral	In the past three years in your jurisdiction, has the population been surveyed for behavioral risk factors?	43
4. Investigation	In the past three years in your jurisdiction, has there been timely investigation of any unusual adverse health events?	65
5. Hospital	In the past three years in your jurisdiction, has there been a review of hospital discharge data to determine age-specific leading causes of hospitalization?	18
6. Work-related	In the past three years in your jurisdiction, has there been a review of work-related morbidity and mortality?	38
7. Immunized	In the past three years in your jurisdiction, has there been an analysis of data on children two years of age who have been immunized with the basic series?	79
8. High-risk	In the past three years in your jurisdiction, has there been an analysis of health services needed by high-risk population groups?	47
Policy Development		53
9. Review	In the past three years, has there been a public review of the public health mission for your agency's jurisdiction?	24
10. Meetings	In the past year, as a part of the job, have you and your senior staff members regularly participated in meetings with other community health organizations?	95
11. Officials	In the past year in your jurisdiction, has there been a formal attempt at informing elected officials about the potential public health impact of actions under their consideration?	91
12. Advocates	In the past year in your jurisdiction, have elected or other government officials been strong advocates for public health?	65
13. Prioritized	In the past three years in your jurisdiction, have community health initiatives been prioritized on the basis of established problems and resources?	56
14. Policy	In the past three years, has your health department published an explicit policy agenda for the department?	25
15. Candidates	In the past year, has there been a formal attempt to inform candidates for elective office about health priorities for your jurisdiction?	56
16. Plan developed	In the past year in your jurisdiction, has a community health action plan developed with shared input from local, regional, and state levels been used?	31
17. Plan used	In the past year in your jurisdiction, has a community health action plan, developed with public participation, been used?	19
18. Agreements	In the past three years, has your health department entered into any written agreements with key health care providers or funding sources to define service roles?	63

continues

Table 4–1 continued

Indicator	Question	% Yes*
Assurance		68
19. Codes	In the past three years in your jurisdiction, have local health codes been reviewed to ensure they were up-to-date?	53
20. Standards	In the past three years in your jurisdiction, have public health services been reviewed to ensure they comply with applicable professional and regulatory standards?	87
21. Safety	In the past year in your jurisdiction, has there been a program to ensure environmental safety?	66
22. Access	In the past year in your jurisdiction, has there been a program to ensure access to basic personal health services for those unable to afford them?	69
23. Effect	In the past year in your jurisdiction, has there been any evaluation of the effect that public health services have on community health?	37
24. Budget	In the past year in your jurisdiction, has there been any evaluation of the effect that budget changes for your health department would have on public health problems?	55
25. Informing	In the past year in your jurisdiction, has there been a formal attempt at informing the public about health problems?	86
26. Media	In the past year in your jurisdiction, have reports on public health problems been provided to the local media?	95
Overall Total		**56**

*n = 370.
Source: Adapted with permission from T.B. Richards et al., "Assessing Public Health Practice: Application of Ten Core Function Measures of Community Health in Six States," *American Journal of Preventive Medicine,* Vol. 11, No. 6, Supplement, pp. 36–40, © 1995, Oxford University Press.

A study in the state of Washington that evaluated the local health department's capacity using APEX reported similar results.[12] They noted that "the strengths reported by the local health departments in Washington reflect the historical strengths of the public health systems in the United States."[13(p.88)] That is, they do a good job carrying out the traditional public health functions. However, the weaknesses noted clearly reemphasize the fact that public health is not well positioned to promote evidence-based decisions. They identified four broad areas that reflect significant weaknesses. They are

1. inadequate health department access to legal counsel, particularly among smaller health departments
2. lack of clarity about their mission and role
3. lack of expertise in data collection and analysis, program evaluation, and community health assessment

4. inability to use data effectively to guide established community public health priorities and program planning and policy[14]

As a result of these identified weaknesses, they call for an increased capacity to collect, analyze, and interpret health data to use the data to guide policy. The suggestion to place epidemiologists, statisticians, and planning and policy officers in local health departments or alternatively request technical assistance and training for present staff is a clear signal that the ability to promote evidence-based decisions for planning and policy is greatly needed. Pratt et al. conclude that the changing nature of public health from the individual focus on clinical-based service to the population-based focus on community services is resulting in confusion and difficulty in adjusting to the new role.[15] They note that "addressing the health problems of the community as a whole is a very different mission from that of providing limited clinical services for the needy."[16(p.91)]

EVIDENCE-BASED PUBLIC HEALTH PRACTICE

This book is an attempt to promote evidence-based decision making, planning, policy, and analysis using the traditional measures of statistics, epidemiology, and methods for assessing healthy communities as well as new applications using quality improvement measurement tools for working with ideas and working with numbers. As evidenced by the previous discussion, public health is not practicing its discipline effectively. The discipline has been in jeopardy recently by not being able to demonstrate that public health programs have been efficient and/or effective in demonstrating improvement in outcome measures or indicators. Lamarche has noted that the public health model is in peril due to limitless spending without health, difficulty adapting to emerging problems, and a diminishing impact on health.[17] The new public health must shift in focus from individuals to populations, use health as a starting point, and rethink resource allocations from curative and hospital care to ambulatory care, primary care, home care, and substituting nonclinical personnel for physicians.[18] These thoughts clearly point to the new role for public health; this is the opportunity to reframe the discipline. However, there is a caution: Evidence is lacking to support this role for public health, and public health practitioners cannot continue to rely on intuition as the basis for making decisions or assessing outcomes. For example, Fox notes that

> Despite progress, we continue to encounter barriers in the struggle to determine effective interventions for troublesome public health problems. The dilemma of where to spend our money only can worsen as we face greater demands on limited local, State, and Federal resources. We cannot ignore the importance of research- [evidence-]based successful interventions. [We must:]

1. Ensure that the research surrounding our interventions is sound and that the data are valid and reliable. This will require vigilant attention to data collection.

2. Assure early buy-in from agency officials, community providers and, most importantly, recipients [customers].

3. Adopt an ongoing epidemiologic approach to program management for continuous evaluation and quality improvement.[19(p.562)]

EVIDENCE-BASED FRAMEWORK FOR PUBLIC HEALTH

To promote evidence-based public health by using evidence-based tools, public health personnel must borrow from the work that has been done in clinical medicine reflecting clinical practice guidelines and clinical pathways. There are five basic elements that can provide the framework for providing evidence-based public health community assessment, including policy development and assurance. These five elements and how they relate to public health practice are embodied in the principles of lifelong learning. The ways to promote lifelong learning in public health practice will be considered in subsequent sections. The elements that provide this evidence-based framework may be thought of as a cycle that begins with *setting priorities* by using assessment tools to determine the importance of the problem being investigated (i.e., what is the evidence or methods used for prioritizing the problem?). Once priorities are determined, it is important to establish public health practice *guidelines* by using quality improvement tools and to answer the question, "how should the problem be managed?" (i.e., what protocols should be followed to ensure a positive outcome?). *Measuring performance* typically uses quality improvement measurement tools to determine how the problem is being managed and to report on the process and variation in the outcomes that have been defined for the community. To complete the cycle of setting priorities, setting guidelines, and measuring performance, it is necessary to focus on *improving performance*. Typically, to improve performance the tools for quality improvement measurement are applied to the problem to determine areas where improvement in outcomes can take place so that public health professionals are better able to manage the problem. The results from this final step lead again to a new determination of setting priorities based on an analysis of how performance might be improved. The key to this evidence-based framework for public health is the embracement of lifelong learning so as to continually be more effective as a learner and problem solver at each of these steps in the process. This cycle of setting priorities, setting guidelines, measuring performance, and improving performance, which is dependent on lifelong learning, is continuous and, therefore, moves the process of evidence-based public health always to the next level of outcome improvement defined by decisions based on evidence. The application of these five evidence-based strategies (lifelong learning, setting priorities, setting guidelines, measuring performance, and improving performance) to a population-based problem has been attempted by Ellrodt and Cho.[20]

Table 4–2 outlines 11 steps to follow for adapting the five evidence-based strategies for a community and/or a population in public health practice.

Evidence-Based Assessment—Setting Priorities

In public health practice, several tools and/or methods for setting priorities [Model Standards, Assessment Protocol for Excellence in Public Health (APEX*PH*), Planned Approach to Community Health (PATCH), Plan-Do-Check-Act (PDCA) cycle] have been outlined in an earlier chapter. In addition to these methods, a public health practitioner must use epidemiologic and statistical skills along with quality improvement measurement and community readiness (Civic Index) to establish population-based priorities.[21] By using these methods of pri-

Table 4–2 Evidence-Based Strategies for Population-Based Health

Evidence-Based Strategies	*Evidence-Based Activities*
Lifelong Learning ↓	• Develop and articulate a succinct problem statement • Implement a thorough literature search • Assess the quality of the article(s)
→ Setting Priorities ↓	• Public health evaluation teams determine the significance of the expected outcomes of the interventions
Setting Guidelines	• Develop Public Health Practice Guideline(s) for each important element of assessment, policy development, and assurance • Utilize guidelines for program community function (e.g., assessment)
Measuring Performance	• Develop a systematic approach to process measurement and reporting—quality improvement measurement • Develop a systematic approach to outcomes measurement and reporting—quality improvement measurement • Implement guidelines
Improving Performance*	• Measure and report process variation and community outcomes • Use process and outcomes measures with updated literature searches and appraisals to continually improve population health status in the community

*At this point, based on level of performance, new priorities are set and the cycle is continuous.

ority setting, various agencies have developed criteria for determining priorities. The criteria range from the potential to change health outcomes, potential to change costs, prevalence of the condition (morbidity, mortality), and the burden of illness. Further, a generic priority setting process for developing public health practice guidelines has been developed by Hayward and Laupacis.[22] This process includes the following steps:

1. Select priority-setting criteria and assign a weight to each.
2. Solicit nominations for topics for guidelines development.
3. Reduce list of topics to a number for which data about criteria can be gathered.
4. Obtain data for priority ranking.
5. For each topic, assign a score for each criterion.
6. Calculate summary priority score and rank topics by this score.
7. Review priority list and schedule guidelines development projects.[23]

These steps address the basic question of the importance of this problem. The answer using this process and the priority setting tools and methods noted above focuses the decision to one based on evidence rather than intuition or hope. For example, the Hanlon method for setting priorities is an attempt to use an evidence-based approach to identify the most important problems to be addressed.[24,25]

A Method for Setting Priorities[*]

The method described here is a modification of a method developed by J.J. Hanlon.

Health problems are prioritized on the basis of size, seriousness, and effectiveness of available interventions. A formula has been developed to assess the relative importance of a problem. The formula is

$$D = (A + 2B)C$$

where A = size of problem
$\quad\quad B$ = seriousness
$\quad\quad C$ = effectiveness of interventions
$\quad\quad D$ = program priority score

This model implies that the seriousness of a health problem is twice as important as its size, and the most important determinant of opportunity is the effectiveness of available interventions.

---

[*]Abridged with permission from *APEXPH: Assessment Protocol for Excellence in Public Health,* © 1991, the National Association of County Health Officials.

Alternatively, the "Size of the Problem" ratings could be established by giving the health problem with the highest frequency a rating of 10, the problems with the lowest frequency a rating of 0 or 1, and the other problems rated according to where they are relative to the most common or least common problems.

Size of the Health Problems

Give each health problem being considered a numerical rating on a scale of 0 through 10 that reflects the percentage of the local population affected by the particular problem—the higher the percentage affected, the larger the numerical rating.

Table 4–3 below is an example of how the numerical rating might be established. The scale shown is for illustrative purposes only and is not based on scientific or epidemiologic data; a community establishing priorities should establish a scale appropriate to the level of the health problems in that community.

Seriousness of the Health Problems

To score the seriousness of a health problem, use a scale between 1 and 10. The more serious the problem, the higher the number. In the priority-setting process, the seriousness of a health problem is considered to have a greater impact than its size; for this reason, in the final calculation, the "Seriousness Rating" given will be multiplied by a factor of 2.

Every community must establish its own criteria for rating the seriousness of health problems. Once criteria for rating the seriousness of health problems have been decided on, the seriousness of every health problem must be judged against the same criteria.

The following questions may be helpful in setting criteria for rating the seriousness of health problems.

- What is the emergent nature of the health problem? Is there an urgency to intervene? Is there public concern? Is the problem a health problem?

Table 4–3 Size of Problem Rating Scale

Percent of Population with the Health Problem	*"Size of Problem" Rating*
25% or more	9 or 10
10% through 24.9%	7 or 8
1% through 9.9%	5 or 6
0.1% through 0.9%	3 or 4
0.01% through 0.09%	1 or 2
less than 0.01% (1/10,000)	0

- What is the severity of the problem? Does the problem have a high death rate or high hospitalization rate? Does the problem cause premature morbidity or mortality?
- Is there actual or potential economic loss associated with the health problem? Does the health problem cause long-term illness? Will the community have to bear the economic burden?
- What is the potential or actual impact on others in the community (e.g., measles spread in susceptible population)?

An example of criteria for scoring for seriousness is shown in Table 4–4.

Effectiveness of Available Interventions for Health Problems

The effectiveness of interventions to reduce the health problem is an important component in priority setting. However, precise estimates are usually not available for specific health problems. It may be helpful to define upper and lower limits of effectiveness and assess each intervention relative to these limits. For example, vaccines are a highly effective intervention for many diseases; those diseases would receive a high "Effectiveness of Intervention Rating." At the other end of the scale are diseases such as arthritis, for which interventions now available are mainly ineffective. With this in mind, each health problem should be scored for the effectiveness of available interventions according to the table (Table 4–5). The best real-world expectations of available interventions, based on evidence of successful intervention programs, should guide this strategy. Three questions may be suggested:

1. How effective is the actual intervention (tools, methodology, devices, drugs, vaccines, etc.)?
2. How effective is the application of the intervention? (What percentage of the population can be reached? Affected?)
3. What is the potential of the intervention (fully funded, staffed, state-of-the-art)?

Table 4–4 Seriousness of Problem Rating Scale

How Serious a Health Problem Is Considered	*"Seriousness" Rating*
Very serious (e.g., very high death rate; premature mortality; great impact on others)	9 or 10
Serious	6, 7, or 8
Moderately serious	3, 4, or 5
Not serious	0, 1, or 2

Table 4–5 Effectiveness of Available Interventions Rating Scale

Effectiveness	Degree of Effectiveness	"Effectiveness" Rating
Very effective	80% to 100% effective	9 or 10
Relatively effective	60% to 80% effective	7 or 8
Effective	40% to 60% effective	5 or 6
Moderately effective	20% to 40% effective	3 or 4
Relatively ineffective	5% to 20% effective	1 or 2
Almost entirely ineffective	Less than 5% effective	0

Calculate Priority Scores for the Health Problems

Calculate priority scores using the Health Problem Priority Setting Worksheet (Figure 4–1). Priority scores are calculated from the scores recorded in columns A, B, and C for each health problem and are recorded in column D. The formula used for this calculation is

$$D = (A + 2B)C$$

Once priority scores have been recorded for all health problems, assign a priority rank for each problem, based on the size of its priority scores, and record it in column E. For example, the health problem with the highest priority score should be given a rank of 1, the problem with the next highest priority score, a rank of 2, and so on. Health problems with the same priority score should be given the same priority rank.

Health Problem*	A Size	B Seriousness	C Effectiveness of Intervention	D Priority Score (A + 2B) C	E Rank

* List the health problems as determined through data collection, community perceptions, or other means.

Figure 4–1 Health Problem Priority Setting Worksheet

Evidence-Based Management—Setting Guidelines

All too often after priorities are determined, health care practitioners are reluctant to establish guidelines for managing or implementing the program identified as a priority. To manage a community program or problem, four steps should be followed.

1. Formulate questions related to the priority that may be answered.
2. Critically review the best available evidence for managing the problem (i.e., locate and synthesize the evidence needed to answer the questions).
3. Evaluate the benefits, risks, and costs for options related to implementing the program.
4. Determine the relative level of the expected outcome to conclude whether benefits outweigh risks and costs.[26]

By assessing effectively these four steps, a public health analyst will be able to base a decision on evidence as to the development of a guideline for the identified priority. If the evidence suggests that public health professionals are unable to set guidelines because they do not have evidence, then they should alter their course or review their priorities.

To obtain evidence to develop community guidelines, the literature must be reviewed to determine the most likely articles to provide valid results. There are several issues to assess at this point, but two of the most important are the grades of recommendation supported by evidence and the type of the community problem to be developing guidelines based on the relevance of the article.

The grades of evidence are based on several approaches as to the quality of evidence supporting a particular recommendation. Table 4–6 lists the types of study designs as to the quality of evidence they support. For instance, a randomized clinical trial is of the highest quality, whereas a single case report would be considered poor quality evidence. Public health analysts must base their programmatic and community-based guidelines on evidence-based studies. The level or grade of evidence based on research designs is but an initial step to developing evidence for developing community or public health practice guidelines.

In addition to the research design issue, Guyett and others have developed guides for selecting articles most likely to provide valid results based on purpose of investigation (therapy or prevention, diagnosis, harm, prognosis) and integration studies (e.g., overview articles, practice guidelines, decision analysis, and economic analysis)[27] (Table 4–7). By combining the grades of evidence for the types of study with the guides for selecting articles, a public health analyst will be able to base the development of the community practice guideline on significant levels of evidence.

Table 4–6 Quality of Evidence Grades by Research Design for Assessing Community Practice Guidelines

Grade	Quality of Evidence—Research Designs
A	Randomized, prospective, community, and/or clinical trial with low false-positive and low false-negative errors
B	Randomized, prospective, community, and/or clinical trial with high false-positive and/or high false-negative errors
C	Nonrandomized prospective, community, and/or clinical trials
D	Cohort studies (incidence studies)
E	Case-control studies
F	Prevalence studies (cross-sectional studies)
G	Descriptive/ecologic studies
H	Case series/case reports
I	Individual evidence (personal experience/expert opinion)
J	One meta-analysis
K	One cost-effectiveness or decision-analysis study
L	One summary study that pools data from other studies

Evidence-Based Programs—Measuring Performance

The Evidence-Based Care Resource Group has noted that they have "frequently been surprised by discrepancies between what they perceived they were doing and what they found when they audited their...records. Because these discrepancies are common it is important to measure physician [and community] performance to ensure that effective care is being provided."[28(p.1575)]

In public health, the same issues occur. However, public health practitioners are more concerned with the performance of community health programs provided by public health agencies than doing community health assessments that are measuring performance. For public health to practice the core functions of assessment, policy development, and assurance, there must be a link and/or a direct connection to the environment of the managed care network that already produces a data set of performance measures. These performance measures are called Health Plan Employer Data and Information Set (HEDIS) and were updated in 1995, with a set of Medicaid HEDIS measurements currently being produced.[29] HEDIS, by some managed care health professionals, has been recommended to be proxy measures for public health measurements as a sort of a backing into population-based health measurement.[30] Most think the fit of HEDIS measurement to popu-

Table 4–7 Guides for Selecting Articles That Are Most Likely To Provide Valid Results

	Primary Studies
Therapy	Was the assignment of patients to treatments randomized?
	Were all the patients who entered the trial properly accounted for and attributed at its conclusion?
Diagnosis	Was there an independent blind comparison with a reference standard?
	Did the patient sample include an appropriate spectrum of the sort of patients to whom the diagnostic test will be applied in clinical practice?
Harm	Were there clearly identified comparison groups that were similar with respect to important determinants of outcome (other than the one of interest)?
	Were outcomes and exposures measured in the same way in the groups being compared?
Prognosis	Was there a representative patient sample at a well-defined point in the course of disease?
	Was follow-up sufficiently long and complete?

	Integrative Studies
Overview	Did the review address a clearly focused question?
	Were the criteria used to select the articles for inclusion appropriate?*
Practice guidelines	Were the options and outcomes clearly specified?
	Did the guideline use an explicit process to identify, select, and combine evidence?*
Decision analysis	Did the analysis faithfully model a clinically/community important decision?
	Was valid evidence used to develop the baseline probabilities and utilities?*
Economic analysis	Were two or more clearly described alternatives compared?
	Were the expected consequences of each alternative based on valid evidence?*

*Each of these guides makes an implicit or explicit reference to investigators' need to evaluate the validity of the studies that they are reviewing to produce their integrative article. The validity criteria one would use in making this evaluation would depend on the area being addressed (therapy, diagnosis, harm, or prognosis) and on whether those that are presented as the part of the table are dealing with primary studies.

Source: Adapted with permission from A.D. Oxman et al., "Users' Guide to the Medical Literature: I. How to Get Started," *Journal of the American Medical Association,* Vol. 270, No. 17, p. 2094, © 1993, American Medical Association.

lation-based health measurement is not exact; in fact, the National Commission for Quality Assurance does not see HEDIS as interchangeable with public health performance targets but as a convergence of interest.[31] Public health benchmarks have been detailed in *Healthy People 2000*[32] and are used by public health practitioners as targets by which to continuously monitor improvement of the targeted outcome indicators.[33] A major problem with the promulgated Year 2000 standards is that they are "implicit rather than explicit"[34] (i.e., they are not based on evidence). An implicit standard or target (such as the Year 2000 objectives) is traditionally based on asking experts what they think, either as individuals or as groups (e.g., consensus panel—such as the Year 2000 objectives). This approach requires processing all information by individuals in their heads and whoever uses the standard must accept the experts' opinion on faith. The presumption is that experts are reasoning in an analytical fashion rather than arriving at their answers intuitively. In a later section on lifelong learning and the learning cube, we see that intuitive knowledge is the weakest form of evidence. Thus, implicit evidence means not formally described or written down.

The alternative approach to the establishment of standards, practice guidelines, performance measures, etc., is the "explicit approach." This approach is characterized by a systematic analysis of evidence (see Tables 4–2 and 4–6), estimation of outcomes and costs, and assessment of preferences. Eddy notes that "explicit" means formally described and written down. Whereas the implicit approach accepts the beliefs of experts—without requiring any explicit descriptions of the evidence considered, the consequences of different options, or the value judgments behind the chosen option—the explicit approach holds that these descriptions are essential to the accurate assessment of a [community], and to the intelligent design and use of a [community—public health practice] guideline."[35(p.138)]

The need for "explicit evidence" changes the demands on the practice of public health and the practitioners who set standards, targets, guidelines, etc. They must change their approach from simple intuition and belief statements to reasoning through a public health program or problem step by step and justifying the conclusions. This change has several consequences:

1. *Setting standard or practice guidelines will be considerably more difficult, take longer, and cost more than the traditional approach of simply asking experts what they think.* Compared with the implicit approach, public health personnel will have to lower their sights on the speed and volume with which guidelines can be designed and raise their sights on the level of investment required.

2. *Most public health experts are not trained to do all the tasks required to understand the consequences of a health practice, to design a guideline for its use, or to develop a standard as an objective outcome measurement.* Although public health knowledge is critical and indispensable, knowledge of statistics, quantitative analysis, epidemiology, quality improvement measurement, economics, and other disciplines is also required. The appropriate model is a team (a grand rounds approach).

3. *Participating as a member of a team requires sharing control.* Experts who are accustomed to providing all the answers and having their recommendations adopted without challenge must understand that their knowledge and insights, although still indispensable, paint only a part of the picture. Their beliefs must be merged with other factors to determine the proper use of a program.[36]

For the measurement of public health performance, a set of guidelines must be established, which, given the gap between perception (implicit evidence) and reality (explicit evidence), appears to be essential for further advancement of evidence-based public health. Six steps are suggested for measuring clinical performances that may be used for public health performance measurement.

1. What is to be measured?
2. Is the needed information available?
3. How is an appropriate sample of community and/or patients identified?
4. How large should the sample be?
5. How will the information be interpreted?[37]

Much of this book has dealt with the statistical questions, and it was not the intent to detail the issues related to each of these questions. However, it is critical for the public health practitioner to realize that these are steps to be followed for developing evidence-based public health performance measures. There are several reports, in addition to the Year 2000 *Healthy People* objectives, that have provided lists of potential performance indicators.[38–40] Each of the lists is primarily a result of implicit-based evidence; however, it is clear that there is much movement toward developing more explicit definitions of performance measurement.

Performance Measurement—How Will the Information Be Collected?

There is considerable debate concerning the issue of how the information will be collected for measuring performance in public health. Much of the controversy is centered around the proposed functions of an information network or system to collect the data. It has been reported there are three functions: (1) to support patient care (a disappearing responsibility in public health—i.e., decline in the process of clinical services), (2) to support administrative and business transactions, and (3) to support outcomes management and performance reporting—including the health status of a community.[41] To respond to these efforts or at least a partial response, there has been the development of Community Health Information Networks (CHIN), Community Health Management Information Systems (CHMIS), and Information Network for Public Health Officials (INPHO), including several independent hospital–community-based systems.[42,43]

Each of these information systems faces the reality of implementing a system that is difficult, time-consuming, and expensive. In a recent report, Wakerly has noted that "you don't have to have a network or electronic superhighway to do community health assessments. But you do have to have agreement on data elements, definitions, how data is reported, and what's meaningful. Getting agreement on this is much harder than accomplishing network building."[44(p.181)]

Recently, it has been noted that some high-profile CHIN and CHMIS initiatives that damaged the reputation of community networks have proponents who believe that integrated delivery systems and the internet will aid the cause of community population-based information systems.[45]

As public health searches to find its niche in the electronics superhighway, it must focus its efforts more on responding to the core public health functions of assessment, policy development, and assurance and not on patient management (a disappearing function) or clinical services from professional providers—these functions will be serviced by the managed care networks. The opportunity for public health in performance measure is to link with managed care networks to provide population-based health information and measurement—a significant need of the managed care providers. Of course, public health must meet its own objectives related to the core functions.

There also has been debate over the nature of these systems (CHIN, CHMIS, INPHO). CHMIS, for example, was envisioned as a centralized data repository. Collected information from other systems in the community would be sent to the CHMIS database (or uploaded). Databases would include health plans, physician groups, and institutional providers (hospitals, nursing homes, business coalitions). CHINs, on the other hand, do not require a central data repository but support an integrated set of applications that connect systems and networks, which allows users to access the other systems and download data they need.[46] It appears the CDC/INPHO system is a cross between these two approaches (e.g., the centralized data repository of the federal government and the attempted connecting of primary care services as proposed by CHMIS).[47]

Certainly, the idea and the importance of a public health information system to meet the core functions are appealing. A major trend that is having an effect on the evolution of population-based health information systems for evaluating the performance of public health is the need for evidence-based public health practice. Certainly, this is not the only factor related to this need of public health systems development. Other trends include

1. growth and spread of managed care plans
2. increasing consumer/community demand for accountability by hospitals, physicians, and health plans during the 1980s
3. growing interest in clinical practice and public health practice focusing on quality improvement, disease management, and population-based assess-

ment, including continuous quality improvement and outcome measures. These efforts require increased and more targeted data collection and data analysis (the major premise of this book)

4. more consumer/community customer demand for and more health plan focus on performance measurement and reporting, including pressure on health plans to demonstrate their ability to manage the care of defined populations (evidence-based population health care)

5. development of HEDIS and other performance data sets (CHINs, CHMIS) and report cards

6. increasing interest on the part of public health specialists in taking these quality improvement tools and using work already being done by health plans and providers to assess the health of entire communities, not just employer groups[48]

Evidence-Based Programs—Improving Performance

The objective of developing evidence-based performance and/or outcomes measures is to evaluate public health programs and be able to show improvement. The use of quality improvement measurement in public health has been detailed in this book for the purpose of managing, analyzing, and improving performance by using quality improvement tools and traditional statistical/epidemiologic methods. The data systems being developed for performance measurement should be designed toward this end of improving outcomes. Table 4–8 suggests the levels of development in a quality improvement process for improving performance in public health practice. The five levels assess the total participation by the organization in the actual improvement of the critical process through the application of improvement tools and methodology. Key concepts are worker involvement, methodology, and use of tools.[49] A public health agency can evaluate the current state of continuous quality improvement (CQI) in its organization by using this benchmarking process and can aid in moving the agency forward to develop standards and/or practice guidelines for evidence-based performance for improving the outcomes in public health programs.[50]

In addition to using this benchmarking guide, the Evidence-Based Care Resource Group has developed strategies for clinical action to improve performance, thereby improving performance and outcome measurement.[51] Figure 4–2, adapted from the Evidence-Based Care Resource Group, outlines the strategies or determinants for community public health action to improve performance using evidence-based guidelines. Thus, the practice environment (community), prevailing opinion, public health attitudes, and evidence-based practice guidelines all contribute to community public health action for improving performance. By improving performance through process measurement, it is possible to determine compliance with guideline recommendations. Compliance with evi-

Table 4-8 A Quality Improvement Process for Improving Performance and Outcomes in Public Health Practice

Improvement Performance Level	Definition	Behavioral Objective	Behavior	Measurement
1. Business as usual	No attempt to allow public health organizations to expand or change	—	A. Programs do not actively support quality improvement measurement B. Inspection or record review is primarily the quality improvement tools C. Quality is only for industrial processes D. Training is provided on an exception basis E. CQI/TQM infrastructure incomplete	None
2. Initiation	Beginning planning and initial actions designed to create a desirable cultural change	• Recognition of the horizontal multifunctional process vs. vertical • Workforce involvement in organizational processes • Organizational performance measures focus on customer needs	A. Organization's mission defined in terms of the primary processes B. Workforce input solicited to identify subprocesses of key process C. Responsibility is determined and accepted for identified processes A. Teams have been formed around selected subprocesses rather than categorical programs A. Primary external customer is identified B. Customer needs/requirements are identified C. Indicators are identified based on customer requirements	A. List of macro/key processes B. Subprocess list C. List of process owners A. Process team charter A. List of customers B. Customer feedback C. List of indicators
3. Implementation	A higher degree of action than has been exhibited in initiation level	• Document baseline organizational subprocesses: assessment, policy, and assurance • Assess program capabilities	A. Document selected processes B. Performance data have been expressed in terms of its central tendency and variability A. An operational definition of the customer requirement has been established B. Program performance is described C. Customer requirement is compared with the process performance	A. Use of quality improvement tools (flowchart, cause and effect, etc.) B. Mean, median range, and standard deviation as applicable A. Customer-defined limits B. Use of quality control charts C. Process performance model

continues

Table 4–8 continued

Improvement Performance Level	Definition	Behavioral Objective	Behavior	Measurement
		• Select program processes to review (interorganizational) (e.g., immunization program)	A. Processes have been selected B. An assessment has been completed on selected processes	A. List of interorganizational processes B. Use quality improvement tools (Pareto, cause and effect, etc.)
		• Increased workforce involvement with organizational processes	A. Teams are identified around all subprocesses	A. Process team charter
		• Start to identify "best-in-class"	A. Survey most likely candidates for leaders	A. Survey of the process
4. Expansion	A wider range of quality improvement efforts and an increasing degree of activity in executing planned strategies	• Document baseline processes and data availability	A. Document selected processes B. Identify customers (internal/external) C. Teams gather pertinent data D. Performance data expressed in terms of central tendency and variability	A. Use of quality improvement tools (flowchart, cause-and effect diagrams, etc.) B. List of customers (internal/external) C. Data D. Mean, median, range, and standard deviation as applicable
		• Make program process changes	A. Assess variation by using comparison analysis to measure special vs. common cause variation B. Process control charts are used to monitor performance C. Process teams use analytical tools to determine root cause of conditions D. Effects of corrective action are monitored to verify the results	A. Percentage assignable B. Control chart interpretation C. Cause-and-effect/ scatter diagrams D. Control chart

5. Integration	Quality improvement is embodied in the way public health does business	• Process capability achieved for customer requirements	A. Process capability studies are processed B. Process teams determine the type and amount of improvement needed C. Fundamental changes to process design are implemented	A. Completed capability studies B. Improvement plan C. Process documentation
		• Participation of communities in continuous process improvement	A. Community performance meets or exceeds requirements B. Community participation in periodic reviews C. Community input is solicited in design/changes	A. Program/service criteria data B. Process team leaders C. Community feedback
		• Establish benchmarks for performance (best-in-class)	A. Measurement criteria are established for performance B. Benchmark assessment instrument is used by public health to develop strategy for continuous quality improvement	A. List of criteria/benchmark matrix B. Benchmark matrix (best-in-class)

Source: Reprinted from *Journal for Healthcare Quality*, 14(1), 8–13, with permission of the National Association for Healthcare Quality, 4700 W. Lake Avenue, Glenview, IL 60025-1485. Copyright © 1992 National Association for Healthcare Quality.

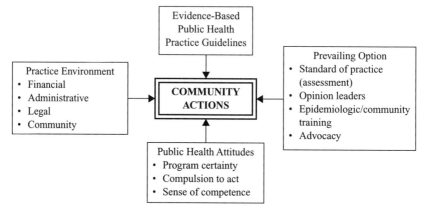

Figure 4–2 Community Action Strategies for Improving Performance. *Source:* Adapted from "Evidence-Based Care: 4. Improving Performance: How Can We Improve the Way We Manage This Problem?" By the Evidence-Based Care Resource Group, by permission of the publisher, *Canadian Medical Association Journal,* 1994, 150 (11).

dence-based practice guidelines by measuring outcomes is the only means by which public health practitioners are able to demonstrate programs and patient care improvement. Thus, in public health practice the goal must be to link the quality improvement process to outcome measurement to provide the opportunity to optimize community and patient health status. Reinertsen has outlined the useful and complementary roles of outcome measurement and quality improvement measurement.[52] In essence, quality improvement focuses on existing variation and complexity in processes to continually improve the process and thereby the outcome. Outcome measurement focuses more on the reported outcomes and not the process that created the outcomes.[53] The public health organization, by adopting these quality improvement strategies for measuring and improving performance, sets the stage for implementing changes and modifications in current public health practice guidelines. As stated previously, many of the current practices in public health are not based on evidence, and it is hoped that by adopting the strategies outlined here the public health practitioner will promote the practice of evidence-based public health practice focusing on the process and the outcome.

EVIDENCE-BASED LEARNING—LEARNING TO BE MORE EFFECTIVE

To promote the evidence-based public health practice model, a new approach for learning is advocated—lifelong learning (evidence-based). To ensure the use of the evidence-based framework as proposed, it is critical for public health offi-cials to base their future decision on evidence. Thus, evidence-based learning is the foundation. To practice evidence-based learning and how to be a more effec-tive learner, it is necessary to be able to critically appraise the public health and medical literature. Further, this learning must occur in an environment in which the public health officials have opportunities to listen, to present, and to evaluate the medical/public health literature. There are at least three ways that public health professionals may learn to be more effective and prepare for lifelong learn-ing so they can base their decisions on evidence. They are:

1. The public health learning cube
2. Public health grand rounds
3. Critical appraisal of the public health/medical literature

The Public Health Learning Cube

This cube was originally put forth by Sackett and others who have promoted the acquisition of critical appraisal skills for advanced lifelong learning in the medical field, specifically by using the materials and methods of clinical epidemi-ology.[54] To further the notion of lifelong learning for evidence-based public health and/or population-based medicine, the cube may also be our model for learning. The basic cube for public health learning is based on clinical/commu-nity evidence, clinical/community problem, and critical appraisal skills (Figure 4–3). The weakest form of learning occurs where there is no clinical/community problem, the community/clinical evidence is supplied, and the critical appraisal level is by intuition only (the lower left cell of the cube). This is considered the "core knowledge" approach and is the least effective way to learn and is based on the weakest form of evidence. This learning cube generates 27 different learning situations (Figure 4–3). The most advanced learning situation would be when the clinical/community problem is an actual program, the level of clinical evidence is an independent and/or guided search, and the critical appraisal level is such that it can be incorporated into the program. This level of learning is highly self-directed and produces an effective public health practitioner. Table 4–9 gives the strengths of public health learning based on the cube elements. In addition to this public health learning cube, the Evidence-Based Care Resource Group has devised a set of guidelines for teaching and learning evidence-based medicine that are valuable for the field of public health practice. They suggest that

1. Learning should be applied and participatory.
2. Learning should be self-directed.

The Public Health Learning Cube

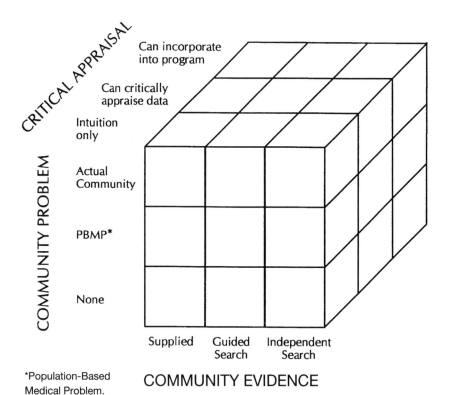

Figure 4–3 The Public Health Learning Cube. *Source:* Adapted with permission from *Clinical Epidemiology: A Basic Science for Clinical Medicine,* D.L. Sackett, © 1985, published by Little, Brown and Company.

Table 4–9 Relationship of Lifelong Learning Concepts to Level of Evidence in Public Health Practice

| Concepts | Evidence | | |
	Weak	Moderate	Strong
Community evidence	Supplied	Guided search	Independent search
Community problem	None	PBMP*	Actual program
Critical appraisal	Intuition only	Can critically appraise data	Can incorporate into program

*Population-based medical problems.

3. Learning should be practice based and practical.
4. Learning should focus on high-priority problems.
5. Efficiency should be emphasized.
6. Expectations should be reasonable.[55]

By applying these guidelines and focusing on the learning cube, the individuals in public health practice can become more effective learners and base their decisions on evidence and not on intuition, rhetoric, or anecdotal information.

Table 4–10 gives the reader an evaluation form for determining where his or her agency may be in the learning cycle. The public health practitioner can substantiate program additions, deletions, or modifications based on their learning levels within the evidence-based model. Obviously, there are situations that are unsatisfactory, and program decisions must not be based on such levels.

A final note on the evidence to support evidence-based medicine or public health practice is that the proof to support would be whether patients and/or communities show improved health status. The authors of evidence-based medicine state:

Table 4–10 Evaluation Form for Assessing Lifelong Learning Skills for Evidence-Based Public Health Practice

	Public Health Practice Learning Domain	
Evidence-Based Rating	*Role Model of Practice of Evidence-Based Population Health/Medicine*	*Leads Practice of Evidence-Based Population Health/ Medicine*
Unsatisfactory	Seldom cites evidence to support community decisions	Never assigns problems to be resolved through literature
Needs improvement	Often fails to substantiate decisions with evidence	Produces suboptimal volume or follow-through of problem resolution through literature
Satisfactory	Usually substantiates decisions with evidence	Assigns problems and follows through with discussion, including methodology
Good	Substantiates decisions; is aware of methodologic issues	Discusses literature retrieval, methodology of papers, application to individual patient and community program
Excellent	Always substantiates decisions or acknowledges limitations of evidence	Discusses literature retrieval, methodology of papers, application to individual patient and community program

Source: Adapted with permission from "Evidence-Based Medicine: A New Approach to Teaching the Practice of Medicine" by the Evidence-Based Medicine Working Group, *Journal of American Medical Association,* Vol. 268, No. 17, p. 2422, © 1992, American Medical Association.

Our advocating evidence-based medicine in the absence of definitive evidence of its superiority in improving patient outcomes may appear to be an internal contradiction. As has been pointed out, however, evidence-based medicine does not advocate a rejection of all innovations in the absence of definitive evidence...and on biologic rationale. The rationale in this case is that physicians [public health practitioners] who are up-to-date as a function of their ability to read the current literature critically, and are able to distinguish strong from weaker evidence, are likely to be more judicious in the...[programs] they recommend. Physicians who understand the properties of diagnostic tests and are able to use a quantitative approach to those tests are likely to make more accurate diagnoses. (Similarly, public health practitioners who understand the programs and are able to use the quality improvement tools are more likely to base outcome measurement on evidence.) While this rationale appears compelling to us, compelling rationale has often proved misleading. Until more definitive evidence is adduced, adoption of evidence-based [public health] medicine should appropriately be restricted to two groups. One group comprises those who find the rationale compelling, and thus believe that use of the evidence-based [public health] medicine approach is likely to improve clinical [program and community] care. A second group comprises those who, while skeptical of improvements in patient [community] outcome, believe it is very unlikely that deterioration in care results from the evidence-based approach and who find that the practice of [public health] medicine in the new paradigm is more exciting and fun.[56(p.2424)]

Public Health Grand Rounds—Tutorial Style

Grand rounds have been traditionally conducted in medicine in the southwest cell of the cube, where clinical evidence is supplied, there is no clinical problem, and critical appraisal is based on intuition (Figure 4–3). In public health practice, public health grand rounds must be introduced first to pursue evidence for programs and for meeting the core functions of assessment, policy development, and assurance. In addition, the grand rounds should become tutorial based where a population-based medical problem (PBMP) is supplied as the community evidence and the critical appraisal of the problem is based on their ability to apply the rules or guides for critically assessing the evidence as proposed in the PBMP. Initially, a major goal of the public health grand rounds would be to review the literature, in a PBMP format, on the issues of how to effectively evaluate the literature from an evidence-based perspective. Thus, articles on causation, therapy, assessment, prognoses of disease, quality of care, and an economic evaluation of a program should all be read to understand the guidelines for evaluating these topics. When this step is accomplished (certainly there are agencies doing this using a similar format to promote evidence-based population health and/or medicine), the next step is to begin, using quality improvement tools, to establish a process by which public health programs are systematically reviewed for evidence-based assessments, policies, and assurances. This approach can be local or at the state/federal level, and the results should be reported and distributed to other agency personnel. Public health must survive the onslaught of attack by legislators and consumers who say that public health practitioners are unable to show in a valid statistical format that the programs are improving outcomes; the response must show that "our results must be based on evidence." The evidence-based learning framework of grand rounds for public health must be adopted and become commonplace in the agency.

Critical Appraisal of the Public Health/Medical Literature

Several articles over a period of the past 15 years have received the attention of the health and medical advocates who see critical appraisal skills as a required subject for graduating physicians and other clinicians. There is no such movement in public health practice. It has been the intention of this book to outline the skills, methods, and knowledge for public health so that the public health practitioner's position for reporting on the health of the public is improved and that decisions are based on evidence using critical appraisal skills. Certainly, agencies may base their recommendations related to the implementation of various community programs on practice guidelines from clinical studies, but the ability to determine if the program worked or had an impact by showing improved outcomes has not been accomplished. Outcomes have not been based on evidence, and recommendations have not been driven by the evaluation of programs by providing evidence for continuation, modification, or termination. The critical appraisal skills outlined here and the evidence-based public health model proposed is offered in the spirit of articulating public health as a major force in the development, planning, and evaluation of population-based medicine in the twenty-first century.

Figure 4–4 outlines the critical appraisal skills for critically evaluating the literature related to four specific intentions: (1) use for a diagnostic test, (2) to learn the clinical course and prognosis of a disorder, (3) to determine etiology or causation, and (4) to distinguish useful from useless or even harmful therapy. Other types of studies and their critical appraisal skills were noted in Table 4–7. Depending on the type of study evaluated, there are three basic questions to be answered that allow the determination of the strengths and weaknesses of an article. The questions are (1) are the study results valid? (2) what were the results? and (3) will the results help in improving the health status of the patients/communities? Practical answers to these three questions related to the critical appraisal guides for primary types of studies are noted in Table 4–7 and Figure 4–4. Specif-

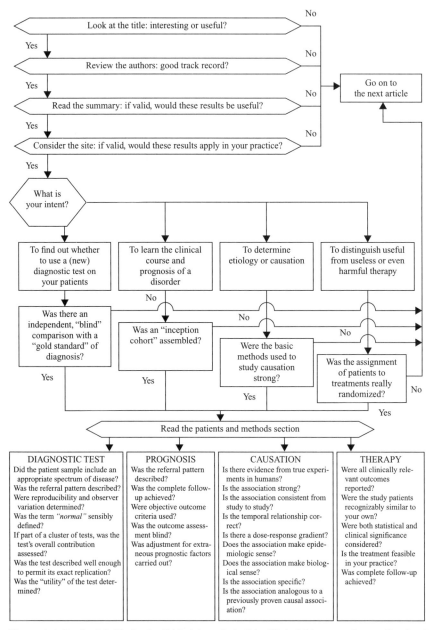

Figure 4-4 Readers' Guide for the Critical Appraisal of the Clinical Literature. *Source:* Reprinted with permission from R.B. Haynes et al., "Problems in Handling of Clinical and Research Evidence by Medical Practitioners," *Archives of Internal Medicine,* Vol. 143, p. 1971, Copyright 1983, American Medical Association.

ically, primary care strategies concerning therapy/prevention, diagnostic tests, harm/benefits, and prognosis are presented. For integrative types of studies to respond to these three questions related to the critical appraisal guides, see Table 4–7 and, in addition, see Users' Guides to the Medical Literature series by the Evidence-Based Medicine Working Group.[57–63] It is suggested that the public health agency, when implementing the tutorial-based grand rounds, begin with these user guides and the basics of critical appraisal as noted in Table 4–7. Although the focus of most of these guides is from a clinical perspective, it takes very little creativity to note how these critical appraisal guides may be adapted for implementing the lifelong learning skills to practice public health from an evidence-based perspective.

CRITICAL APPRAISAL GUIDES FOR PUBLIC HEALTH

In addition to the critical appraisal guides noted in Table 4–7 and Figure 4–4, critical appraisal guides have been developed for the evaluation of articles based on assessment, planning, and policy for public health practice. These guides were developed for evaluating the public health literature as part of a public health learning series.[64] Specifically, three critical appraisal guides are presented for evaluating the public health literature.

1. articles based on rates and ratios—used in assessment and policy analysis
2. articles based on numbers and percentage—used in health status and resource allocation problems
3. articles based on measures of central tendency, used for assessing program performance and improvement

The appraisal guides are shown in Exhibits 4–1 to 4–3.

CONCLUSION

Evidence-based public health practice is essential to meet the challenges being faced by the health industry in terms of scarce resources, government downsizing, improved performance, improved health outcomes, and decisions based on evidence and not intuition, opinion, or anecdotal information. This chapter has provided a framework for developing evidence-based decisions in public health. A case was made for public health to refocus its approach in areas of assessment (setting priorities), management (setting guidelines), programs (measuring and improving performance), and lifelong learning (grand rounds, the cube, and critical appraisal) and develop these areas by promoting evidence-based public health practice. Several assessment tools were outlined that may be used for critically

Exhibit 4–1 Appraisal Guide: Rates and Ratios

Critical Appraisal Guides
Evaluating the Public Health Literature
Measures Based on Rates and Ratios

Citation: _____

1. Purpose of investigation (What is the research question? What is measured?)
   _____
   _____
   _____
   _____

2. Community research designs (evidence-based policy and planning):
   ❑ Randomized community trial
   ❑ Cohort study (community)
   ❑ Control community vs study community
   ❑ Cross-sectional (prevalence survey)
   ❑ Ecological (comparison analysis)
   ❑ Community series
   ❑ Descriptive profile (county, state, national)

3. Evidence-based evaluation—does this study represent or report problems related to:
   ❑ Ecological fallacy
   ❑ Variations in the base (i.e., per 100; 1,000; 10,000)
   ❑ False associations
   ❑ Small denominators and variation of rates
   ❑ Advantages and disadvantages of the rate

4. Is this study about rates and/or ratios?
   ❑ Yes   ❑ No

5. Do you understand the type of frequency measure being used (rate/ratio/proportion)?
   ❑ Yes   ❑ No

6. What is the data source used in this study?
   ❑ Vital statistics   ❑ Program data
   ❑ Census data–U.S.   ❑ Clinical data
   ❑ Survey data   ❑ Unable to tell

7. Do the data for the study represent:
   ❑ Residence data   ❑ Other (i.e.,
   ❑ Occurrence data   workplace)

8. The analysis involves:
   ❑ Counts   ❑ Ratios
   ❑ Rates   ❑ Indexes
   ❑ Proportions

9. Determine the specific rate being used.
   ❑ Mortality (death) ❑ Natality (births)
   ❑ Morbidity (illness)

10. What type of rate is being used?
    ❑ Crude   ❑ Specific
    ❑ Adjusted
    ❑ Standardized Mortality Ratio (SMR)
    ❑ Proportionate Mortality Ratio (PMR)
    ❑ Risk or rate ratio
    ❑ Incidence/prevalence
    ❑ Other

11. What is the constant (k) used to calculate the rate/ratio/proportion? Determine what could be used. Is there a standard? What is that standard for this type of rate?
    Type of rate _____

Constant (k)	Used*	Standard
100		
1,000		
10,000		
100,000		

*What constants are used in this study?

12. Are the numbers and rates both provided in the study?
    ❑ Yes   ❑ No

13. Has the proper conversion of rates to numbers and numbers to rates been presented?
    ❑ Yes   ❑ No

14. What is the geographic level of the data?
    ❑ Household   ❑ District
    ❑ Block   ❑ State

Exhibit 4–1 continued

❏ Census tract ❏ Region
❏ Zip code ❏ National
❏ County

15. What time period does this study cover?
 ❏ <1 year ❏ 4–5 years
 ❏ 1 year ❏ >5 years
 ❏ 2–3 years ❏ Specified period

16. What does the numerator represent (i.e., the type of event)?
 ❏ Birth ❏ Demographic
 ❏ Death variables
 ❏ Marriage ❏ Social variables
 ❏ Divorce ❏ Hospital discharge
 ❏ Abortion ❏ Hospital admission
 ❏ Death by cause ❏ Cases
 ❏ Other

17. What is the source of the numerator?

_____
_____
_____

Is this information reliable?
 ❏ Yes ❏ No

18. What time period is considered for the numerator?
 ❏ <1 year ❏ 4–5 years
 ❏ 1 year ❏ >5 years
 ❏ 2–3 years ❏ Specified period

19. How was the denominator (i.e., population-at-risk) derived in this study?
 ❏ Estimate ❏ Total count (U.S. census)
 ❏ Projection ❏ Other

20. What is the source of the population-at-risk (denominator) data?
 ❏ Census data ❏ Program/clinic
 ❏ State documents ❏ records
 ❏ Other
 Is this information reliable?
 ❏ Yes ❏ No

21. Is the numerator data from the same time period as the denominator data?
 ❏ Yes ❏ No

22. What is the standard or basis for comparison to determine if the rate is high or low?
 ❏ District ❏ National
 ❏ State ❏ 2000 objective
 ❏ Region

23. Is the rate high or low?*
 ❏ Yes ❏ No

24. Has statistical significance been determined for the rate?
 ❏ Yes ❏ No
 Is it necessary to determine significance?
 ❏ Yes ❏ No

25. Determine the significance of the rate using the following formula:

$$SE = \frac{R}{\sqrt{d}}$$

where SE = standard error
 R = rate per population
 $\sqrt{}$ = square root
 d = number of events on which rate is based

26. Are the confidence intervals for the rates given? If not, calculate using the following formula:

$$CI = R \pm 1.96\frac{R}{\sqrt{d}}$$

where CI = confidence interval
 R = rate
 $\sqrt{}$ = square root
 d = number of events on which rate is based
 1.96 = two standard errors

27. Has statistical significance been determined for the count (event)?
 ❏ Yes ❏ No
 Is it necessary to determine significance?
 ❏ Yes ❏ No

28. Determine the significance of the event using the following formula:

$$SE_d = \sqrt{d}$$

where SE = standard error
 $\sqrt{}$ = square root
 d = number of deaths (counts or events)

_____

*The rate must be compared with a standard (i.e., above or below the selected standard).

continues

Exhibit 4–1 continued

29. The results from this evaluation analysis suggest program:
    - ❒ Change   ❒ Contraction
    - ❒ Expansion   ❒ No change
30. What program change or modification would be a practical application of this analysis? _____
    _____
    _____
31. Is there strong evidence as indicated by the results to influence policy?
    - ❒ Yes   ❒ No

32. Is there evidence to warrant further investigation?
    - ❒ Yes   ❒ No
33. What programs in community/public health could be influenced by the results of this study?
    1. _____
    2. _____
    3. _____
    4. _____
    5. _____
    6. _____

Exhibit 4–2 Appraisal Guide: Numbers and Percentages

Critical Appraisal Guides
Evaluating the Public Health Literature
Measures Based on Numbers and Percentages

Citation: _____

1. Purpose of investigation (Why are the data presented? What is measured?)

    _____
    _____
    _____
    _____
    _____
    _____

2. Is this study about numbers and/or percents?
    ❒ Yes   ❒ No
3. Do the data for the study represent (i.e., data source):
    ❒ Clinical data   ❒ Program data
    ❒ Census data   ❒ Unable to tell
4. Evidence-Based Evaluation—does this study represent:
    ❒ Arithmetical errors
    ❒ Percentage errors
    ❒ Improbable precision
    ❒ Misleading presentation
    ❒ Incomplete data
    ❒ Improper or faulty comparisons
    ❒ Improper sampling
    ❒ Failure to allow for the effect of chance
5. Are the data:
    ❒ Qualitative   ❒ Quantitative
6. What type of variable is being measured?
    ❒ Discrete   ❒ Continuous
7. Arithmetical error evaluation.
    Did we accept the value because it appears in print?
    ❒ Yes   ❒ No
    Is the subject matter important to you?
    ❒ Yes   ❒ No
    Did you check the author's calculations before accepting them?
    ❒ Yes   ❒ No

Did you find mistakes?
❒ Yes   ❒ No
If yes, list problems. If no, proceed with appraisal.

_____
_____
_____
_____
_____
_____
_____
_____
_____

8. Percentage error evaluation.
    What type of percent was determined?
    ❒ Simple percent
    ❒ Percentage change
    ❒ Percentages points of change (relative change)
    Were percentages computed correctly?
    ❒ Yes   ❒ No
    Were percentages based on levels rather than based on change in the level?
    ❒ Yes   ❒ No
    Were adding or subtracting of percentages calculated?
    ❒ Yes   ❒ No
9. Selection of base value for percentage calculations.
    How is the base value selected?
    Is the base value small?
    ❒ Yes   ❒ No
    Is the base value representative of the period of comparison?
    ❒ Yes   ❒ No
10. False percentages.
    Were the percentages added (beware of adding percentages)?
    ❒ Yes   ❒ No

continues

Exhibit 4–2 continued

Do results show decreasing percentages (beware of decreasing percentages)?

☐ Yes   ☐ No

Do numbers accompany percentages (beware of percentages unaccompanied by the actual numbers)?

☐ Yes   ☐ No

Do percents show huge differences (beware of huge percentages)?

☐ Yes   ☐ No

11. Precision.

Is the result (number or percent) presented to several decimal points (if not, be skeptical)?

☐ Yes   ☐ No

Is the degree of precision warranted by the evidence?

☐ Yes   ☐ No

Did you ask "how could anyone have found that out?"

☐ Yes   ☐ No

Did you approach results with a healthy skepticism?

☐ Yes   ☐ No

12. Misleading presentation.

Are accompanying numbers presented?

☐ Yes   ☐ No

Are percentages calculated appropriately?

☐ Yes   ☐ No

Are there attempts to misinform the audience?

☐ Yes   ☐ No

13. Incomplete data.

Are all data provided to make an accurate evaluation?

☐ Yes   ☐ No

Are you able to check the original measurement and make appropriate calculations?

☐ Yes   ☐ No

14. Faulty comparisons.

Were the proper comparisons made?

☐ Yes   ☐ No

Did the two groups being compared represent like characteristics?

☐ Yes   ☐ No

Is chance an effect that was not properly assessed?

☐ Yes   ☐ No

15. You used your "Statistical Guides" to:

☐ Calculate the error of number

☐ Calculate the significance of the number

☐ Calculate the error of the percentage

☐ Calculate the significance of the percentage

16. The results from this "critical thinking" evaluation suggest?

☐ Information   ☐ Contraction

☐ Change   ☐ No change

☐ Expansion

17. Is program change or modification a potential application of this analysis?

☐ Yes   ☐ No

18. Is there strong evidence as indicated by the results to influence policy?

☐ Yes   ☐ No

19. Is there evidence to warrant further information and/or investigation?

☐ Yes   ☐ No

Exhibit 4–3 Appraisal Guide: Measures of Central Tendency

Critical Appraisal Guides
Evaluating the Public Health Literature
Measures Based on Central Tendency

Citation: _____

1. Purpose of investigation (What is the question? What is measured?)
   _____
   _____
   _____

2. What type of community research design is being prepared? (Evidence-based policy and planning)
   ❒ Randomized community trial
   ❒ Cohort study (community)
   ❒ Control community vs study community
   ❒ Cross-sectional (prevalence survey)
   ❒ Ecological (comparison analysis)
   ❒ Community series
   ❒ Descriptive study (county, state, national)

3. Evidence-based evaluation—does this study reflect or report problems related to:
   ❒ Ecological fallacy
   ❒ Variations in the base (i.e., per 100; 1,000; 10,000)
   ❒ False associations
   ❒ Small denominators
   ❒ Advantages/disadvantages of the measures (mean, median, mode, range, variance, standard deviation)

4. Is this study or report about averages and/or dispersions?
   ❒ Yes   ❒ No

5. Do you understand the type of measure being used (mean, median, mode, range, variance, standard deviation)?
   ❒ Yes   ❒ No

6. What is the data source used in this study?
   ❒ Vital statistics   ❒ Program data
   ❒ Census data–U.S.   ❒ Clinical data
   ❒ Survey data   ❒ Unable to tell

7. Do the data for the study represent:
   ❒ Residence data
   ❒ Other (e.g., workplace)
   ❒ Occurrence data

8. Does the analysis involve:
   ❒ Means   ❒ Ranges
   ❒ Medians ❒ Variances
   ❒ Modes   ❒ Standard deviations

9. Is the level of measurement appropriate for the statistic?

	Yes	No
Nominal ...mode	❒	❒
Ordinal .....median	❒	❒
Interval .....mean standard deviation	❒	❒
Ratio.........mean standard deviation	❒	❒

10. Does this study commit any statistical sins?

	Yes	No
The mean of the means	❒	❒
Skewed distributions (used appropriate statistics)	❒	❒
Level of measurement	❒	❒
Data distortion problem— mean	❒	❒

11. Are the numbers (counts) and the measurements (statistics) both provided in the study?
    ❒ Yes   ❒ No

12. What is the geographic level of the data?
    ❒ Household   ❒ District
    ❒ Block   ❒ State
    ❒ Census tract ❒ Region
    ❒ Zip code   ❒ National
    ❒ County

13. What time period does this study cover?
    ❒ <1 year   ❒ 4–5 years
    ❒ 1 year   ❒ >5 years
    ❒ 2–3 years   ❒ Specified period

continues

Exhibit 4–3 continued

14. What does the numerator represent (i.e., the type of event)?
    - ❑ Birth
    - ❑ Death
    - ❑ Marriage
    - ❑ Divorce
    - ❑ Abortion
    - ❑ Death by cause
    - ❑ Demographic variables
    - ❑ Social variables
    - ❑ Hospital discharge
    - ❑ Hospital admission
    - ❑ Cases
    - ❑ Other

15. What is the source of the numerator data?

    _____
    _____
    _____
    _____
    _____
    _____
    _____
    _____

    Is this information reliable?
    - ❑ Yes
    - ❑ No

16. What time period is considered for the numerator?
    - ❑ <1 year
    - ❑ 1 year
    - ❑ 2–3 years
    - ❑ 4–5 years
    - ❑ >5 years
    - ❑ Specified period

17. With what are the computed measures being compared?
    - ❑ Program/clinic
    - ❑ District
    - ❑ State
    - ❑ National
    - ❑ 2000 objective

18. The results from this "evaluation analysis" suggest program:
    - ❑ Change
    - ❑ Expansion
    - ❑ Contraction
    - ❑ Further study
    - ❑ No change

19. What program or modification would be a practical application of this analysis?

    _____
    _____
    _____
    _____
    _____
    _____

20. Is there strong evidence as indicated by the results to influence policy?
    - ❑ Yes
    - ❑ No

21. Is there evidence to warrant further investigation?
    - ❑ Yes
    - ❑ No

appraising the medical and public health literature. By wisdom and not convention public health practitioners will begin to make progress toward creating healthy communities. This will take shape and begin to happen as they adopt the public health practice guidelines for basing decisions on evidence. In the subsequent chapters (Part II—Basic Methods), the focus is on the tools for quality improvement to bring the rhetoric of evidence-based public health practice into the mainstream of epidemiology, statistics, and quality measurement. Thus, the quality improvement tools for problem identification and problem analysis are detailed. The basis for these tools is predicated on sound epidemiologic and statistical methods, which are also highlighted as appropriate for the application of the quality improvement tools. Finally, a chapter on small area analysis is presented in the context of developing quality improvement measurement.

NOTES

1. "Koop Urges Public Health to 'Take the High Road,' " *The Nation's Health* December (1995): 1, 8.

2. E.R. Brown, "President's Column: Advocacy and Public Health," *The Nation's Health* December (1995): 2.

3. " 'Marketing Our Value' Is Public Health's Challenge, Says Evans," *The Nation's Health* December (1995): 8.

4. Ibid.

5. Ibid.

6. "Koop Urges Public Health to 'Take the High Road,'" *The Nation's Health*, 8.

7. G.M. Christenson and S. Dandoy, eds., *American Journal of Preventive Medicine* 11, no. 6 Supplement (1995).

8. A.S. Handler et al., "A Strategy for Measuring Local Public Health Practice," *American Journal of Preventive Medicine* 11, no. 6 Supplement (1995): 29–35.

9. T.B. Richards et al., "Assessing Public Health Practice: Application of Ten Core Function Measures of Community Health in Six States," *American Journal of Preventive Medicine* 11, no. 6 Supplement (1995): 36–40.

10. C.A. Miller et al., "A Screening Survey To Assess Local Public Health Performance," *Public Health Reports* 109 (1994): 659–664.

11. C.A. Miller et al., "A Proposed Method for Assessing the Performance of Local Public Health Functions and Practices," *American Journal of Public Health*, 84 (1994): 1743–1749.

12. M. Pratt et al., "Local Health Departments in Washington State Use APEX to Assess Capacity," *Public Health Reports* 111, no. 1 (1996): 87–91.

13. Ibid., 88.

14. Ibid., 90.

15. Ibid., 91.

16. Ibid.

17. P.A. Lamarche, "Our Health Paradigm in Peril," *Public Health Reports* 110, no. 5 (1995): 556–560.

18. Ibid.

19. C.E. Fox, "Why We Fail To Replicate Pilot Results: Adopting Realistic Expectations," *Public Health Reports* 110, no. 5 (1995): 562.

20. A.G. Ellrodt and M. Cho, "Introduction to Evidence-Based Practice," in *Patient-Focused Care in the Hospital: Restructuring and Redesign Methods to Achieve Better Outcomes*, vol. 4, eds. C.E. Aydin et al. (New York: Faulkner & Gray, 1995), 301–328.

21. M.E. Lara and C. Goodman, eds., *National Priorities for the Assessment of Clinical Conditions and Medical Technologies: Report of a Pilot Study* (Washington, DC: National Academy Press, 1990), 77–81.

22. R.S.A. Hayward and A. Laupacis, "Initiating, Conducting and Maintaining Guidelines Development Programs," *Canadian Medical Association Journal* 148, no. 4 (1993): 507–512.

23. Ibid., 508.

24. J.J. Hanlon, "The Design of Public Health Programs for Underdeveloped Countries," *Public Health Reports* 69 (1954): 1028–1033.

25. G.E. Pickett and J.J. Hanlon, *Public Health Administration and Practice*, 9th ed. (St. Louis: CV Mosby, 1990), 226–227.

26. Evidence-Based Care Resource Group, "Evidence-Based Care: 2. Setting Guidelines: How Should We Manage This Problem?" *Canadian Medical Association Journal* 150, no. 9 (1994): 1417–1423.

27. A.D. Oxman et al., "Users' Guide to the Medical Literature: I. How to Get Started," *JAMA* 270, no. 17 (1993): 2093–2095.

28. Evidence-Based Care Resource Group, "Evidence-Based Care: 3. Measuring Performance: How Are We Managing This Problem?" *Canadian Medical Association Journal* 150, no. 10 (1994): 1575–1579.

29. M.R. Traska, *Managed Care Strategies 1996* (New York: Faulkner & Gray, 1995), 66.

30. Ibid., 67.

31. Ibid.

32. U.S. Department of Health and Human Services, *Healthy People 2000: National Health Promotion and Disease Prevention Objectives*, DHHS Pub. (PHS) 91-50212 (Washington, DC: Government Printing Office, 1991), GPO Stock No. 017-001-0474-0.

33. Ibid.

34. Traska, *Managed Care Strategies 1996,* 67.

35. Eddy, "Practice Guidelines: What Are They, and How Are They Designed?," 138.

36. Ibid., 140.

37. Evidence-Based Care Resource Group, "Evidence-Based Care: 3," 1576.

38. D.R. Nerenz and B.M. Zajac, *Ray Woodham Visiting Fellowship Program Project Summary Report* (Chicago: Hospital Research and Educational Trust, 1991).

39. "Measuring the Quality of Health Care," *Employee Benefit Research Institute (EBRI) Issue Brief* 159 (1995), 15.

40. B.M. Zajac et al., "Health Status of Populations as a Measure of Health System Performance," *Managed Care Quarterly* 3, no. 1: 29–38.

41. Traska, *Managed Care Strategies 1996,* 174.

42. Ibid.

43. E.L. Baker et al., "CDC's Information Network for Public Health Officials (INPHO): A Framework for Integrated Public Health Information and Practice," *Journal of Public Health Management Practice* 1, no. 1 (1995): 43–47.

44. Traska, *Managed Care Strategies 1996,* 181.

45. F. Bazzoli, Restoring the Image of Networks, *Health Data Management* 4, no. 11 (1996): 38–50.

46. Traska, *Managed Care Strategies 1996,* 174.

47. Baker et al., "CDC's Information Network for Public Health Officials (INPHO)," 43–47.

48. Traska, *Managed Care Strategies 1996,* 169–170.

49. Headquarters Air Force Logistics Command, "Benchmark Matrix and Guide: Part III," *Journal for Healthcare Quality* 14, no. 1 (1992): 8–13.

50. Ibid., 8.

51. Evidence-Based Care Resource Group, "Evidence-Based Care: 4. Improving Performance: How Can We Improve the Way We Manage This Problem?" *Canadian Medical Association Journal* 150, no. 11 (1994): 1793–1796.

52. J.L. Reinertsen, "Outcomes Management and Continuous Quality Improvement: The Compass and the Rudder," *QRB* January (1993): 5–7.

53. Ibid., 6.

54. D.L. Sackett et al., *Clinical Epidemiology: A Basic Science for Clinical Medicine* (Boston: Little, Brown and Company, 1985).

55. Evidence-Based Care Resource Group, "Evidence-Based Care: 5. Lifelong Learning: How Can We Learn to Be More Effective?" *Canadian Medical Association Journal* 150, no. 12 (1994): 1971–1973.

56. Evidence-Based Medicine Working Group, "Evidence-Based Medicine: A New Approach To Teaching the Practice of Medicine," *JAMA* 268, no. 17 (1992): 2420–2425.

57. Evidence-Based Medicine Working Group, "Users' Guides to the Medical Literature: II. How To Use an Article About Therapy or Prevention, A. Are the Results of the Study Valid?" *JAMA* 270, no. 21 (1993): 2598–2601.

58. Evidence-Based Medicine Working Group, "Users' Guides to the Medical Literature: III. How To Use an Article about a Diagnostic Test, A. Are the Results of the Study Valid?" *JAMA* 271, no. 5 (1994): 389–391.

59. Evidence-Based Medicine Working Group, "Users' Guides to the Medical Literature: IV. How To Use an Article about Harm," *JAMA* 271, no. 20 (1994): 1615–1619.

60. Evidence-Based Medicine Working Group, "Users' Guides to the Medical Literature: V. How To Use an Article about Prognosis," *JAMA* 272, no. 3 (1994): 234–237.

61. Evidence-Based Medicine Working Group, "Users' Guides to the Medical Literature: VI. How To Use an Overview," *JAMA* 272, no. 17 (1994): 1367–1371.

62. Evidence-Based Medicine Working Group, "Users' Guides to the Medical Literature: VII. How To Use a Clinical Decision Analysis, B. What Are the Results and Will They Help Me in Caring for My Patients?" *JAMA* 273, no. 20 (1995): 1610–1613.

63. Evidence-Based Medicine Working Group, "Users' Guides to the Medical Literature: VIII. How To Use Clinical Practice Guidelines, A. Are the Recommendations Valid?" *JAMA* 274, no. 7 (1995): 570–574.

64. G.E.A. Dever, *Creating Critical Thinkers* (Atlanta, GA: Georgia Department of Human Resources, 1993).

Part II

Basic Methods

Chapter 5

Public Health Practice— Epidemiologic Measurement and Quality Improvement

In the previous chapters, the foundation was laid for evidence-based public health practice by focusing on the quality improvement concepts of performance. Thus, some basic concepts of continuous quality improvement (CQI) were outlined for moving forward toward a healthy public health, from understanding the assessment process in community analysis to outlining the basic quality improvement models to be used in public health practice. The message was that public health practitioners must move with haste toward practicing their discipline by using evidence-based methods. When the agency has reached the latter level, it must begin to use and understand the basic epidemiologic, biostatistical, and statistical methods to evaluate the progress of the selected program or programs on a continuous basis. The present chapter is most concerned with basic epidemiologic measurement that uses rates, ratios, and proportions. In analyzing the outcomes using quality improvement methods, public health agencies must grasp the most fundamental concepts of epidemiologic measurement so they may apply these concepts to the understanding of a process by describing and evaluating the variation.

RATES AND RATIOS—GENERAL CONSIDERATIONS

This chapter is designed to evaluate rates and ratios so that the reader is not misled by the presentation of data in articles, reports, and presentations. Further, most major health planning data represent rates and/or ratios that must be evaluated for making health planning and policy decisions as proposed by the core public health functions of assessment, policy development, and assurance. Specifically, in Chapter 4, critical appraisal guides were developed for evaluating the public health literature in reference to numbers and percents, rates and ratios, and measures of central tendency. These guides were proposed to facilitate the public health evaluation process and to further evidence-based decision making.

Rates and ratios provide the basis for most analysis and are certainly used for assessing community health status. No matter the sophistication of analysis, rates and ratios usually reflect the basics of community-based analysis and assessment and are integral to analyzing process and outcomes measures using quality improvement methods and understanding variation. Further, in public health, ratios and proportions are used to characterize populations by age, sex, race, exposure, and other variables. Ratios, proportions, and most important, rates are used to describe three aspects of the human condition: morbidity (injury, illness), mortality (death), and natality (birth). The focus on this chapter is the evaluation and interpretation of data in the community health setting that uses basic rates and ratios.

Frequency Measures (Proportions, Ratios, Rates)

To use the quality improvement tools for managing a process and targeting priorities, we must understand the differences between basic counts (attribute data) and the measures of rates, ratios, and proportions (variables data). Also, before studies that contain specific measures can be interpreted or critically appraised, it is likewise important to understand the relationship among these three basic types of measures and how they differ (Table 5–1).

The three measures (proportions, ratios, rates) operationally defined are

$$(1) \text{ Proportion (part to whole): } \frac{a}{a + b}$$

Table 5–1 Proportions, Ratios, and Rates for Frequency Measures

Measures	Numerator	Denominator
Proportion	People with the disease, condition, or event	All people (with and without the disease, condition, or event)
Ratio	People with the disease, condition, or event	People without the disease, condition, or event
Rate	People with the disease, condition, or event in a given period	All people (with and without the disease, condition, or event)

Source: Reprinted from G.E.A. Dever, Rates and Ratios Module, in *Creating Critical Thinkers,* Public Health Learning Series Monograph prepared for the Georgia Department of Human Resources, p. 6, © 1993.

(2) Ratio (part to part): $\frac{a}{b}$ and

(3) Rate (part to whole over time): $\frac{a}{a+b} \times k$

Proportion

A proportion is the expression of one part to the whole. The numerator is always included in the denominator (e.g., sex of children participating in a WIC program may be expressed as $\frac{female}{(all)male\ and\ female}$. Thus, in a proportion, the numerator is the count of the number of persons or events that satisfy specified criteria, whereas the denominator is the maximum number of individuals or events that could satisfy the numerator criteria. Mathematically, a proportion is expressed as $\frac{a}{(a+b)}$. Both counts are determined for the same time interval. For example, in a public health clinic, there were 30 female and 10 male visits during the week. The proportion of female clients is $\frac{30}{40} = 0.75$. If we convert this to a percentage, we multiply by 100 giving us 75 percent. *It should be noted that a percentage is a proportion multiplied by 100 percent.* In the needs assessment data on motor vehicle deaths, the proportion of male deaths is $\frac{12}{16} = 0.75$, multiplied by 100 results in 75 percent (i.e., 75 percent of all deaths due to motor vehicle accidents are male).

Ratio

A ratio is always defined as a part divided by another part. The numerator is not included in the denominator, and the two parts are usually independent (e.g., sex of children participating in a Women's, Infants and Children's (WIC) program may be compared as $\frac{female}{male}$). Thus, a ratio contains a numerator (a) that represents the count of the number of events that meet a specified criterion and a denominator (b) that represents the count of the number of events that satisfy a different criterion. Mathematically, a ratio is expressed as *a:b*, where *a* is a count of one variable and *b* is a count of another. Both counts are taken during the same time interval. For example, in a public health clinic there were 30 females and 10 males, the female-to-male ratio is 30:10 or 3:1 (i.e., there are three females for every one male in the clinic). In analyzing data for a community needs assessment, it was noted that the number of deaths due to motor vehicle accidents in the community for ages 15 to 24 was 16 (12 male and 4 female). Therefore, the male-to-female ratio is 12:4 or 3:1 (i.e., three male deaths for every one female in the community).

Rate

A rate measures the occurrence of an event in a population over time. Simply, a rate is $\frac{events}{population\ at\ risk} \times 1,000.$ *Numerators of rates are just the number of indi-*

viduals or things (events) something happened to in the *population-at-risk,* whereas *denominators* of rates are made up of people or things called collectively the *population-at-risk.*

There are some very basic points to remember about a rate. They are

1. Cases in the numerator must come from the population-at-risk.
2. The denominator must be the population-at-risk for the event (i.e., it should have been possible for them to experience the event).
3. The numerator and denominator should cover the same time period.
4. All rates are multiplied by an appropriate constant (i.e., 100; 1,000; 10,000; or 100,000).

Using the motor vehicle accident deaths as an example and given that the community has a total population of 9,200, and a population for age 15 to 24 of 2,100, the mortality rate for males would be $\frac{16}{2,100} \times 10,000 = 76.2$ per 10,000 population. Questions to ask about a rate should include the following: (1) what kind of rate is it? (2) of what is it a rate? (3) to what population or group does the rate refer? and (4) how was the information obtained?[1] In addition, use the critical appraisal guide in Chapter 4 to extensively evaluate the use of rates and ratios in the public health literature.

Proportions, Ratios, and Rates—Again!

As evidenced from this brief discussion, proportions, ratios, and rates are not three distinctly different kinds of frequency measures. They are all ratios: proportions are a particular type of ratio, and some rates are a particular type of proportion. In epidemiology, however, the terms for these measures are often shortened in a way that makes it sound as though they are completely different. For instance, when a measure is called a ratio, a nonproportional ratio is usually meant *(compare a part with another part)*; when a measure is called a proportion, a proportional ratio that does not measure an event over time is usually meant *(compare a part with the whole)*; and when the term *rate* is used, a proportional ratio that does measure an event in a population over time is frequently meant *(compare a part with the whole over time).*[2] Therefore, all rates are ratios, calculated by dividing a numerator (e.g., the number of deaths in a given period) by a denominator (e.g., the average population during this period). The result is usually multiplied by 100, 1,000, or some other convenient figure and expressed as a rate per 100, per 1,000, and so on. Some rates are proportions (i.e., the numerator is contained within the denominator). The correct use of the term *rate* has unfortunately become controversial. For simplicity's sake, this controversy will be ignored, and the term *rate* will be used for all measures that are commonly called rates, even in instances in which some epidemiologists regard this as incorrect.[3]

To Convert or Not To Convert

Numbers are converted into rates—or ratios or proportions—to generate comparable indices. For example, if we look at the number of deaths for two different groups of people or for a group at two different times, that number may differ only because the size of the population-at-risk differs. By converting to a rate such as deaths per 100,000 persons, the size effect is removed and the rates become comparable indices. So numbers are converted to rates for making comparisons. In CQI, when statistical analysis is applied, not all data will be converted to rates. There are many instances when using quality improvement methods in which basic counts (attribute data) may be used for assessing variation—either special or common cause.

Rates and Numbers—More on Conversion

Rates are used to develop comparable indices. Researchers will automatically convert all numbers to rates or even to adjusted rates to make inferences about differences or changes (i.e., to assess the health status of the population). In public health practice using quality improvement methods, numbers, not rates, are of interest to those concerned with the output of a program or the demand for services—that is, the health events themselves. The public health program practitioner will need numbers to estimate the magnitude of a problem and to project resource (dollar) need. Rates are not important in the allocation of resources but are important for health status measurement. So public health practitioners do not always convert. It is important to recognize that although converting fractions to a base number (thus creating rates) makes *comparing* them easier, the *significance* of any difference really depends on the *real* numbers (the population-at-risk) used to *derive* the rates.

Guidelines for Using Rates

Ecologic Fallacy

The ecologic fallacy (EF) consists of generalizing the data collected in a particular area to all the individuals living in that area (i.e., associating an indicator with persons who were not included in its calculation). An example is the use of a "normal family life index," which is the percentage of children younger than 18 who live with their parents. The denominator is the total number of persons younger than 18. The rationale is that if there are many single-parent homes in an area, this characterizes an undesirable social condition. For instance, if a survey was completed in which the neighborhood consisted of mostly older retired couples, young newly married couples, or single people, the results could reflect an EF if there were very few children younger than 18, in which the social condition could be classified as undesirable because of single-parent homes. Similarly, any index whose denominator is "families with children" might be based on too small a group for use in characterizing neighborhoods. The guidelines are (1) derive indicators from a denominator that includes the entire population group or most of it, and (2) apply indicators with subgroup denominators only to the persons in that subgroup.

Variations in Base

Variations in base may cause some problems in comparing rates. A proportion (say, 5/100) is multiplied by 100 to become a percentage (5 percent) or by 1,000 to become an infant mortality rate (of 50) or perhaps by 10,000 to become a disease rate (of 500). A rate must be accompanied by an indication of its base to be meaningful. A statement that "the rate has doubled" should be answered with the question, "rate per what?"

False Association

False association comes about by forgetting that rates apply to aggregates and not to individuals. A neighborhood may have a high unemployment rate and a high alcoholism rate, and statistical tests would show an association between these factors. Yet the unemployed and the imbibers could be two different groups of people.

Small Denominators and Variance of Rates

Rates based on very large populations may be interpreted as fixed numbers for purposes of comparison. But as the population base becomes smaller, statistical variation becomes more prominent as an explanation of differences. For instance, the graph showing infant mortality rates based on single-year numbers versus the five-year moving average numbers clearly shows how small numbers may lead to large variations (Figure 5–1). A rate has implications of a probabilistic or predictive statement. For example, the statement that two infants died out of 75 born is simply a statement of fact. To convert this to an infant mortality rate of 26—meaning 26 deaths per 1,000 live births—is by implication a statement of a long-run trend or a prediction. Yet, if during the following year only one infant died out

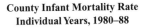

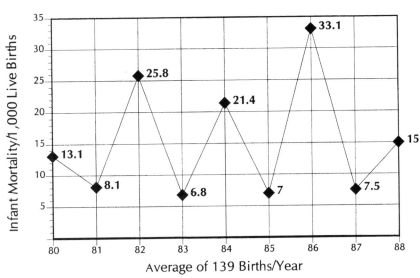

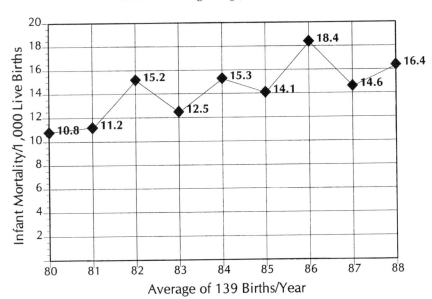

Figure 5–1 Variation in County Infant Mortality Rates Based on One- and Five-Year Periods

of 75 born (again a statement of fact), the infant mortality rate is only 13. This so-called "large decrease" is a result of statistical variation, and the magnitude of the decrease is exaggerated because of the use of a base of 1,000. The problem of small-denominator rates arises in any statistical analysis in which numbers are converted to percentages (rates per hundred). It is common practice to stratify data by age, race, morbidity, or other factors and to compare percentages of some phenomena for the different strata. However, the resulting information may be meaningless. Most statisticians use guidelines to determine when percentages should or should not be computed—for example, calculating confidence limits. Later in this chapter, a more thorough discussion of this statistical variation is presented under Data Issues—Technical Considerations.

Rate Interpretation

Crude Death Rate

Crude death rate is defined as total deaths divided by the population at risk multiplied by a constant, usually 1,000 (Table 5–2). It measures the average risk of death in the population at large. It is easy to compute. Its level reflects not only mortality risks but also the age and sex composition of the population. Hence, it can only be used to compare relative mortality in two populations if they have a similar age/sex composition. It is often used for comparing mortality in a given area between two time periods that are not too far apart. Crude rates should be considered with caution. Because crude rates are calculated using the entire population in a given community or geography, important variables such as age, gender, and race are not taken into consideration. In cases in which such variables play an important role, crude rates can be misleading. Such is the case when one considers various chronic diseases that are more prevalent in elderly populations than in younger populations. For example, crude rates representing groups with a high percentage of young persons would be misleading, and the fact that the rate is very high among the group's elderly would not be apparent.[4]

Age- and Sex-Specific Death Rate

An age/sex-specific death rate measures risk of death among persons in a specific age and sex group (Table 5–2). It is simple to calculate. It does not summarize total mortality in a single figure; however, it can be used to compare the mortality of two populations of the same specific age and sex group, even when the age and sex compositions of these populations are different. It takes no account of differences in the population structure in terms of race, occupation, religion, etc. It provides the essential components for constructing life tables.

Table 5-2 Measuring Death

Measure	Numerator (x)	Denominator (y)	Expressed per Number at Risk	You May Want To Know This
Crude death rate	Total number of deaths reported during a given time interval	Estimated mid-interval population	1,000 or 100,000	Beware of the "Confounders," Age, Sex, and Race.
Cause-specific death rate	Number of deaths assigned to a specific cause during a given time interval	Estimated mid-interval population	100,000	The Age, Sex confounder is at work here too! Don't compare Lung Cancer rates unless you get your confounders analyzed.
Proportionate mortality	Number of deaths assigned to a specific cause during a given time interval	Total number of deaths from all causes during the same interval	100 or 1,000	Beware this is not what it seems; check the numerator and denominator. This is not the risk you want to take. In fact, is this based on a "population-at-risk?"
Death-to-case ratio	Number of new cases of that disease reported during the same time interval	Number of new cases of that disease reported during the same time interval	100	This is similar but not the same as the "Case Fatality Ratio." Tells us how good or poor we are at plugging the dike—Do we stop the disease or does the dike break—AIDS case fatality rate is high.
Neonatal mortality rate	Number of deaths under 28 days of age during a given time interval	Number of live births during the same time interval	1,000	A good indicator of health status in 1950 when Neonatal Mortality was a significant problem. In 1995 re-evaluate the contribution of this problem to the overall health of the area—you may be surprised.

continues

Table 5-2 continued

Measure	Numerator (x)	Denominator (y)	Expressed per Number at Risk	You May Want To Know This
Postneonatal mortality rate	Number of deaths from 28 days to, but not including, 1 year of age, during a given time interval	Number of live births during the same time interval	1,000	The second part of the total infant mortality issue. Re-evaluate its contribution to improving the health status of your area.
Infant mortality rate	Number of deaths under 1 year of age during a given time interval	Number of live births reported during the same time interval	1,000	Infant Mortality (including Neo and Post) is statistically tricky. Small Areas and Small Numbers present Large Errors. Know when to Fold them (i.e., to calculate or not to calculate). Also know that all infants dying in one calendar year were not born in the same year—still a widely accepted measure as is.
Maternal mortality rate	Number of deaths assigned to pregnancy-related causes during a given time interval	Number of live births during the same time interval	100,000	An important indicator in the early part of this century. Maternal mortality is disappearing as a major issue. Check Maternal Morbidity.
Case-fatality rate	Number of specific deaths among the incident cases	Number of incident cases	100 or 1,000	Beware there are not twins in this list. This is not the Death-to-Case Ratio. This offspring requires that deaths in the numerator be limited to the number of cases in the denominator. The other is simply the ratio of specific deaths to cases during a specified time.

Source: Data from G.E.A. Dever, Rates and Ratios Module, In Creating Critical Thinkers, Public Health Learning Series Monograph prepared for the Georgia Department of Human Resources, pp. 18–19, © 1993 and Principles of Epidemiology, 2nd ed., p. 100, 1992, Centers for Disease Control and Prevention.

Comparison of overall mortality conditions in the two populations is cumbersome because of the need to compare rates for all the different age groups and for males and females.

Age-Adjusted Rates

When comparing death rates between two populations, the age composition of the populations must be taken into account. Older people have a higher number of deaths per 1,000 people. Therefore, if a population is heavily weighted by older people, then a comparison between two population groups might just reflect the age discrepancy rather than an intrinsic difference in mortality experience. One way to deal with this problem is to compare age-specific death rates (i.e., death rates specific to a particular age group). Another way that is useful when an overall summary figure is required is to use *age-adjusted* rates. These are rates adjusted to what *would be* if the two populations being compared had the same age distributions as some arbitrarily selected standard population.

Crude and Age-Adjusted Rates Compared

As noted in Exhibit 5–1, both crude and age-adjusted rates have decreased since 1940; however, the decrease in the age-adjusted rate is much greater. The

---

Exhibit 5–1 Crude and Age-Adjusted Rates Compared

- The table below shows the crude and age-adjusted mortality rates for the United States at five time periods.
- The adjustment is made to the age distribution of the population in 1940 (the standard).
- In 1987 the age-adjusted rate was 5.4/1,000, and the crude mortality rate was 8.7/1,000.

INTERPRETATION

- This means that if in 1987 the age distribution of the population was the same as it was in 1940, then the death rate would have been only 5.4/1,000 people.
- The crude and age-adjusted rates for 1940 are the same because the 1940 population serves as the "standard" population whose age distribution is used as the basis for adjustment.

Year	Crude Mortality Rate per 1,000 People	Age-Adjusted Rate (to population in 1940)
1940	10.8	10.8
1960	9.5	7.6
1980	8.8	5.9
1983	8.6	5.5
1987	8.7	5.4

Source: Reprinted from G.E.A. Dever, Rates and Ratios Module, in *Creating Critical Thinkers,* Public Health Learning Series Monograph prepared for the Georgia Department of Human Resources, p. 23, © 1993.

percentage change in crude mortality between 1940 and 1987 was $(10.8 - 8.7)/$ $10.8 = 19.4$ percent. Whereas the percentage change in the age-adjusted rate was $(10.8 - 5.4)/10.8 = 50$ percent. The reason for this difference is that the population is growing older. For instance, the proportion of persons 65 years and older doubled between 1920 and 1960, rising from 4.8 percent of the population in 1920 to 9.6 percent in 1969. The age-adjusted rates are actually fictitious numbers—they do not tell you how many people actually died per 1,000, but how many *would have* died if the age compositions were the same in the two populations. However, they are appropriate for comparison purposes. A recent study demonstrated that the selection of the standard (gold standard is 1940) using 1940 to 1990 affected the size of the age-adjusted rates but hardly changed the proportional mortality by age, sex, cause of death, and geographic area. It concluded that the 1940 standard is still a valid and appropriate measure to use.[5] A comparison of crude, specific, and adjusted rates showing advantages and disadvantages of each type of rate is illustrated in Table 5–3. Also, Table 5–4 demonstrates how to make a community diagnosis by comparing the relative status of the crude and adjusted rates.

Prevalence Rate

Prevalence rates measure the number of individuals with the disease in a population at a given point in time. Therefore, cause and effect (e.g., smoking and lung cancer) are studied simultaneously, making it impossible to establish a time

Table 5–3 Advantages and Disadvantages of Using Crude, Specific, and Adjusted Rates for Community Health Assessment

Health Status Indicators	Advantages	Disadvantages
Crude rates	Easy to calculate. Summary rates. Widely used for international comparisons (despite limitations)	Because population groups vary in age, sex, race, etc., the difference in crude rates is not directly interpretable
Specific rates	Applied to homogeneous subgroups. The detailed rates are useful for epidemiologic and public health purposes	Comparisons can be cumbersome if many subgroups are calculated for two or more populations
Adjusted rates	Represents a summary rate. Differences in composition of groups reviewed allowing unbiased comparison	Not true rates (fictional). Magnitude of rates is dependent on the standard million population chosen. Trends in subgroups can be masked

Source: Adapted with permission from J.S. Mausner and A.K. Bahn, *Epidemiology—An Introductory Text*, p. 138, © 1985, W.B. Saunders Company.

Table 5–4 Community Health Diagnosis Using Crude and Adjusted Rates

Relative Status of

Crude Rate	Adjusted Rate	*Community Diagnosis*
Low	Low	Low mortality is not due to age, race, and sex factors; other mortality conditions are favorable.
Low	High	Low mortality is due to favorable age, race, and sex factors; other mortality conditions are unfavorable.
High	Low	High mortality is due to unfavorable age, race, and sex factors; other mortality conditions are favorable.
High	High	High mortality is not due to age, race, and sex factors; other mortality conditions are unfavorable.

Source: Courtesy of North Carolina Vital Statistics, 1977.

sequence for a presumed cause. A prevalence rate is important in determining workload—particularly for chronic disease. It is useful for planning of facilities regarding hospital beds, for determining clinic visits, and for determining health personnel needs. High prevalence does not usually signify high risk but may reflect increased survival because of improved medical care or behavioral change (i.e., long duration). Low prevalence may reflect a rapid fatal process or rapid cure (i.e., short duration). The prevalence rate is often determined by means of a special study, such as a survey. Prevalence data are easier to obtain than incidence data because only one examination of a population is necessary.[6]

Incidence Rate

Incidence rates provide a measure of the number of new cases of a disease in a population during a specified period of time. It is a fundamental tool for etiologic studies—acute and chronic illnesses. Incidence is a direct indicator of risk: high incidence = high risk of disease. Low incidence rates are synonymous with low risk of disease. Incidence rate is often grossly underestimated because of incomplete reporting. If incidence is not subject to seasonal variation, annual rates may be estimated on the basis of observations over a fraction of a year.[7]

Incidence and Prevalence Rates

Incidence refers to the number of new cases of a disease during a specific period of time; prevalence refers to the number of existing cases of a disease at a particular point in time. Incidence rates provide a measure of the number of new cases of a disease in a population during a specified period of time. Prevalence rates measure the number of individuals with the disease in a population at a given point in time.

An incidence rate is a measure of risk. It is a dynamic concept that tells the rate at which new cases of disease occur in a given population over a period of time. By combining information on incidence rates with other variables, factors that may affect the risk of acquiring disease may be determined.

By contrast, the prevalence rate is a static concept; it indicates the amount of disease prevailing in a given population at a given point in time, allowing public health professionals to assess the burden of a particular disease in the community. A prevalence rate is an essential measure for planning health care resources.

Prevalence depends on two factors: the number of individuals who have become ill in the past (previous incidence) and the duration of their illnesses. With chronic diseases such as diabetes mellitus, the prevalence will accumulate even if only a few individuals in a population develop the disease each year. If, however, the disease is acute because of either recovery or death, prevalence will be relatively low even if incidence is high. Influenza exemplifies a disease with a fairly high incidence but relatively low prevalence. Another example is the acute and fatal sudden infant death syndrome, which leaves no residual disease or prevalence in a population.

If the incidence and duration of a disease are fairly stable, their relationship can be expressed as

$$\text{Prevalence} = \text{Incidence} \times \text{Duration}$$

When the prevalence and duration are known, incidence can be estimated.

Summing Up—Rates

Rates have been discussed and detailed for mortality and morbidity. Tables 5–2, 5–5, and 5–6 give the specifics for mortality (death), morbidity (illness), and natality (births) as to the measures, numerators, and denominators. Further, a column called "You May Want To Know This" gives some insight into the evaluation and interpretation of each of these rates.

DATA ISSUES—TECHNICAL CONSIDERATIONS

While using epidemiologic measurement, it is important to recognize that any given variable, indicator, or benchmark statistic may vary due to several influences.[8] In CQI, variation is usually considered as common cause or special cause. However, variation in data must be minimized by being aware of and overcoming the influences that may lead to technical problems. The sources of these influences that can cause variation are

Table 5-5 Measuring Illness

Measure	Numerator (x)	Denominator (y)	Expressed per Number at Risk (10^n)*	You May Want To Know This
Incidence rate	Number of new cases of a specified disease reported during a given time interval	Population at start of time interval	varies: 10^n where $n = 2,3,4,5,6$	This is similar to and many times equated to mortality rates. Over the long haul they become very close—in fact even epidemiologists use incidence and mortality interchangeably. How many new friends did you acquire during 1997?
Attack rate	Number of new cases of a specified disease reported during an epidemic period	Population at start of the epidemic period	varies: 10^n where $n = 2,3,4,5,6$	This sounds like a Crime Rating. How many attacks have you had this week. However, during an epidemic period—oh say 2 weeks, how many of the people who attended the "ant rally" really reported ant fever?
Secondary attack rate	Number of new cases of a specified disease among contacts of known cases	Size of contact population at risk	varies: 10^n where $n = 2,3,4,5,6$	These criminals won't give up nor will the ants—more fever is on the way. Now my family is involved. An expanded contact population-at-risk.
Point prevalence	Number of current cases, new and old, of a specified disease at a given point in time	Estimated population at the same point in time	varies: 10^n where $n = 2,3,4,5,6$	Point/Period Prevalence—you tell me the difference—is a week, a point, or an interval. In any event prevalence is the "state of affairs" (i.e., disease for a defined time period). Define: Friendship Prevalence—add up all your friends—what do you get?
Period prevalence	Number of current cases, new and old, of a specified disease identified over a given interval	Estimated population at mid-interval	varies: 10^n where $n = 2,3,4,5,6$	

*$10^2 = 100$; $10^3 = 1,000$; $10^4 = 10,000$; $10^5 = 100,000$; $10^6 = 1,000,000$.

Source: Data from G.E.A. Dever, Rates and Ratios Module, in *Creating Critical Thinkers*, Public Health Learning Series Monograph prepared for the Georgia Department of Human Resources, p. 20, © 1993 and *Principles of Epidemiology*, 2nd ed., p. 91, 1992, Centers for Disease Control and Prevention.

Table 5-6 Measuring Births

Measure	Numerator (x)	Denominator (y)	Expressed per Number at Risk	You May Want To Know This
Crude birth rate	Number of live births reported during a given time interval	Estimated total population at mid-interval	1,000	The U.S. growth indicator—how many babies are "born in the U.S.A." Good for international comparisons—very weak for state-by-state or other geographies with wildly fluctuating population—confounders.
Crude fertility rate	Number of live births reported during a given time interval	Estimated number of women age 15–44 years at mid-interval	1,000	Some of the confounders are eliminated—namely "men" and "women not able to reproduce." A good additional measure would be Age Specific or Age Adjusted Fertility Rates.
Crude rate of natural increase	Number of live births minus number of deaths during a given time interval	Estimated total population at mid-interval	1,000	Given all those who were born, take away all those who died, and you have the "teeter-totter" of population change. Of course, migration must be counted—who moved in and who moved out.
Low birth weight ratio	Number of live births under 2,500 grams during a given time interval	Number of live births reported during the same time interval	100	Low birth weight babies (<5^1/2 lbs or <2500 gms) contribute to huge health care costs. How do you propose we reduce our low birth weight ratio?

Source: Data from G.E.A. Dever, Rates and Ratios Module, in *Creating Critical Thinkers*, Public Health Learning Series Monograph prepared for the Georgia Department of Human Resources, p. 21, © 1993 and *Principles of Epidemiology*, 2nd ed., p. 116, 1992, Centers for Disease Control and Prevention.

1. *Local demographic characteristics,* which include age distribution, socio-economic status, and racial distribution peculiar to a community. Many statistics/indicators are heavily influenced by these characteristics. It has been well documented that for such a measure as an infant mortality rate, the rates will vary considerably among populations of different socioeconomic and racial characteristics.

2. *Validity and comparability of the denominator* may vary, depending on whether the population data for the denominator stem from data obtained during a particular decennial census year, such as 1990. For example, rates calculated for 1990 will be more accurate than rates calculated for 1995, a mid-census year. Clearly, by 1995, the characteristics of the population are likely to have changed, and justification for using decennial census data decreases. Thus, it is important to be familiar with reliable and valid sources of local population projections or estimates.

3. *Methodology used for obtaining population projections or estimates* to be used as denominators for rates can vary. Such variation stems from the source and use of factors for calculating the projections or estimates. Estimates may be derived from decennial census data and from additional data such as births, deaths, and migration. As one moves away from the census year, estimates may depart from the "true" population values. Hence, estimates of the 1999 population based on projections from 1990 may differ considerably from estimates of the 1999 population based on the 2000 census. Many demographic "vendors" are very capable of providing valid, reliable, and accurate population estimates and projections.

4. *Validity and comparability of the numerator* may vary for several reasons, including the underreporting or, less frequently, overreporting of events and increased reporting of events identified by community-specific surveys or screening programs.[9]

Statistical Instability

A common problem experienced by community health agencies is how to develop and analyze rates when the event in question is an infrequent occurrence. A detailed explanation of this problem and a procedure to address it follow.[10]

Traditionally, a community health standard is determined as a target that is to be obtained at a certain point in time.* For example, by the year 2000, the infant

---

*However, the CQI process uses the Plan-Do-Check-Act cycle to standardize and then moves forward to continually monitor and improve the process but does not allow the process to slip below the standard. Remember that by applying the CQI methodology, the objective is to continually improve even beyond a stated Year 2000 objective.

mortality target objective is 7.0 per 1,000 live births. For geographic areas that have a large number of events, the process is a matter of comparing the observed rate with the previously established standard or expected rate. However, for areas where the event is infrequent, consideration needs to be given to the statistical instability of the rate under consideration. For example, if a county selected an infant mortality rate of 9.0 as its standard for 1990 and actually achieved a rate of 11.0 in 1990, one might assume the county did not reach its target goal. However, if the rate was based on 50 deaths, then the rate has a 95 percent confidence interval of ±3 or from 8.0 to 14.0, which includes the goal of 9.0 (Table 5–7). Even though the rate of 9.0 was not reached that specific year, the rate of 11.0 is not statistically significantly different from the standard that was set. In setting standards, one must not only decide what the standard will be and when it is to be reached but also determine what degree of confidence to use as a measure of

Table 5–7 95 Percent Confidence Intervals for Selected Number of Events

Number of Events	Confidence Interval* (C.I.)
20	C.I. = Rate ± (0.44 • Rate)
30	C.I. = Rate ± (0.36 • Rate)
40	C.I. = Rate ± (0.31 • Rate)
50	C.I. = Rate ± (0.28 • Rate)
75	C.I. = Rate ± (0.23 • Rate)
100	C.I. = Rate ± (0.20 • Rate)
150	C.I. = Rate ± (0.16 • Rate)
200	C.I. = Rate ± (0.14 • Rate)
300	C.I. = Rate ± (0.11 • Rate)
400	C.I. = Rate ± (0.10 • Rate)
800	C.I. = Rate ± (0.07 • Rate)
1,600	C.I. = Rate ± (0.05 • Rate)

*Derivation of Confidence Interval ($n = 50$):

Standard Error of a Number $= \sqrt{n}$ using $n = 50$ (number of events)

$$= \sqrt{50}$$

$$= 7.07 \times 1.96 = 13.86$$

$$= 13.86 \div 50 = 0.28$$

Thus, given 50 events and to obtain a 95 percent interval, the length would be ±28 percent of the rate. Or C.I. = ± (1.96 • Rate)/$\sqrt{n}$ would be used if one had the rate to determine the 95 percent confidence intervals.

Source: From *Healthy Communities 2000: Model Standards,* 3rd edition. Copyright 1991 by the American Public Health Association. Adapted with permission.

whether the standard has actually been met. When using point estimates (such as the number of cases or deaths), it is desirable to report the standard error of the statistics so that the reader has some conception of the possible error. The confidence interval specifies the discrepancy between the estimate and actual or true value. Although one can never be absolutely sure that this value is not outside the range of tolerated error, we can specify to what degree we are confident the estimate is reliable (95 or 99 percent). If it is decided that more precision is needed than knowing that the true rate falls within a 6-point spread (±3), as in the previous infant mortality example, then the standard may be changed, but this would not be the most appropriate approach.[11] The approach to investigate is how to increase the number of events on which the observed rate is based. There are at least two ways of addressing this problem.

1. Expand the geographic area so more events will be counted. For example, rather than using the one small county, zip code, or census tract, expand the geographic area to include one or more of the adjoining counties, zip codes, or census tracts.
2. Aggregate the time period being investigated. Rather than investigating the infant mortality rates for 1990, it would be more prudent to expand the time period to a three- or five-year aggregation. Also aggregation as a method is appropriate for age groups, socioeconomic groups, etc.[12]

These approaches do have obvious drawbacks: (1) in the first instance, a geographic area that is not under the control of the same jurisdiction may have to be included, and (2) the second option requiring adding data years together may limit the ability to determine the success of program interventions and also test the validity of time trends.[13]

Unfortunately, the alternative to these approaches is to use a rate that is very unstable, fluctuates widely from one year to the next, and does not adequately represent the true rate. In public health practice, the use of quality improvement statistical tools will provide additional approaches to deal with these technical issues.

Another statistical question is how many events should be used to establish a stable rate. There is no single answer to this question. Obviously, the larger the number of events, the more stable the rate. Unfortunately, a very large number of events is required to create a rate with a small confidence interval. For example, it requires 1,600 events to obtain a 95 percent confidence interval whose length is ±5 percent of the rate. Although one would prefer to have such a small confidence interval, rare health events and small geographic areas generally preclude such precision.[14] It is recommended that most analysis be based on 20 or more expected events (infant deaths, low-birth-weight infants, etc.). *Regardless of the number of events, the confidence interval for the rate should be computed when comparing the observed rate with the standard (expected rate).* If the standard falls within the confidence interval range, then the observed rate and the standard (expected rate) are not statistically different. Table 5–7 shows the length of confidence intervals based on the number of events in the numerator of the rate.[15] Further, Table 5–8 suggests a minimum number of events per year or the aggregate number of years to be analyzed to achieve or develop a confidence interval less than or equal to the rate ±20 percent.

Infant Mortality—An Example

To illustrate the application of using confidence intervals for epidemiologic assessment, infant mortality rates will be evaluated. In a state, for example, infant mortality is an important cause of death; in fact, it is a national indicator. Between 1986 and 1990 (5 years), there were 11,830 births in County A, as compared with 427,973 in the state. In the county, 201 infant deaths occurred (rate = 17/1,000 births), whereas in the state there were 6,649 (15.5/1,000 births). The significance of these values can be estimated using the standardized mortality ratio (SMR).

$$\text{SMR} = \frac{\text{Observed infant deaths}}{\text{Expected infant deaths}} \times 100$$

Table 5–8 Number of Years and Events Needed To Develop a Standard with a Confidence Interval Less Than or Equal to the Rate ±20 Percent

Number of Events per Year	Aggregate Number of Years
100	1
50–99	2
33–49	3
25–32	4
20–24	5
17–19	6
15–16	7
13–14	8
11–12	9
10	10
0–9	*

*Standard not recommended for fewer than 10 events per year.
Source: From *Healthy Communities 2000: Model Standards,* 3rd edition. Copyright 1991 by the American Public Health Association. Adapted with permission.

Therefore to determine the expected deaths, we calculate the following:

$$\text{Expected infant deaths} = \frac{P_1}{P_2} \times \text{deaths in state}$$

$$= \frac{11,830}{427,973} \times 6,649$$

$$= 183.8$$

$$\text{Where } P_1 = \text{population in the county}$$
$$P_2 = \text{population in the state}$$

$$\text{SMR} = \frac{201}{183.8} \times 100 = 109.4$$

The standard error (SE) is

$$\text{SE} = \frac{\text{SMR}}{\sqrt{d}}$$

$$= \frac{109.4}{\sqrt{201}}$$

$$= 7.7$$

Where d = number of observed deaths in the county

The confidence interval is

$$\text{CI} = \pm 7.7 \times 1.96 = \pm 15.1$$

$$\text{Upper limit} = 109.4 + 15.1 = 124.5$$

$$\text{Lower limit} = 109.4 - 15.1 = 94.3$$

$$\text{CI} = 94.3 \text{ to } 124.5$$

Because the confidence interval includes 100, it can be concluded that there is no significant difference in infant mortality between the county and state rate.[16]

If, for example, the same problem was analyzed but only one year of information was available to evaluate, the results would be quite different. In 1995, there were 157 births in a county, as compared with 101,423 births in the state. In the county, four infant deaths occurred (rate = 25.5/1,000 births), whereas in the state there were 1,186 deaths (11.7/1,000 births). The significance of this one-year rate can be evaluated using the SMR.

$$SMR_{1995} = \frac{\text{Observed infant deaths}}{\text{Expected infant deaths}} \times 100$$

Where

$$\text{Expected infant deaths} = \frac{P_1}{P_2} \times \text{deaths in state}$$

$$= \frac{157}{101,423} \times 1,186$$

$$= 1.84$$

Thus

$$SMR = \frac{4}{1.84} \times 100 = 217.4$$

The (SE) is

$$SE = \frac{SMR}{\sqrt{d}}$$

$$= \frac{217.4}{\sqrt{4}}$$

$$= 108.7$$

The confidence interval is

$$CI = \pm 108.7 \times 1.96 = \pm 213.1$$

$$\text{Upper limit} = 217.4 + 213.1 = 430.5$$

$$\text{Lower limit} = 217.4 - 213.1 = 4.3$$

$$CI = 4.3 \text{ to } 430.5$$

Because the confidence interval includes 100, it can be considered that there is no significant difference. However, the width of the confidence interval clearly indicates wide statistical variability and renders the result meaningless (i.e., the rate is based on too few events; however, this would have never been known if the confidence interval had not been calculated).

If we use the value of 4 (infant deaths) and calculate our value based on Table 5–7, we have the following:

$$\text{SE of a Number} = \sqrt{n} \qquad \text{using } n = 4 \text{ (infant deaths)}$$

$$= \sqrt{4}$$

$$= 2 \times 1.96 = 3.92$$

$$= 3.92 \div 4 = 0.98$$

Thus, given four events and to obtain a 95 percent confidence interval, the length would be 98 percent of the rate, obviously an unstable situation. In fact, the result is subject to such wide statistical variation that the rate is meaningless. However, from a policy perspective in public health practice, it allows one to make a sound evidence-based decision about the need for a program or allocating resources to a problem that, in this case, needs more study before action.

It also is of value to calculate the confidence interval of rates, allowing the comparison with the year 2000 standard or goal. For example, is the county five-year rate (17.0 deaths per 1,000) significantly higher than a goal of 13 deaths per 1,000 births? The confidence interval is given by

$$\text{CI} = \text{rate} \pm 1.96 \times \text{SE}$$

Where

$$\text{SE} = \frac{\text{rate}}{\sqrt{\text{deaths}}}$$

$$\text{SE} = \frac{17.0}{\sqrt{201}} = 1.2$$

$$\text{CI} = 17.0 \pm (1.96 \times 1.2) = 17.0 \pm 2.35$$

$$\text{Upper limit} = 17.0 + 2.35 = 19.35$$

$$\text{Lower limit} = 17.0 - 2.35 = 14.65$$

This means that, just by chance, the county rate may vary between 14.65 and 19.35, 95 percent of the time. It thus is significantly higher than a target value of 13.0.[17]

In summary, public health practitioners can identify the significance of a specific health problem in their area by calculating the rate and determining the confidence intervals.

The importance of confidence intervals should *NOT* be underestimated in the analysis and interpretation of rates for the public health practice of assessment. Confidence intervals are also critical to analyzing a process, and the quality improvement tools discussed later further elaborate on confidence intervals related to control charts for monitoring and assessing a process.

Validity

Validity is the ability to measure accurately the event a public health analyst intends to measure (i.e., to what extent the measurement reflects the true value of an event). Validity is threatened by many factors, such as the manner in which data are collected, the sampling design used, the natural history of the condition under study, and the point in that natural history at which the data are obtained.[18] The following examples illustrate how these factors can influence validity.

1. *The manner in which data are collected* may greatly affect the completeness of the data. For example, incidence rates of communicable diseases may vary depending on the reporting system used. Some states and local areas use only the reports received from private physicians; other areas may add data they receive from laboratories or hospitals. Still other areas have a sentinel reporting system in which they contact key physicians and/or hospitals to determine the number of events. Thus, each reporting system will provide a different level of completeness.

2. *The sampling design used* can threaten validity in the study of conditions and/or causes of death for which high-risk groups such as the elderly do not have the same probability of being sampled. If a condition that is prevalent in elderly populations is studied in the general community and nursing homes or retirement communities are not in the sampling frame, an undercount is likely to occur.

3. *The natural history of the disease* can affect the validity of data obtained to assess the effectiveness of a program. For example, to evaluate the impact of a screening program on mortality due to cancer of the cervix, one would have to wait 10 years to observe a decrease in mortality rates, as it can take approximately this long for an in situ lesion to progress to an invasion lesion.[19]

Reliability

Reliability is the relation of the true value to the observed value. The goal is to ensure that the observed value is as accurate as possible to the true value at each measurement. Questions regarding reliability of data may arise for several reasons. For example, undernumeration of certain population groups in the census may result in higher rates for these groups. Furthermore, population projections based on the undercount of certain population groups will result in correspondingly higher rates.[20] One should also be cognizant of residence allocation differences between numerator and denominator. In a community with a large long-term-care institution, the morbidity rates for a specific condition may vary depending on whether

1. the residents of the institution are considered as community residents and are therefore included in the denominator for the entire community
2. the cases of the specific condition in the institutionalized population are included in developing community-specific morbidity rates.[21]

Finally, reliability in assigning codes should be considered. Terminology used to describe specific conditions may vary or change over time or by geographic location. Training of coders and standardization of rules and definitions can minimize this source of error.[22]

CONCLUSION

Two of the major problems facing all decision makers, including public health practice professionals, is the identification of a problem and the resulting difficulty of determining priorities. This chapter shows how the various rates and the SMR, a simple but reliable method, can be used to identify various problems from an epidemiologic perspective.[23]

Each rate, among others to be discussed later, is useful and valid for priority setting in health management. Certainly, all techniques and methods are subject to variability and errors, so for this reason the concepts of validity and reliability are discussed.[24] It is contended here that public health practitioners using these epidemiologic measures will be better equipped for focusing on the evaluation of outcomes utilizing quality improvement methods in the community health setting.

NOTES

1. U.S. Department of Health and Human Services, Public Health Service, Centers for Disease Control and Prevention, *Principles of Epidemiology*, 2d ed. (Atlanta: CDC, 1992), 73–143.

2. Ibid.

3. Ibid.

4. American Public Health Association, *Healthy Communities 2000: Model Standards,* 3d ed. (Washington DC: Government Printing Office, 1991) 460.

5. F. Seltzer, "Choosing a Standard for Adjusted Mortality Rates," *Statistical Bulletin* 77, no. 1 (1996): 13–19.

6. U.S. Department of Health and Human Services, *Principles of Epidemiology*, 73–143.

7. Ibid., 81–84.
8. APHA, *Healthy Communities 2000*, 73–143.
9. Ibid.
10. Ibid.
11. Ibid.
12. Ibid.
13. Ibid.
14. Ibid., 458–459.
15. Ibid., 459.
16. G.E.A. Dever, *Epidemiology in Health Services Management* (Gaithersburg, MD: Aspen Publishers, Inc., 1984), 115.
17. Ibid., 116.
18. APHA, *Healthy Communities 2000*, 460.
19. Ibid.
20. Ibid.
21. Ibid., 461.
22. Ibid.
23. Dever, *Epidemiology in Health Services Management*, 131.
24. Ibid.

Chapter 6

Measures of Central Location and Dispersion

In the previous chapter, the focus was on epidemiologic measurement, which is essential to the assessment function of public health practice. By understanding the nature of rates—their uses, advantages, disadvantages, and limitations—one is able to appropriately use these rates for independent evaluation or in conjunction with the basic quality improvement tools. Likewise, the statistical analysis of a process in continuous quality improvement (CQI) is heavily dependent on measures of central location—mean, median, and mode—and measures of dispersion—the range and standard deviation. The construction of control charts is generally used with 4 of the 12 steps. They are (1) measuring and analyzing data, (2) implementing a trial run, (3) evaluating the results, and (4) monitoring the process to hold the gain. All four of these steps require the use of the measures of central location and dispersion. You may recall that these four steps were noted in Chapter 3 when we discussed the CQI improvement model and the Plan-Do-Check-Act (PDCA) cycle, which represents a 12-step process for improvement. As discussed later, each of the 12 process improvement steps of the PDCA cycle requires the use of specific management tools for collecting and displaying data and specific tools for targeting quality improvements. However, suffice for now, it is important to know that all of the tools require a basic understanding of measurement, and many of the tools are dependent on calculations based on measures of central location and dispersion.

A FIRST STEP: DO WE KNOW OUR LEVELS OF MEASUREMENT?

To use or calculate a statistic or use a quality improvement process tool, it is necessary to be aware of the level of measurement of the data. Further, to use these

147

process tools, data must be collected. The data collected are usually actual measurements or counts of some process or characteristic of the process being studied. Levels of measurement range from assignments of attributes and events, such as the number of infant deaths in a geographic area, to assessments of numerical scores. The level of measurement used is critical in that only certain methods may be used on data measured at different levels. Thus, the level of measurement of our data determines what we may do in the analysis of the data and what type of control charts (quality improvement tools) should be considered in the quality improvement process. There are *four* levels of measurement (Table 6–1). Also see Table 6–1 for examples and appropriate descriptive statistics to use based on the level of measurement. In quality improvement, knowledge about the levels of measurement is important. As many are aware, the data encountered in most statistical applications represent counts (attributes and events), rankings (ordered data), and measurements (every observation is a value on a numerical scale). In quality improvement, measurement ranking or ordinal level of measurement rarely occurs. However, one such application discussed in Chapter 8 would be the use of a Pareto chart. Basically, in CQI two main classes of distribution occur. One class that uses the properties of the normal distribution (i.e., measures of central location and dispersion) deals with observations that vary along a continuous numerical scale. These measurements represent interval or ratio level. The other class represents data obtained by counting and, therefore, deals with events or nominal measurement. In CQI, some of the control charts used for understanding variation measure events (i.e., counts or counts reflecting rates of occurrence—it occurred or did not occur). Further, Table 6–1 illustrates the relationship of the measures of central location and dispersion to the levels of measurement.

MEASURES OF CENTRAL LOCATION

We calculate a measure of location when we need a single value to summarize a set of data. Traditionally, in public health practice, professionals are usually faced with two situations in which a measure of central location is important, epidemiology and health planning. For example, if public health practitioners were presenting information on suicide deaths in Georgia for a particular year, they might describe this as, "The median age of persons in Georgia who committed suicide in the selected year was 35.7 or the average age was 43 and the mode was 34." Also, measures of central location are often used for further calculations. Moreover, for quality improvement methods related to public health practice, these measures of location are pertinent to the analysis of variation using control charts.

The measure that is best for use in a particular instance depends on the characteristics of the distribution, such as its shape, and on the intended use of the mea-

Table 6–1 Levels of Measurement

Level of Measurement*	Definition	Let's Ask Al and Bob	Example	Appropriate Statistics
Nominal: (Classify)	Pertains to naming. We assign subjects or units of analysis to a particular category or variable. These categories represent differing ATTRIBUTES, not qualities. The categories can be interchanged without altering the essential information. "What is your name? Is it Peggy or Sue?"	Do A and B differ?†	• Name • Blood type • Disease list • Psychiatric diagnosis • Sex • Race • Marital status	Individual counts Classifications Mode
Ordinal: (Rank)	Refer to order or ordering. A ranking from most to least or some logical sequence of a variable category. It represents a sequence, not an exact amount. "Who are the five best-dressed women and men in the country?"	Is A bigger (better) than B?	• Best/worst • Patient satisfaction • High/low risk • Patient condition • Acceptable/unacceptable • Functional health status (COOP/WONCA)	Mode Median Range Interquartile range
Interval: (Difference)	Refers to a numerical score, not a ranking. Zero is an arbitrary point. Equal differences between values represent equal amounts, but ratios have no meaning because of the arbitrary location of the zero point (e.g., temperature). The difference is the same even if we didn't stand at zero.	How much do A and B differ?	• Temperature on two scales; however, it is not twice as hot • Dates of birth	Mode Median Mean Range Standard deviation Interquartile range
Ratio: (Bigger)	Refers to a numerical score, where zero is an absolute zero—meaning a complete lack of the variable being measured—scale has equal intervals. Equal differences between values represent equal amounts. Equal ratios of values are also equivalent because of a genuine zero point (e.g., weight scale). Heart disease is twice as high in males compared to females. Your height to weight ratio is 2:4.	How many times is A bigger than B?	• Diseases • Distances • Dollars • Ages • Inches	Mode Median Mean Range Standard deviation Interquartile range

*Event level of measurement (i.e., counts or occurrences) is suggested by some CQI experts. To apply the use of control charts for measuring variation, one uses events (nominal level of measurement) or continuous variables (interval, ratio, levels of measurement). This will become more relevant when the use and application of control charts are discussed.

†A = Al; B = Bob.

Source: Reprinted from G.E.A. Dever, The Main Highway Module, in *Creating Critical Thinkers*, Public Health Learning Series Monograph prepared for the Georgia Department of Human Resources, p. 7, © 1993.

sure. On the following pages, the selection, calculation, and use of several measures of central location for measuring the quality improvement process in public health practice are described.

The Mean (Average)

The average is simply the average of a set of observations where

$$\text{Mean} = \frac{\text{the sum of all values}}{\text{number of observations}}$$

$$\text{or } \overline{X} = \frac{\Sigma x_i}{n}$$

which is read as "X-bar equals the sum of all the x's divided by n." This is defined as the arithmetic mean of a sample.

Example

Consider the following birth weights in grams of 10 newborn babies in a rural county hospital.

1. To calculate the numerator, sum the individual observations:

   $\Sigma x_i = 2541 + 2521 + 2522 + 2539 + 2530 + 2516 + 2538 + 2519 + 2525 + 2514$

   $\Sigma x_i = 25{,}265$

2. For the denominator, count the number of observations:

   $$n = 10$$

3. To calculate the mean, divide the numerator (sum of observations) by the denominator (number of observations):

   $$\overline{X} = \frac{2541 + 2521 + 2522 + 2539 + 2530 + 2516 + 2538 + 2519 + 2525 + 2514}{10}$$

   $$\overline{X} = \frac{25{,}265}{10}$$

   $$\overline{X} = 2526.5 \text{ g}$$

Therefore, the mean birth weight for babies born in this rural county was 2,526.5 g.

However, in assessing process and outcome variables using quality improvement methods, the data may be viewed in a different light. Although the method of compilation is the same as the one illustrated above, different arithmetic means can be identified that are associated with different segments of data. As a result, these are introduced here to distinguish among them conceptually for later application.

Mean of Means (Equal Subgroups)

To illustrate, consider the first five observations in the previous example as a sample of five babies born during evening hours. The corresponding mean equals

$$\bar{X}_1 = \frac{2541 + 2521 + 2522 + 2539 + 2530}{5}$$

$$\bar{X}_1 = \frac{12{,}653}{5}$$

$$\bar{X}_1 = 2530.6 \text{ g}$$

Repeating the process for the second five observations or sample of five babies born during daylight hours, we get

$$\bar{X}_2 = \frac{2516 + 2538 + 2519 + 2525 + 2514}{5}$$

$$\bar{X}_2 = \frac{12{,}612}{5}$$

$$\bar{X}_2 = 2522.4 \text{ g}$$

Another mean that will be used at a later point is the mean of the individual sample means (this assumes the subgroups are equal). This is given as

$$\bar{\bar{X}} = \frac{\Sigma \bar{X}}{k}$$

where $\bar{\bar{X}}$ = the arithmetic mean of a set of sample means (based on samples selected from a process being analyzed)

k = the number of samples selected from a process

Using the result of the previous illustration, we have the mean of means:

$$\overline{\overline{X}} = \frac{2530.6 + 2522.4}{2}$$

$$\overline{\overline{X}} = 2526.5 \text{ g}$$

Note this is no different from the original mean based on 10 observations. When subgroup samples are the same size, the mean of the means will equal the original mean.

Average Advantages

The mean is the most commonly used, easily understood, and recognized measure. Computation is quite simple—only total values (Σx_i) and number of observations (n) are needed for calculation. It may be treated algebraically; however, beware the *mean of means*. When subgroups are averaged, there must be an equal number of observations in each group; if not, weighted averages are in order. The sum of the deviations about the mean is always zero.

Average Disadvantages

The average may be distorted by extreme values and therefore not typical (i.e., beware the *skewed distribution*—discussed later in this chapter). Means cannot be computed with "open-ended" class intervals (i.e., greater than or less than). Means can only be used for data at the interval or ratio level of measurement. Means cannot be used for event, nominal, or ordinal level of measurement. Means computed for event, nominal, or ordinal level data are meaningless.

How To Calculate the Mean of Means (Unequal Subgroups)

To calculate the average age (when the subgroups are unequal) of patients attending a hypertension clinic given the data in Table 6–2, which represents the average age at three clinics reflective of unequal subgroups, we must weight the average by the number in each subgroup. Therefore, we determine the mean of the patients based on the fact that each clinic had a different number of patients.
Therefore, is the average

$$120 \div 3 = 40$$

which is the sum of the average ages ($\overline{X}$) divided by the number of the clinics, or

$$1,250 \div 35 = 35.7$$

which is the sum of average ages weighted by the number of patients attending the clinics?

Table 6–2 Average Age of Patients Attending a Hypertensive Clinic (1990)

	Average Age ($\overline{X}$)	n^*	($\overline{X}$) (n)
Clinic 1	25	10	250
Clinic 2	35	20	700
Clinic 3	60	5	300
Totals	120	35	1,250

$^*n$ = number of patients attending the clinic.
   Source: Reprinted from G.E.A. Dever, The Main Highway Module, in *Creating Critical Thinkers,* Public Health Learning Series Monograph prepared for the Georgia Department of Human Resources, p. 10, © 1993.

If the subgroups were equal, the mean would be 40. However, to calculate a mean of means, we must know more information—specifically, how many observations there were for each individual mean. The mean of means for unequal subgroups in this example is 35.7.

Average Facts

When averages are compared, the distributions should have the same basic shape. For symmetric distributions, the mean, median, and mode are equal. The mode is not affected by skewness, whereas the mean is affected most by skewness. Averages can be misleading and are not always used correctly. When using averages, it is important to consider the pattern of variability.

The Median

Another common measure of central location is the median. It is especially useful when data are skewed.

Median means middle, and the median is the middle of a set of data that has been put into rank order. Specifically, it is the value that divides a set of data into two halves, with one half of the observations being larger than the median value and one half smaller. For example, suppose we had the following set of systolic blood pressures (in mmHg) obtained from a public health hypertension clinic: 110, 120, 122, 130, 180. In this example, two observations are larger than 122 and two observations are smaller; thus, the median is 122 mmHg, the value of the third observation. Note that the mean (662 ÷ 5 = 132.4 mmHg) is larger than four of the five values.

Identifying the Median from Individual Data

1. Arrange the observations in increasing or decreasing order.
2. Find the middle rank with the following formula:

$$\text{Middle rank} = \frac{n+1}{2}$$

    a) If the number of observations (n) is odd, the middle rank falls on an observation.
    b) If n is even, the middle rank falls between two observations.
3. Identify the value of the median:
    a) If the middle rank falls on a specific observation (that is, if n is odd), the median is equal to the value of that observation.
    b) If the middle rank falls between two observations (that is, if n is even), the median is equal to the average (i.e., the arithmetic mean) of the values of those observations.

Example with an Odd *Number of Observations*

In this example, we demonstrate how to find the median infant mortality rate for five zip codes in a northside community from the following set of data with $n = 5$:

$$13, 7, 9, 15, 11$$

1. Arrange the infant mortality rates in increasing or decreasing order. We can arrange them as either

$$7, 9, 11, 13, 15$$

or

$$15, 13, 11, 9, 7$$

2. Find the middle rank:

$$\text{Middle rank} = \frac{(n+1)}{2} = \frac{(5+1)}{2} = 3$$

Therefore, the median lies at the value of the third observation.
3. Identify the value of the median. Because the median is equal to the value of the third observation, the median infant mortality rate is 11.

Example with an Even *Number of Observations*

In this example, we demonstrate how to find the median infant mortality rate from six zip codes in a northside community from the following set of data with $n = 6$:

15, 7, 13, 9, 10, 11

1. Arrange the infant mortality rates in increasing or decreasing order:

7, 9, 10, 11, 13, 15

or

15, 13, 11, 10, 9, 7

2. Find the middle rank:

$$\text{Middle rank} = \frac{(n+1)}{2} = \frac{(6+1)}{2} = 3.5$$

3. Identify the value of the median. Because the median is equal to the average of the values of the third and fourth observations, the median infant mortality rate is 10.5:

$$\text{Median} = \frac{(11+10)}{2} = 10.5$$

The Mean of Sample Medians

For reasons that become more apparent later, we may also use the mean of sample medians. This is accomplished with the following formula:

$$\bar{\bar{X}} = \frac{\Sigma \tilde{X}}{k}$$

where $\bar{\bar{X}}$ = the arithmetic mean of a set of sample medians (based on repeated samples drawn from a process)
  $\Sigma \tilde{X}$ = sum all the sample medians
  k = the number of samples

Median Advantages

The median is easy to calculate and is not distorted by extreme values (i.e., it is most stable). Sometimes it is more typical of the data than other measures because of its independence of unusual values. The median may be calculated when the class intervals of the distribution are "open-ended." The relationship of percentiles to median measures is as follows: (1) 25th percentile is the lower quartile, (2) the 50th is the median, and (3) the 75th is the upper quartile. Also, note that the median divides a distribution into two parts, the quartile divides a distribution into four parts, and the decile divides a distribution into 10 parts.

Median Disadvantages

The median is not a familiar statistic. All items must be arranged according to size before calculation. It has a larger "standard error" than the arithmetic mean. The median cannot be manipulated algebraically. There is no "median of the medians." Data of at least an ordinal level of measurement are required.

The Mode—The Style (What Is Popular)

The mode is the value that occurs most often in a set of data. For example, in the following parity data, the mode is 1, because it occurs four times, which is more than any other value:

$$0, 0, 1, 1, 1, 1, 2, 2, 2, 3, 4, 6$$

We usually find the mode by creating a frequency distribution in which we check how often each value occurs. If we find that every value occurs only once, the distribution has no mode. Or if we find that two or more values are tied as the most common, the distribution has more than one mode.

Example

In this example, we demonstrate the steps you use to find the mode of the following set of data for prenatal care visits: 11, 8, 12, 14, 15, 12, 9, 10, 11, 13, and 11.

1. Arrange the data into a frequency distribution, showing the values of the variable (x) and the frequency (f) with which each value occurs (Table 6–3).
2. Identify the value that occurs most often.

Mode = 11 prenatal care visits

Table 6–3 Distribution of Prenatal Care Visits

x (Number of Visits)	f (Frequency of Visits)
8	1
9	1
10	1
11	3
12	2
13	1
14	1
15	1

In certain situations all values may have the same frequency, in this instance, there would be no mode for the distribution of data analyzed. Further, when there are two values that each occur twice, the distribution would have two modes. This type of distribution is called bimodal.

Mode Advantages

The mode is the most typical and therefore the most descriptive value. It is quite easy to approximate when observations are few (are you watching 10 people or 1,000 people?). If only a few items, it is not essential to arrange to determine. Its use is appropriate for data of the nominal level of measurement or higher. It is the most unrestricted (i.e., has the fewest assumptions). It is independent of extreme values and is an average of position. The mode is used primarily for bimodal distributions.

Mode Disadvantages

The mode can only be approximated with a limited data set. Significance is limited when a large number of values is not available. If none of the values are repeated, the mode does not exist. There may be no mode, one mode, or more than one mode.

Summary: Which Measure Do We Use?

The mean (the average) is used for numerical data and for distributions that are symmetrical. The median (the middle) is used for ordinal data or for numerical data whose distribution is skewed. The mode is used for nominal data representing the typical or bimodal distributions. If the mean and the median are equal, the distribution of our observations is nicely shaped. If the mean is larger than the median, the distribution is skewed to the right. If the mean is smaller than the median, the distribution is skewed to the left. See Table 6–1 for a detailed summary.

MEASURES OF DISPERSION

When we look at the graph of a frequency distribution, we usually notice two primary features: (1) the graph has a peak, usually near the center, and (2) it spreads out on either side of the peak. Just as we use a measure of central location to describe where the peak is located, we use a measure of dispersion to describe how much spread there is in the distribution. Several measures of dispersion are available. Usually, we use a particular measure of dispersion with a particular measure of central location. The measures of the central location (averages, medians, modes) are not sufficient to summarize the data. For instance, the average or typical value is not very useful unless the variation is given. Further, if the variation about the mean is large, then the average is not typical. To compensate for this, we must measure the degree of variation or dispersion about the average. To completely describe data points, we need a summary measure of the variation or dispersion. The need for measures of variation is demonstrated by the figure below (Figure 6–1), in which (a) has the same mean but very different variation, (b) has a different mean but the same variation, and (c) has a different mean and a different variation.

In this section on measures of dispersion, we will review the properties of the range and the standard deviation. The simplest measure of variation is the range.

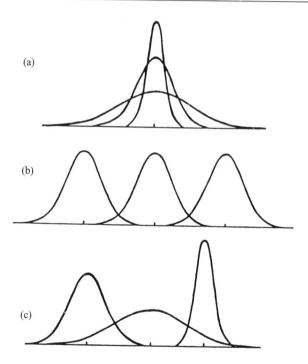

Figure 6–1 Graphical Representation of Measures of Variation. *Source:* Reprinted with permission from S.K. Kachigan, *Statistical Analysis*, p. 55, © 1986, Radius Press.

Range, Minimum Values, and Maximum Values

The range of a set of data is the difference between its largest (maximum) and smallest (minimum values). In the statistical world, the range is reported as a single number, the difference between maximum and minimum. In the epidemiologic community, the range is often reported as "from (the minimum) to (the maximum)" (i.e., two numbers). The range is also used to determine percentiles, quartiles, and interquartile ranges. In using quality improvement methods, the range allows us to interpret the magnitude of the variation.

Example

Using data on prenatal care visits, we demonstrate how to find the minimum value, maximum value, and range of the following data:

$$11, 8, 12, 14, 15, 12, 9, 10, 11, 13, 11$$

1. Arrange the data from smallest to largest:

$$8, 9, 10, 11, 11, 11, 12, 12, 13, 14, 15$$

2. Identify the minimum and maximum values:

$$\text{Minimum} = 8; \text{maximum} = 15$$

3. Calculate the range:

$$\text{Range} = \text{maximum} - \text{minimum} = 15 - 8 = 7$$

Thus, the range for prenatal care visits is 7.

Range Advantages

The range can be computed quickly and easily. The ease of computation makes it the preferred dispersion statistic for practical applications involving small data sets ($n \leq 15$). However, because the techniques of process control emphasize small sets of numbers, the range is a valuable statistic. The range delimits the distribution of scores for constructing a frequency distribution. It helps in determining the number of intervals and the appropriate interval class and is dependent on only two values—the highest and lowest. The range does not require knowledge of the other values between the extremes.

Range Disadvantages

The range is greatly affected by the two extremes if not representative. It gives no information on how the other values are distributed between the two extremes and tends to be larger when the sample size is larger.

Percentiles, Quartiles, and Interquartile Range[*]

We can consider the maximum value of a distribution in another way. We can think of it as the value in a set of data that has 100 percent of the observations at or below it. When we consider it in this way, we call it the 100th percentile. From this same perspective, the median, which has 50 percent of the observations at or below it, is the 50th percentile.

The most commonly used percentiles other than the median are the 25th percentile and the 75th percentile. The 25th percentile demarcates the first quartile, the median or 50th percentile demarcates the second quartile, the 75th percentile demarcates the third quartile, and the 100th percentile demarcates the fourth quartile.

The interquartile range represents the central portion of the distribution and is calculated as the difference between the third quartile and the first quartile. This range includes about one-half of the observations in the set, leaving one-quarter of the observations on each side.

How To Calculate the Interquartile Range from Individual Data

To calculate the interquartile range, you must first find the first and third quartiles. As with the median, you first put the observations in rank order, then determine the position of the quartile. The value of the quartile is the value of the observation at that position, or if the quartile lies between observations, its value lies between the values of the observations of either side of that point.

1. Arrange the observations in increasing order.
2. Find the position of the first and third quartiles with the following formulas:

$$\text{Position of 1st quartile } (Q_1) = \frac{(n+1)}{4}$$

$$\text{Position of 3rd quartile } (Q_3) = \frac{3(n+1)}{4} = 3 \times Q_1$$

3. Identify the value of the first and third quartiles. If a quartile lies on an observation (i.e., if its position is a whole number), the value of the quartile is the value of that observation. For example, if the position of a quartile is 20, its value is the value of the 20th observation. If a quartile lies between

---

[*]Many of the examples for this section are to be found in U.S. DHHS, PHS, CDC, Epidemiology Program Office, *Principles of Epidemiology: An Introduction to Applied Epidemiology and Biostatistics*, Self Study Course 3030-G, 2nd ed., December 1992, Atlanta, GA 30333; pp. 145–204.

observations, the value of the quartile is the value of the lower observations. For example, if the position of a quartile is $20^{1}/4$, it lies between the 20th and 21st observations, and its value is the value of the 20th observation, plus 1/4 the difference between the value of the 20th and 21st observations.

4. Calculate the interquartile range as Q_3 minus Q_1.

Example

1. Arrange the following observations in increasing order:

   Given these data   13, 7, 9, 15, 11, 5, 8, 4

   We arrange them like this   4, 5, 7, 8, 9, 11, 13, 15

2. Find the position of the first and third quartiles. Because there are eight observations, $n = 8$:

$$\text{Position of } Q_1 = \frac{(n+1)}{4} = \frac{(8+1)}{4} = 2.25$$

$$\text{Position of } Q_3 = \frac{3(n+1)}{4} = \frac{3(8+1)}{4} = 6.75$$

Thus, Q_1 lies one-fourth of the way between the second and third observations, and Q_3 lies three-fourths of the way between the sixth and seventh observations.

3. Identify the value of the first and third quartiles:

Value of Q_1: The position of Q_1 was $2^{1}/4$; therefore, the value of Q_1 is equal to the value of the second observation plus one-fourth the difference between the values of the third and second observations:

Value of the third observation (see step 1): 7

Value of the second observation: 5

$$Q_1 = 5 + \frac{1}{4}(7 - 5) = 5 + \frac{1(2)}{4} = 5 + \frac{2}{4} = 5.5$$

Value of Q_3: The position of Q_3 was $6^{3}/4$; thus, the value of Q_3 is equal to the value of the sixth observation plus three-fourths of the difference between the value of the seventh and sixth observations:

Value of the seventh observation (see step 1): 13

Value of the sixth observation: 11

$$Q_3 = 11 + \frac{3}{4}(13 - 11) = 11 + \frac{3(2)}{4} = 11 + \frac{6}{4} = 12.5$$

4. Calculate the interquartile range as Q_3 minus Q_1:

$$Q_3 = 12.5 \text{ (see step 3)}$$

$$Q_1 = 5.5$$

Interquartile range $= 12.5 - 5.5 = 7$

Generally, we use quartiles and the interquartile range to describe variability when we use the median as the measure of central location. We use the standard deviation, which is described in the next section, when we use the mean.

Figure 6–2 illustrates a normal distribution that shows the summary of a distribution that consists of the following: (1) smallest observation (minimum), (2) first quartile, (3) median, (4) third quartile, (5) largest observation (maximum), and (6) the interquartile range. Together these values provide a very good description of the center, spread, and shape of a distribution.

Standard Deviation

The standard deviation is the most commonly used measure of dispersion to describe epidemiologic and health planning data and is a statistic used extensively in quality improvement measurement. It is the measure of the spread of data about the mean. It is a special form of average deviation from the mean, and it is affected by the value of every item. No matter how the observations are distributed, at least 75 percent of the values are always between the mean and plus or minus two standard deviations. If the observations are distributed normally, however, then the so-called bell-shaped distribution follows specific rules:

1. 68 percent of the observations will be between plus or minus one standard deviation.
2. 95 percent of the observations will be between plus or minus two standard deviations.
3. 99.7 percentage of the observations will be between plus or minus three standard deviations.

The variance and standard deviation are measures of the deviation or dispersion of observations around the mean of a distribution. Variance is the mean of the squared differences of the observations from the mean. It is usually represented in formulas as s^2. The standard deviation is the square root of the variance.

It is usually represented in formulas as s. The following formulas define these measures:

$$\text{Variance} = s^2 = \frac{\sum (x_i - \bar{x})^2}{n-1}$$

$$\text{Standard deviation} = s = \sqrt{\frac{\sum (x_i - \bar{x})^2}{n-1}}$$

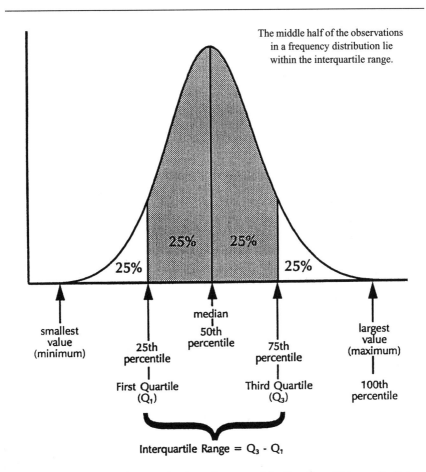

The middle half of the observations in a frequency distribution lie within the interquartile range.

Figure 6–2 A Normal Distribution Showing a Summary of the Quartile and Interquartile Ranges. *Source:* Reprinted from U.S. DHHS, PHS, CDC, Epidemiology Program Office, *Principles of Epidemiology: An Introduction to Applied Epidemiology and Biostatics,* Self Study Course 3030-G, 2nd ed., p. 170, 1992.

Example

Given the following data (Table 6–4), we calculate the variance and the standard deviation.

$$\text{Variance} = s^2 = \frac{\sum (x_i - \bar{x})^2}{n - 1}$$

$$\text{Standard deviation} = s = \sqrt{s^2}$$

1. Calculate the mean (Column 1, Table 6–4):

$$\bar{X} = \frac{\sum x_i}{n} = \frac{55}{11} = 5.0$$

2. Subtract the mean from each observation to find the deviations from the mean (Column 2, Table 6–4).
3. Square the deviations from the mean (Column 3, Table 6–4).

Table 6–4 Example Data To Calculate Variance and Standard Deviation

Column 1 x_i	Column 2 $x_i - \bar{x}$	Column 3 $(x_i - \bar{x})^2$	Column 4 x_i^2
0	$0 - 5.0 = -5$	25	0
1	$1 - 5.0 = -4$	16	1
2	$2 - 5.0 = -3$	9	4
3	$3 - 5.0 = -2$	4	9
4	$4 - 5.0 = -1$	1	16
5	$5 - 5.0 = 0$	0	25
6	$6 - 5.0 = 1$	1	6
7	$7 - 5.0 = 2$	4	49
8	$8 - 5.0 = 3$	9	64
9	$9 - 5.0 = 4$	16	81
10	$10 - 5.0 = 5$	25	100
55	0	110	385

Source: Reprinted from U.S. DHHS, PHS, CDC, Epidemiology Program Office, *Principles of Epidemiology: An Introduction to Applied Epidemiology and Biostatics,* Self Study Course 3030-G, 2nd ed., p. 175, 1992.

4. Sum the squared deviations (Column 3):

$$\sum (x_i - \bar{x})^2 = 110$$

5. Divide the sum of the squared deviations by $(n-1)$ to find the variance:

$$\sum \frac{(x_i - \bar{x})^2}{n-1} = \frac{110}{11-1} = \frac{110}{10} = 11.0$$

6. Take the square root of the variance to calculate the standard deviation:

$$s = \sqrt{s^2} = \sqrt{11.0} = 3.3$$

Standard Deviation Advantages

Interval level data must be used to calculate the standard deviation. If scores to be analyzed are below the interval level of measurement (nominal or ordinal), the standard deviation cannot be used in any meaningful fashion. When assumptions are met, the standard deviation is used frequently—tables are available for ease in interpretation. Standard deviations are always used in relation to a mean. Standard deviations are used in other statistical procedures.

To illustrate the relationships of the standard deviation and the mean to the normal curve, consider data that are normally distributed, as in the following figure (Figure 6–3). More than 68 percent of the area under the normal curve lies between the mean and plus or minus one standard deviation (i.e., from 1 standard deviation below the mean to 1 standard deviation above the mean). Also, 95.5 percent of the area lies between the mean and plus or minus two standard deviations, and 99.7 percent of the area lies between the mean and the plus or minus three standard deviations. Further, 95 percent of the area lies between the mean and plus or minus 1.96 standard deviations.

WHICH STATISTICS? WHICH MEASURE TO USE?

1. *Mean* is used for numerical data and for bell-shaped (not skewed) distributions.
2. *Median* is used for ordinal data for data whose distribution is skewed.
3. *Mode* is used mostly for nominal data or when bimodal distributions are encountered.
4. *Range* (specifically percentiles and interquartiles) is used in two situations:
   a) When the median is used—with ordinal data or with skewed numerical data.

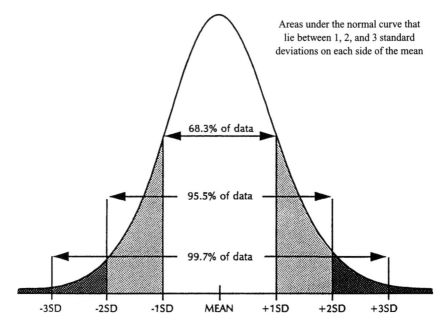

Figure 6–3 Areas under the Normal Curve That Lie between 1, 2, and 3 Standard Deviations on Each Side of the Mean. *Source:* Reprinted from U.S. DHHS, PHS, CDC, Epidemiology Program Office, *Principles of Epidemiology: An Introduction to Applied Epidemiology and Biostatics,* Self Study Course 3030-G, 2nd ed., p. 177, 1992.

---

  b) When the purpose is to emphasize extreme values.
 5. *Interquartile range* is used to describe the central 50 percent of a distribution regardless of shape.
 6. *Standard deviation* is used when the *mean* is used (i.e., with the bell-shaped—not skewed—distribution).

A REVIEW OF FACTS

 1. When averages are compared, the distributions should have the same basic shape.
 2. For symmetric distributions, the mean, median, and mode are equal.
 3. The mode is not affected by skewness, whereas the mean is affected most by skewness. The median is the measure of choice for a skewed distribution.
 4. A percentile is a number such that a certain percentage of the observations are below it and the remaining observations are above it.

5. Averages, unqualified, have little meaning as descriptive measures. "The simplest question to ask when confronted by an average is 'Which Average?'"

6. When averages corresponding to two sets of data are compared, the meaning of the comparison may be meaningless unless the underlying distributions are similar in shape.

7. When using averages, it is important to consider the pattern of variability.

8. Beware the *"average" of "averages."*

FREQUENCY DISTRIBUTIONS—HISTOGRAMS

A histogram is a pictorial representation or a graphic summary of variation in a set of data. The picture that the histogram presents (i.e., the pattern) makes it easier to understand patterns than what a simple table of numbers presents. The corresponding continuous distributions reflective of the data in a histogram aid in relating the histogram to the continuous distribution. Histograms may be used to compare two sets of data visually and draw conclusions about differences in the underlying processes. Histograms/variations of the bell-shaped curve may be used to portray different patterns of health program data. The commonly used numeric summaries include the average, median, range, standard deviation, and quantile boundaries that can be used as summaries to enhance comparisons of sets of data. When there is a need to discover and display the distribution of data, a histogram is a method or tool that is appropriate for this task. In a CQI process, when using a histogram, we are looking for distributions that are not normal but probably should be normal (i.e., the shape of the histogram). Further, we review the histogram for the spread or variation in addition to the shape. The spread (variability) may be small or large. In Figure 6–4, four normal curve graphic representations of performance related to CQI are shown. In graph A, the normal curve of performance is displayed; in B, the mean rises: raising the mean level of performance; in C, variation around the mean decreases: reducing variation around the mean, thereby reducing variation in the process; and in D, mean rises and variation decreases: in the CQI process, both B and C are pursued (i.e., improve performance and reduce variation). The benefits of D are higher standards (quality) and greater consistency (less variation in quality) and predictability in product, personnel, and organizational performance of delivering the service.[1] This approach leads to a more satisfied community, clinic, program, customer, client, and patient. Typically in public health practice, the histogram is used very little to solve problems or to understand a process. The evaluation of a histogram and the resulting frequency distribution by the public health practitioner are essential parts of applying quality improvement methods to public health programs for assessing outcomes.

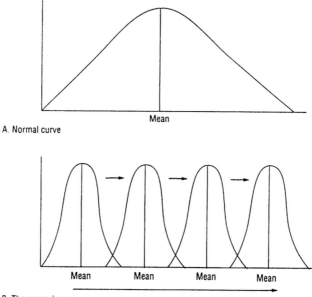

A. Normal curve

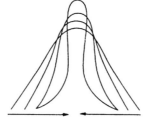

B. The mean rises

C. Variation around the mean decreases

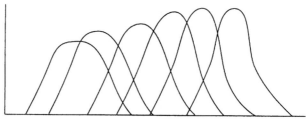

D. Mean rises and variation decreases

Figure 6–4 Graphic Representations from Normal Curve of Performance to Continuous Improvement. *Source:* Reprinted with permission from *The Health Care Manager's Guide to Continuous Quality Improvement,* by Wendy Leebov, EdD, and Clara Jean Ersoz, MD, published by American Hospital Publishing, Inc., copyright 1991.

SHAPES OF FREQUENCY DISTRIBUTIONS—QUALITY IMPROVEMENT EVALUATION IN PUBLIC HEALTH PRACTICE

Figure 6–5 compares the most common types of histograms and the corresponding continuous distributions as illustrated by patterns found in data that may represent specific situations. It is the shape or patterns of these distributions that aid in an analysis of trying to understand the cause of a problem—common or special cause.

Bell-Shaped Distribution (Also Called Normal or Gaussian Distribution)

Figure 6–5A shows the "typical" bell-shaped distribution. This distribution is the normal natural distribution of data from a process. Deviation from the natural process may indicate the presence of complicating factors or outside influences.[2] Generally, this distribution forms the basis for all quality improvement efforts in an organization, and all other distributions that may occur are evaluated against this standard. In public health, this distribution may be typical of (1) the distribution of causes of death by age group, or (2) the number of communities involved in assessing community needs.[3]

Uniform Distribution (Also Called Plateau Distribution)

Figure 6–5B shows a uniform distribution. This is a flat top with no distinct peak. This shape occurs with a mixture of several distributions having different mean values. In public health, this distribution may be typical of (1) month of occurrence of a disease with no seasonal patterns, (2) patient visits to a clinic during a week, or (3) organizationally, may indicate many different processes are at work.[4] Wide variability in a process leads to the wide variability observed in the data. Defining and implementing standard procedures will reduce variability.

Skewed Distribution

Figure 6–5C shows a skewed or a non-normal distribution. This is an asymmetrical shape in which the peak is off-center in the range of data and the distribution tails off sharply on one side and gently on the other. The illustration in Figure 6–5C is called a "positively skewed" distribution because the long tail extends rightward, toward increasing values. Additionally, for this type of distri-

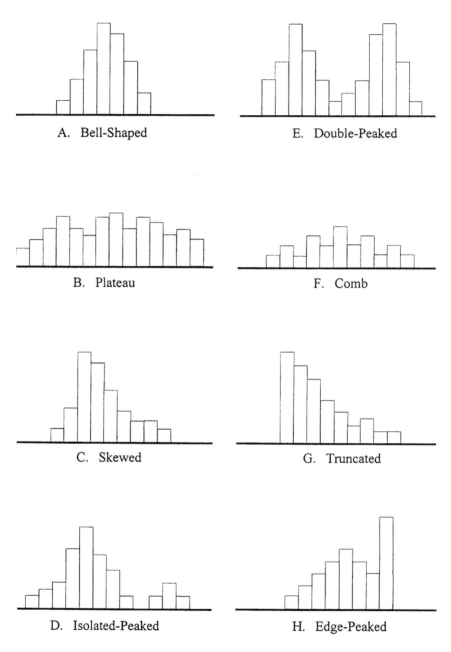

Figure 6–5 Common Histogram Patterns To Assess Variations and Cause. *Source:* Adapted from *Quality Improvement Tools®: Problem Solving Glossary* by P.E. Plsek and A. Onnias, © 1989, Juran Institute, Inc., p. 23.

bution, the mean is greater than the median or mode. A "negatively skewed" distribution would have a long tail extending leftward, toward decreasing values, and the mean is smaller than the median and mode.

The skewed pattern typically occurs when a practical limit, or a specification limit, exists on one side of the distribution. In these cases, there simply are not as many values *available* on one side as there are on the other side. Practical limits occur frequently when the data consist of time measurements or counts of things.

For example, tasks that take a very short time can never be completed in zero or less time. So those occasions when the time task takes a little longer than average to complete, a positively skewed tail on the distribution would result.[5]

Such skewed distributions are not inherently bad, but a public health professional should question the impact of the values in the long tail. Could they cause customer dissatisfaction (e.g., long waiting times)? Could they lead to higher health care costs? In public health, this distribution may be typical of (1) distributions of clinical tests, (2) disease patterns of rare occurrences, or (3) attendance at clinics for immunizations during the flu season.

Isolated-Peaked Distribution

Figure 6–5D shows an isolated-peaked distribution. Note that there is a small separate group of data in addition to the larger distribution. Like the double-peaked distribution, this pattern is a combination and suggests that two distinct processes are at work. But the small size of the second peak indicates an abnormality, something that does not happen often or regularly.[6]

It is recommended that you evaluate closely the conditions surrounding the data in the small peak to see if you can isolate a particular time, office, program, procedure, operator, etc. Such small isolated peaks in conjunction with a truncated distribution may result from the lack of complete effectiveness in screening out nonconforming items.[7] It is also possible that the small peak represents errors in measurements or in transcribing the data. Recheck your measurements and calculations. In public health, this distribution could be typical of (1) distribution of a disease pattern by county in a state, (2) distribution of requests for vital statistics birth records, or (3) variation in clinic attendance for prevention programs.[8]

U-Shaped Distribution (Also Called Bimodal or Double-Peaked Distribution)

Figure 6–5E shows a bimodal distribution, a valley in the middle of the range of the data with peaks on either side. This pattern is occasionally seen and usually indicates that the data are mixtures of two separate (bell-shaped normal) distributions and suggests two distinct processes are at work. To isolate the two patterns, stratification of data is appropriate. In public health, this distribution may be typical of (1) the age distribution of patients attending a clinic, (2) the mortality patterns of the very young (infants) and the older population in a community, (3) high- and low-risk communities analyzed by disease category, (4) clinically, the hormone levels of males and females, (5) the number of patients attending a daily clinic, or (6) the times the population may show up to pick up food vouchers (i.e., the Women's, Infant's, and Children's Nutrition program).[9]

Comb Distribution

Figure 6–5F shows a comb distribution (which resembles the teeth in a comb). There are high and low values alternating in a regular fashion. This pattern typically indicates measurement error, errors in the way the data were grouped to construct the histogram, or a systematic bias in the way the data were rounded off. This might also be a type of plateau distribution, but the regularity of alternating highs and lows is a warning of possible errors in data collection or in histogram construction.[10]

Review the data collection procedures and the construction of the histogram before considering possible process characteristics that might cause the pattern. In public health, this distribution may be typical of (1) errors in coding causes of death by two different coders (nosologists), (2) block-time appointment schedules at a public health clinic, or (3) monthly attendance at community forums to improve the health status of the populations.[11]

Reverse J-Shaped Distribution (Also Called Truncated Distribution)

Figure 6–5G shows the typical reverse J-shaped distribution. Usually the distribution ends or starts very abruptly on one side and falls off gently on the other. Reverse J-shaped distributions are often smooth, bell-shaped distributions with a part of the distribution removed—by some action. In public health, this distribution may be typical of (1) the screening of a population for identifying high-risk groups—diabetes, pap smear, blood pressure, etc., (2) survival time after diagnosis of various types of cancer—specifically, lung cancer, or (3) the availability of immunizations to school-aged children—high use initially then use falls off slowly.[12]

Edge-Peaked Distribution

Figure 6–5H shows the typical edge-peaked distribution. This is a large peak that is appended to an otherwise smooth distribution. This shape occurs when the extended tail of the smooth distribution has been cut off and lumped into a single category at the edge of the range of data. This shape very frequently indicates inaccurate recording of the data (e.g., values outside the "acceptable" range are reported as being just inside the range).[13] In public health, this distribution may be typical of (1) errors in ordering data, or (2) aggregating several categories into one final category creating the peak or the edge (e.g., patients attending a clinic after 5 PM versus patients attending the clinic categorized by hour).

QUICK REVIEW—HISTOGRAM INTERPRETATION

The number of bars in a histogram will determine how much of the pattern is revealed (e.g., if measurement is in hours as opposed to half-hour segments, then clearly half the pattern is hidden). As noted, not all distributions are bell-shaped or normal, so do not be alarmed or jump to conclusions without further investigations into your skew. If there is an abrupt end to the data limits, be cautious and check the accuracy of the data. If you cannot explain or understand the shape of the distribution, be sure to look for explanations (e.g., twin peaks may indicate that the data represent two different sources). Before conclusions are reached, be sure data are representative of typical or current conditions (e.g., are the data old, is there bias or incompleteness in the data). Sometimes it is best to collect new data or develop a system that enables the organization to continuously monitor the situation. Beware of the conclusions based on a small sample. The larger the sample, the more confidence we have that the resulting histogram (peaked, spread, or shaped) is representative of the process. One may want a consultation on what is an appropriate sample size for the current situation. The interpretation of a histogram is only a possible explanation—most times, additional analysis or direct observation may be needed to confirm your results. Thus, an analysis of a histogram requires two steps: your quality improvement team must (1) identify and classify the pattern of variation presented by the distribution of data in the histogram, and (2) develop a plausible and relevant explanation for the revealed pattern. The result is an analysis of how the process is operating and of the reason or possible cause of variation in the problem under investigation. Histograms are used in the third step of the 12-step CQI/PDCA cycle process. This third step of measuring and analyzing data may be accomplished using a histogram. Further, histograms may be used to identify root causes, evaluate results, implement a trial run, monitor the process, and hold the gains (see Table 8–2).

CONCLUSION

Measures of central location and dispersion are important to the application and use of the quality improvement methods to be described in Chapters 8, 9, and

10. These measures (mean, median, mode, range, and standard deviation) are in themselves important quality improvement methods to describe the pattern in the data obtained from a process being monitored and evaluated by the public health practitioner. A common product produced from data analysis using measures of central location and dispersion is the frequency distribution known as the histogram. It has been suggested that the histogram be used for solving problems and to understand a process as well as just describing the distribution of the data. In Chapter 8, the steps on how to understand a histogram are outlined, including how to use the histogram as a quality improvement method. Measures of central location and dispersion (including the histogram) form the foundation of assessing public health programs by using quality improvement methods that focus on continuous measurement. This is discussed in detail in Chapter 10.

NOTES

1. W. Leebov and C.J. Ersoz, *The Health Care Manager's Guide to Continuous Quality Improvement* (Chicago: American Hospital Publishing, 1991), 8.
2. P.E. Plsek and A. Onnias, *Juran Institute Quality Improvement Tools: Histograms*, (Wilton, CT: Juran Institute, Inc., 1989), 21–22.
3. G.E.A. Dever, "The Main Highway" module, in *Creating Critical Thinkers* (Atlanta, GA: Georgia Department of Human Resources, 1993), 25.
4. Ibid., 24.
5. Plsek and Onnias, *Juran Institute Quality Improvement Tools*, 21–22.
6. Ibid., 23.
7. Ibid.
8. Dever, "The Main Highway," 24–25.
9. Ibid.
10. Plsek and Onnias, *Juran Institute Quality Improvement Tools*, 21.
11. Dever, "The Main Highway," 24–25.
12. Plsek and Onnias, *Juran Institute Quality Improvement Tools*, 21.
13. Ibid., 23.

Chapter 7

Measurement for Quality Improvement in Public Health Practice—Problem Identification

Several attempts have been made to classify the quality improvement tools into specific categories.[1-6] The categories range from management tools, quality control tools, tools for collecting and displaying data, tools for making improvements, tools for problem solving, and tools for monitoring quality. All of these classifications of quality improvement tools are used to eventually focus measurement on outcomes. Each of these categories shows overlaps in what tools should be reserved for what category. In fact, as a result of these various classifications, it is probably more realistic to illustrate the tools, their use, and their application in public health practice by correlating the core functions of public health to the use of the various continuous quality improvement (CQI) tools. Most of the tools are to be used in any process of the Plan-Do-Check-Act (PDCA) cycle (see Exhibit 2–2)—assessment of community needs, development of policy, and assurance of service and programs—but clearly certain tools are more pertinent to specific steps in the process. Table 7–1 shows the relationship of the 12 steps of the CQI process (which includes the PDCA cycle) to the tools used for problem identification. Also, note that recommendations are made as to the frequency of use of each of the tools.

You may recall that a comparison of assessment approaches (see Exhibit 2–2) revealed similarities to the CQI process and the PDCA cycle. One of the core functions of public health, assessment, is clearly linked to the methods used in quality improvement for determining the identification of problems and the analysis of problems of public health programs. Certainly, many of these quality improvement measurements for problem identification and problem analysis of public health programs are not new to the public health practitioner. However, the concept of using these tools in a continuous and ongoing evaluation of outcomes

175

Table 7–1 Relationship of the 12 Steps in the Quality Improvement Process to the Tools Used for Problem Identification

Steps in the Continuous Quality Improvement Process

Problem Identification Tools for Public Health Practice*	Plan						Do		Check/Act			
	(1) Identify outputs, customer's expectations	(2) Describe current process	(3) Measure and analyze	(4) Focus on an improvement opportunity	(5) Identify root cause	(6) Generate and choose solutions	(7) Map out a trial run	(8) Implement a trial run	(9) Evaluate the results	(10) Draw conclusions	(11) Standardize the change	(12) Monitor; hold the gains
Surveys			●		◗	◗			●			●
Interviews	●	●		○	◗	◗	◗		◗	◗	◗	○
Check sheets			●						◗			●
Logs		●	●					●	◗			◗
Focus groups	●			○	●	●	◗	●	●	●	◗	◗
Brainstorming				●	●	●	◗				●	
Multivoting					○							
Flowcharts				●	●	◗	●				●	

Legend: ● = often used; ◗ = used less often; ○ = used rarely.
*Not all these CQI tools are described in this book.
Source: Reprinted with permission from *The Health Care Manager's Guide to Continuous Quality Improvement,* by Wendy Leebov, EdD, and Clara Jean Ersoz, MD, published by American Hospital Publishing, Inc., copyright 1991.

and monitoring of public health programs has certainly been lacking. Further, many of the problem analysis-type tools have seen little and in some instances no use or application in public health practice. This chapter specifically focuses on the tools used for problem identification:

- surveys
- checksheets/logs
- focus groups
- brainstorming
- nominal groups
- flowcharts

The problem identification (working with ideas) and problem analysis (working with numbers) tools and those tools that may be used for both problem identification and analysis are shown in Figure 7–1. The problem analysis tools are discussed in the next chapter.

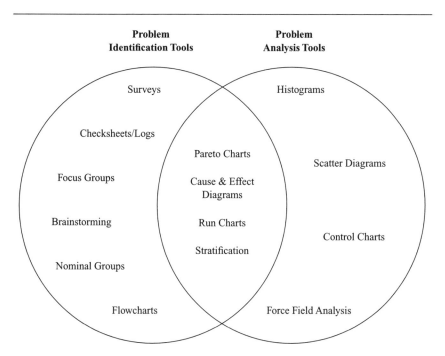

Figure 7–1 Problem Identification Analysis Tools Used for Continuous Quality Improvement in Public Health Practice. *Source:* Adapted with permission from *The Memory Jogger™*, copyright 1989 by GOAL/QPC, 13 Branch Street, Methuen, Massachusetts.

SURVEYS—MEASURING QUALITY

In public health practice, the survey is used frequently to collect, measure, and analyze data but seldom with the intent to measure the quality or outcome of a program. This is not to say surveys are nonessential to public health practitioners but that the survey is a quality improvement tool that is very underused for measuring customer satisfaction (patients, clinics, communities, etc.) or for monitoring and evaluating program outcomes. Certainly, the Behavioral Risk Factor Survey designed by the Centers for Disease Control and Prevention (CDC) and that is used by most state health agencies is characteristic of the measurement and analytical use of a survey.[7] Of course, this use should continue, and the advanced quality improvement tools for problem analysis should be used for subsequent survey data analysis.

Surveys are questionnaires used to collect quantitative data. Each question represents a snapshot or a cross section of information at a point in time that you can compare with another snapshot or cross section of information when you survey at a later point to ensure a continuous monitoring of the issue or problem. They are particularly useful and efficient in population-based health for assessing lifestyle and behavioral risk factors from public health customers when the need is to identify trends and patterns for large numbers of people.

A survey is one of the most widely used and yet maybe the least understood and least used technique in public health to collect data. Using a survey to collect data from a public health program population is a simple and fairly accurate process to measure attributes of the target population that relate to risk factors or behavioral characteristics. There are, however, basic questions that must be asked when conducting a survey to ensure adequate and true representation of the population under study. Questions include (1) should a sample of the population be selected? and (2) what method should be used to select the sample?[8]

Sample

The population sample is defined according to the type and size of the target population. First, the target population must be defined and identified. The next step is to determine if this population is accessible and determine the nature and extent of existing data for the targeted population. This allows the researcher to isolate the target population, to determine what data to collect, and to define the sample size. Of course, each of these issues must be tempered and based on available resources and the logistics of completing the survey.

If the decision is to survey the total target population, then this type of survey attempts to enumerate all individuals in the targeted area and would be considered a complete census of the population. This is obviously the least biased sample. If, however, a smaller number of individuals in a population is surveyed, then it would be necessary to determine two major elements: sampling method and sample size.

Sampling Method

Methods of sampling may be classified as probability or nonprobability. A probability sample can be a simple random sample, a stratified random sample, or a systematic sample. Examples of nonprobability samples are a convenience sample, a purposive sample, or a quota sample. The following is a brief explanation of each of these methods:

- *Simple random sampling* is a process in which the required sample size is selected at random from the total population under study. This type of sampling methodology produces a simple but unbiased sample. Every subject has an equal chance of being selected. For example, to assess the quality of a high-risk pregnancy program in a public health clinic that has 500 clients, a sample of 60 records is required. The 60 records could be selected from the original 500 records by using a table of random numbers. Once the 60 records are selected and the analysis is completed, the results can be generalized to the 500 high-risk mothers.
- *Stratified random sampling* requires the determination of a sample based on groups called "strata." The objective is to divide the population into smaller comparable groups (e.g., age, gender, socioeconomic status) to get a more accurate representation of the population. Once a stratum has been defined, a simple random sample is selected. A common practice in public health is to divide a population up according to location (i.e., urban or rural).
- *Systematic sampling* begins by generating one random number—starting the process with that number and then selecting the remainder of the records using a constant interval. Thereafter, every record that falls at that interval will be selected. For example, if the beginning random number was 6 and the constant interval was 11, the sixth birth record first and then every eleventh birth record registered in the county thereafter (i.e., 17th, 28th, 39th, etc.) would be selected.

    The other type of sampling method is nonprobability. For nonprobability sampling techniques, we must keep in mind that samples selected by these methods may not be representative of the target population. Therefore, inferences should be strictly related to the sample studies alone, and conclusions should be interpreted with caution due to potential nonrepresentation.
- *Convenience sampling* is structured to capitalize on readily available data. For example, only those community health clinics who served greater than

25 percent of their teenage population in a family planning program could be selected. This method is statistically weak, and the results certainly do not represent the population as a whole. Obviously, a very biased sample results. Because of the nonrepresentation of the sample produced, it is recommended to avoid this type of sampling altogether.

- *Purposive sampling* is a technique used to select a sample for a specific purpose and is usually based on the experience and judgment of the practitioner. For example, during a 10-day family planning clinic, the health department decided to sample two days to determine the quality of care given to the patients. Or if a state health policy office decided to ask three health districts about the status of their planning and assessment efforts in public health, this represents a purposive sample.

- *Quota sampling* is usually chosen to select a sample based on an arbitrary quota. For example, only 5 percent of the target population to be included in the sample is selected.[9]

Survey Methodology

Once a sample size[*10] and a sampling technique have been selected, the individual members of the sample can be identified by surveying the population either by mail, telephone, or interview.

A mail survey will be able to reach a large number of individuals with the least amount of expenditure and human resources. It is essential that mail surveys be pilot-tested before mailout. This method provides honest (especially if identity is anonymous) and the least biased answers. The major problem with this type of survey is the response rate. A low response rate renders the responses nonrepresentative of the total population. It is extremely difficult to get a high response rate unless one is willing to do a second and third follow-up. Additionally, misinterpretation of the questions or not completing all the questions may cause a problem in accurately analyzing the results. Mail surveys typically require at least six to eight weeks to complete and analyze. Probably the most frustrating aspect to conducting a mail survey is the waiting for the responses to return and the usually low response rate. In fact, mail surveys for collecting information from the general population should be used minimally.

A telephone survey is very accurate, but some answers could be biased in response due to leading questions. Further, because individuals are recruited to do the telephone survey for collecting the data over the phone, specific training and coaching are required to record and extract data accurately from the respondents. This method has the advantage of getting a very high response rate and can be completed within a relatively short time period. Some respondents do not care to answer the more personal questions on demographic and socioeconomic issues. Also, cooperation by the respondents has recently begun to decline, mainly due to time and mistrust.[11]

The face-to-face interview (direct administration) is the most accurate method but again could be biased because the identity of the respondent is not anonymous. It is very important the interviewer (researcher) does not engage in behavior that may affect a subjective response. For example, dress, language, and location of survey could alter responses; therefore, there must be every attempt to thoroughly train all interviewers to ensure consistency in data collection efforts. Interview surveys usually have much higher response rates than other survey

---

*Sample size determination can be a rather complex issue and is not discussed in this book; however, the public health practitioner need only consult a text on biostatistics or epidemiology for information on determining sample size. For instance, a good book on surveys, sample size, sampling design, etc., is *Field Epidemiology* by M.B. Gregg, ed. (New York: Oxford University Press, 1996). In a section of this book entitled "Surveys and Sampling" by Peavy, a very simple explanation of determining a sample size based on proportion is provided. He notes that "the size of the sample must be sufficient to accomplish the purpose but should not be more than necessary, or it becomes wasteful."[(p.155)]

In public health practice a very common approach in sampling is to determine what proportion of a population has some characteristic (e.g., diabetes, smoking, stress). To estimate a sample size for a proportion, use the following formula:

$$n = \frac{t^2 pq}{d^2}$$

where n = sample size estimate
t = confidence (for 95 percent use 1.96)
d = precision (0.05 or 0.10 usually)
p = proportion in the target population with the characteristic (if proportion is unknown, maximize sample size by letting $p = 0.5$)
$q = 1 - p$

Peavy notes that the above formula may be altered to calculate a final sample size. He states that "Once n is calculated, compare n with the size of the target population (N). If n is less than 10 percent of N, then use n as the final sample size. However, if n is greater than 10 percent of N, then use the following formula to adjust for a small target population:

$$n_f = \frac{n}{1 - \frac{n}{N}}$$

where n_f = final sample size
N = size of target population

Then n_f must be appraised to see whether it is consistent with the resources available to take the sample. This demands an estimation of the cost, labor, time, and materials required to obtain the proposed sample size. It sometimes becomes apparent that n_f has to be drastically reduced. If this happens, you are faced with a hard decision: whether to proceed with a much smaller sample size, thus reducing precision, or to abandon efforts until more resources can be found."[(p.155)]

types, but can be expensive and inconvenient due to scheduling and availability of respondents. If possible, all responses should be anonymous.[12]

In public health, the telephone and face-to-face interview (direct administration) types of surveys are more common and in many instances may be combined. However, these two types of surveys tend to cost more than mail surveys due to expenses associated with training, surveying, and supporting the interviews.

Uses of Surveys in Quality Improvement

In quality improvement from a public health practice point of view, a survey becomes a basic tool for identifying problems. In fact, to meet the number one concern in quality improvement measurement—the customer—the survey becomes a most essential tool. In some instances, the survey may be used for collecting data based on an isolated problem. However, this is not the usual application of a survey. The following are examples of how surveys might be used in quality improvement for public health:

- to identify public health customer or employee expectations and needs. Patients/clients can be asked to rank the importance they place on various elements of the service offered. For example, surveying food service facilities with non-English-speaking employees to determine who may need food handling training. Thus, a survey is used as a basic measure of customer satisfaction (community, clinic, patient, programs)
- to monitor customer satisfaction. Survey results can be graphed on trend charts that show, for example, "ratings that must be improved" or "ratings that are laudatory of the employees." These results may be used to communicate results to staff for improving the negative ratings and applauding the positive ratings
- to identify the difference between *observed* and *expected* performance (based on Year 2000 objectives) to target problems or improvement opportunities. Survey results may be analyzed using a Pareto chart, which may be used for problem analysis or problem identification
- to screen population groups for treatment of important diseases (e.g., pregnant mothers, young children, school children, or factory workers)
- to evaluate how effective the health services are (e.g., prenatal care attendance, immunization coverage, use of outpatient clinics)
- to provide health information about households and their members (e.g., water supplies, food habits, lifestyles)

- to measure the effects of a public health outcome indicator
- to estimate the incidence or prevalence of important diseases and lifestyle characteristics (e.g., hypertension, diabetes, smoking, alcohol use)
- to find out about local beliefs, customs, and health behavior (e.g., use of local foods, breast- and bottlefeeding, smoking)
- to show public health customers or employees that you care about what they think[13]

How To Develop and Conduct a Survey

Five main stages are involved in developing and conducting a public health survey or investigation:

1. Clarification of the need for the survey and statement of objectives. What exactly do you want to find out? The percentage of satisfied patients? What service is most important to most of the communities? Determine the relative strengths and weaknesses of your department on the quality or service delivery of the programs.
2. Determination of the sample and methods.
   - *Size of sample.* Selected communities for one week? A five percent sample of patients each day? A 10 percent sample of programs at randomly selected times.
   - *Design questions that relate to the specific purpose of the survey.* It helps to brainstorm possibilities with a group of people who understand your purpose.
   - *Use focus groups to fine-tune the questions.* Do this by carefully selecting people who are similar to groups you wish to survey.
   - *Use appropriate survey methodology* so that you will have confidence in the results. For example, how frequent, type of interviewers, and kind of survey (mail, telephone, face-to-face).
   - *Standardize the survey process (the instrument and the interview).*
   - *Provide training for the interviewers* who are involved in the survey distribution and data collection.
3. Organization and implementation of the survey.
4. Analysis, interpretation, and presentation of findings and recommendations.
5. Use of findings in quality improvement, health planning, disease control, policy development, assurance activities, and assessment.

These five steps are illustrated in detail in Figure 7–2.

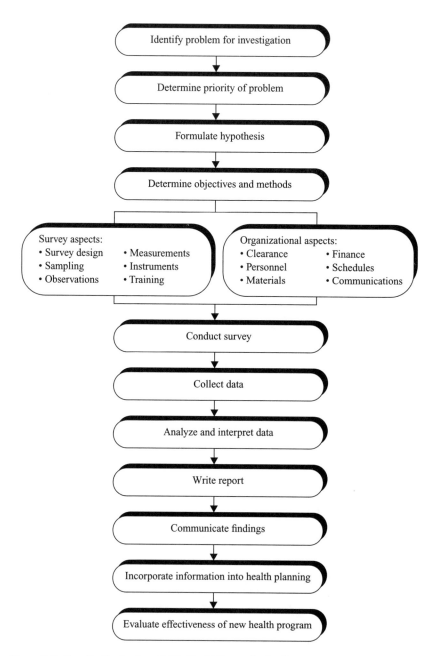

Figure 7–2 Steps for Conducting a Public Health Survey for Quality Improvement. *Source:* Adapted with permission from J.P. Vaughan and R.H. Morrow, *Manual of Epidemiology for District Health Management*, p. 73, © 1989, World Health Organization.

Prevention/Risk Factor Surveys and Quality Improvement in Public Health Practice—An Example

One survey instrument available from the Pennsylvania Department of Health, Division of Health Promotion is *The 1991 Behavioral Risk Factor Survey* developed by the CDC and adapted for use in Pennsylvania. Table 7–2 presents a listing of the various categories of personal health behaviors that are surveyed by the instrument. To increase accuracy and effectiveness, it is suggested that communities think about using a random telephone survey.[14] As noted previously, a mailout instrument used for identifying risk factors would not be recommended due to the high potential for a low response rate.

All completed telephone surveys must be coded and entered into a computerized database and analyzed using standard statistical tests. A combination of presentation graphics and survey research should be used to develop a statistical profile of current levels of health care attainment, provide an assessment of needs that are not being fulfilled, and identify subpopulations that are at particular risk. Key findings from this survey need to be presented in a concise document with tables and graphics. The survey results may be used to provide questions for focus group discussions and in the establishment of community health care priorities.[15]

Further, the Pareto chart (a quality improvement tool discussed in detail in Chapter 8) organizes and displays the data that have been collected and helps to illustrate the relative order of importance for the behaviors being evaluated (Figure 7–3). For example, unhealthy behaviors involving untreated hypertension,

---

Table 7–2 Behavioral Risk Factor Survey: Health Behaviors

	Health Behaviors
1	Seat belt use
2	Hypertension
3	Exercise
4	Weight control
5	Tobacco/smokeless tobacco use
6	Preventative health measures
7	Health insurance
8	Demographics
9	Women's health
10	AIDS
11	Foods: fruits & vegetables

Source: Adapted with permission from *A Guide for Assessing and Improving Health Status: Community...Planting the Seeds for Good Health*, p.14, © 1993, The Hospital Association of Pennsylvania.

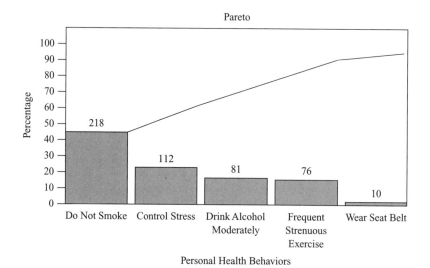

Figure 7–3 Sample Pareto Chart Featuring Personal Health Behaviors

smoking, and poor diet are very commonly (about 80 percent of all responses) reported and that the responding individuals are seeking ways to modify their behaviors. However, they may not know how to access services or know what is available locally to assist in their efforts.[16] The results from this survey analysis may be used to focus attention on high-risk behavior, but more important, repeating the survey provides a process by which these behaviors are continuously monitored. An example of this latter approach is The Prevention Index.[17] This index and information are based on randomly selected adults from across the country and collected by telephone. All 12 years of this project (1983–1994) followed the same procedure. Table 7–3 shows the results of the 1995 Prevention Index by health behavior, whereas Table 7–4 shows the trends across time in the change of the Prevention Index score. Although improvement has been shown, change has come very slowly. This index should be used regularly in public health practice for quality improvement measurement—it is a benchmark. Comparisons can be made on a community basis. Standards are available to be measured against when CQI is the goal (i.e., monitor the progress, hold the gains—standardize the process—and then continue to strive to improve the outcome).

In addition to the Behavioral Risk Factor Survey and the Preventive Index survey, a two-part survey prepared by the author was given to focus groups (Exhibit 7–1). The survey was used to elicit responses about major concerns in a community setting along with collecting the demographics of the respondents who participated in the focus group. This example illustrates the simplicity of a survey instrument that was used in a face-to-face interview or focus group setting.

Table 7–3 Prevention Index, 1995

Health-Promoting Behavior	Adults Practicing (%)	Experts' Rating, Scale 1–10	Value Contributed to Index
1. Do not smoke	74	9.78	4.4
2. Avoid smoking in bed	93	9.24	5.2
3. Wear seat belt	73	9.16	4.0
4. Avoid driving after drinking	85	9.03	4.6
5. Have smoke detector in home	93	8.53	4.8
6. Socialize regularly	86	8.31	4.3
7. Participate in frequent strenuous exercise	37	8.20	1.8
8. Drink alcohol moderately	89	8.15	4.4
9. Avoid home accidents	75	8.07	3.6
10. Limit fat in diet	53	7.82	2.5
11. Maintain proper weight	18	7.71	0.8
12. Obey speed limit	48	7.65	2.2
13. Have annual blood pressure test	84	7.62	3.8
14. Control stress	70	7.58	3.2
15. Consume fiber	54	7.41	2.4
16. Limit cholesterol in diet	45	7.15	1.9
17. Intake adequate vitamins/minerals	59	7.12	2.5
18. Have annual dental examination	73	7.08	3.1
19. Limit sodium in diet	47	7.04	2.0
20. Limit sugar in diet	40	6.90	1.7
21. Sleep 7–8 hours/night	59	6.71	2.4
PREVENTION INDEX			65.6

Source: Adapted with permission from *The Prevention Index: A Report Card on the Nation's Health*. 1995 Summary Report. p. 4, © 1995, Rodale Press, Inc.

Table 7–4 Prevention Index Scores

Year	Prevention Index Score
1984	61.5
1985	63.2
1986	64.1
1987	65.2
1988	64.8
1989	65.4
1990	66.2
1991	66.2
1992	66.5
1993	67.3
1994	66.8
1995	65.6

Source: Adapted with permission from *The Prevention Index: A Report Card on the Nation's Health*, 1995 Summary Report, p. 4, © 1995, Rodale Press, Inc.

Exhibit 7–1 A Focus Group Survey To Determine Rank Order of Concerns in a Community and Their Corresponding Demographic Characteristics

---

Part I Community Concerns

Please rank the top five concerns of those listed below in order of preference. Place the number 1 next to the one issue that concerns you most, number 2 by your second most important concern, number 3 by your third most important concern, and so forth. RANK ONLY YOUR TOP FIVE CONCERNS FROM ONE TO FIVE. Thank you.

Concerns	Rank
1. CRIME (Law Enforcement)	11. _____
2. DEFENSE	12. _____
3. DRUG CRISIS	13. _____
4. ECONOMY	14. _____
5. EDUCATION	15. _____
6. ENERGY	16. _____
7. ENVIRONMENT	17. _____
8. HEALTH	18. _____
9. HOUSING	19. _____
10. TRANSPORTATION	20. _____

Part II Demographics

1. Age ❏ 18–24 ❏ 25–34 ❏ 35–44 ❏ 45–64 ❏ 65+   2. Sex ❏ Male ❏ Female

3. Race ❏ Black, not Hispanic ❏ Hispanic ❏ Indian   ❏ White, not Hispanic ❏ Asian ❏ Other

4. Employment status ❏ Working full time ❏ Unemployed, looking for work ❏ Unemployed, lack of child care ❏ Retired   ❏ Working part time ❏ Unemployed, due to health ❏ Retired, due to health

5. Education ❏ Grade school ❏ Some high school ❏ High school   ❏ Some college ❏ College graduate

6. Marital status ❏ Married ❏ Divorced ❏ Separated   ❏ Never married ❏ Widowed

7. Income (Annual) ❏ 15,000 or less ❏ 15,000–25,000   ❏ 25,000–50,000 ❏ 50,000 or more

8. Health status ❏ Excellent ❏ Good   ❏ Fair ❏ Poor

CHECKSHEETS/LOGS

Checksheets and logs must be considered as a continuously monitoring tool for measurement in public health practice and not to be used only as a basis for collecting information on a one-time basis. In quality improvement, the main objective is to solve problems, and to solve problems, you must obviously identify a problem and subsequently analyze the problem to determine what can be done to have an effect on the problem and then to monitor the process to be sure you hold the gains you have implemented toward resolving the problem. A checksheet or log if used in this fashion becomes a significant tool for identifying a problem and monitoring a process.

Checksheets

To detect patterns in data, a sample of observations is needed. In most problem-solving processes, this is a fundamental starting point. A *checksheet* is a form designed to make it easy to record data. All you do is place a checkmark to reflect an observation. A checksheet enables you to count the frequency of an event or action within specified time periods. It enables you to record these facts in a systematic way and later summarize results, extract patterns, or draw conclusions.[18]

For example, checksheets can be used to track the following:

- the number of nurses present at the immunization clinics held on every Friday
- the number of restaurants having a specific failure/problem/complaint
- the reason for clinic visits
- the number of complications associated with each high-risk mother
- the number of patient complaints recorded biweekly
- the number of charts monitored for quality improvement

Table 7–5 illustrates a sample checksheet formatted to collect data on the birth order of the child by age, and another typical checksheet (Table 7–6) tracks frequency of visits by type in a public health clinic.

Checksheets can be used for a variety of purposes. For example, Leebov and Ozeki have suggested the following:

- *to discuss performance and results.* Once you total results, you can discuss the trends, the frequencies of key events, and the distribution or spread of the data that might suggest theories about causes.

Table 7–5 Example Checksheet Analyzing Birth Order

	Birth Order of Child					
Age (Years)	1	2	3	4	5	Total
0–19						
10–14						
15–19						
20–24						
TOTAL						

Table 7–6 Example Checksheet Used To Track Visits to a Public Health Clinic, by Type

	Frequency of Visits												
Type of Visit	Jan.	Feb.	Mar.	Apr.	May	June	Jul.	Aug.	Sept.	Oct.	Nov.	Dec.	TOTAL
Family planning													
Early intervention program													
Hypertension													
Immunization													
TOTAL													

- *to search for key causes.* Structured well in advance, checksheets can reveal how individuals, places, methods, and procedures influence a problem.

- *to measure the results of a solution or improvement.* Like other measurement tools, checksheets can be used to check up on the results of improvements.

- *ongoing monitoring.* Use checksheets to monitor performance, ensuring that you hold your gains and checking that previous problems do not reappear.[19,20]

Logs

This tool is both simple to construct and easy to use. It is used to keep track of a sequence of events or the period of time during which certain data occurred to chart trends or frequency analyses. Logs are constructed by identifying the data to be captured, as well as other associated elements. For example, one may want to keep a log of all the patients attending a clinic by date, program code, and visit code. Such a format may be used to track patients on a daily basis to link to other administration and management attributes such as time and costs of delivering direct clinic services. Exhibit 7–2 is a sample of such a log sheet. It is important to keep in mind that logs should be designed to be simple and user friendly. Logs are usually drawn as rows and columns. Recorders should be given a brief orientation session on using the logs. They should be encouraged to record only the raw data requested and discouraged from trying to identify or elicit a trend in the data. Logs must be translated into a summary format to reveal their meaning or the patterns within the recorded data.[21]

To develop a log, the following steps and issues should be addressed:

- Identify the basic elements necessary to record (e.g., from an epidemiologic or public health perspective, you could collect data on person, place, and time).
- Engage employees in designing the log because logs must be easy to complete and user friendly.
- Set up a chart with elements as column titles (Exhibit 7–2).
- Train staff about data collection and how to record the appropriate information in each column.
- Develop a format for synthesizing and summarizing the data recorded in the log (e.g., a table, histogram, or checksheet).
- At periodic intervals, use a checksheet, histogram, or Pareto chart to show the patterns in the raw data.[22] This allows the continuous monitoring of the information.

FOCUS GROUPS

The *focus group* is a powerful information-gathering technique that uses small group discussion to identify the views of individuals in the group about a certain subject. A facilitator leads the discussion using a question guide. Focus groups work best when questions are open ended and the facilitator encourages substantial discussion of each question.

The advantage of focus groups over written surveys is that you can probe and follow up for more information. In addition, the discussion tends to achieve depth because the interaction among participants triggers additional thoughts.

Uses of Focus Groups in Quality Improvement

Leebov and Ersoz have suggested six uses for focus groups in quality improvement efforts.[23] From a public health perspective these uses include:

Exhibit 7–2 Sample of Daily[1] Master Patient Tracking Log

_____   (___)_____   ___/ ___/1994
Clinic Name   Phone   Date

Patient ID #	Patient Name	Visit Code[2]	Program Code
1			
2			
3			
4			
5			
6			
7			
8			
9			
10			
11			
12			
13			
14			
15			
16			
17			
18			
19			
20			
21			
22			
23			
24			
25			

VISIT CODES

New Patient
1. Problem focused history/ exam
2. Expanded problem focused history/exam
3. Detailed history/exam, low complexity
4. Comprehensive history/ exam, moderate complexity
5. Comprehensive history/ exam, high complexity

Established Patient
11. Presenting problem(s) minimal
12. Problem focused history/ exam
13. Expanded problem focused history/exam, low complexity
14. Detailed history/exam, moderate complexity
15. Comprehensive history/ exam, high complexity

••• Special Notes •••

[1] Use a new set of forms (beginning with patient #1) for each new day. DO NOT combine different days onto the same tracking sheet.
[2] Primary provider MUST decide the visit code for each patient and either enter the code on the tracking sheet or inform the clerk of the appropriate code to be entered on the tracking sheet.

Source: Reprinted with permission from *Public Health Service Cost Study Training Manual*, p. 44, © 1994, Department of Human Resources, Division of Public Health, Office of Resource Development, Atlanta, Georgia.

1. Identification of program requirements and customer expectations for the public health programs (customers include staff and communities)
2. Solicitation of ideas, perceptions, and needs of the program's performance for meeting requirements (with customers, staff, communities, and clinics)
3. To understand the interaction of one public health program with other programs in a department of clinic in order to focus on improvements (with customers, staff, communities, and clinics)
4. To brainstorm opportunities and ideas for improvement (with customers, staff, communities, and clinics)
5. Field-test suggested changes, potential solutions, or options identifying brainstorming efforts in order to refine or select among the possibilities for program improvement
6. Develop community-based surveys to determine community expectations related to developing a healthy public health (with customers and staff)

Focus Group Design

Identifying Participants and Composition of the Group

The focus group approach requires that the group be homogeneous in terms of the demographic characteristics that the group represents. Therefore, each group included in the project should represent a particular socioeconomic class, race, or other description of lifestyle or stage.

An appropriate sampling strategy would be to recommend a two-stage design in which communities representative of a set of characteristics are selected and then followed by a process called "snowball sampling" to select participants within the community. The cost of randomly selecting a sample of communities in the first stage can be controlled, but random selection of participants from the community will probably be prohibitive. "Snowballing," a low-cost method used in focal group selection, involves identification of participants through reference. Using this method, local facilitators contact key persons who are representative of local characteristics; these persons, in turn, contact friends and neighbors and invite them to attend the meeting. This approach can increase the probability of homogeneity in the focus group; however, it is not a probability sample that allows the researcher to make statements about this subpopulation as a whole. Generalization is not the intent of focus groups; rather, the purpose is to determine the range of values and beliefs and to gain insights regarding "feelings," for example, about the health care system.

The only continuous and successful linkage of focus groups to follow up surveys has been achieved by the marketing industry, the major user of focus group technique in collecting product and service information from the public. This history suggests the usage of marketing segment characteristics as the demographic features to be used in developing the sample. Clusters of people with similar backgrounds, means, and consumer behaviors have been geographically identified by several marketing data firms; however, the most comprehensive is the PRIZM Cluster System by Claritas Corp. in Fairfax, WV.[24] Using a complex statistical analysis that incorporates social rank, ethnicity, degree of urbanization, household composition, mobility, and housing data, PRIZM assigns every American neighborhood to 1 of 62 basic lifestyle clusters. Neighborhood levels can be aggregated by ZIP code, postal carrier routes, census blocks and tracts, and minor civil divisions. Although the use of this approach to identify communities or a sampling base can be expensive, it is highly recommended because it is an ideal way to get representation of all demographic groups in an area with minimal resources and effort.

This two-stage design is very powerful for the following reasons:

- It will ensure community heterogeneity in the information being collected because the sample is derived from a comprehensive inventory of different lifestyle clusters. (Stage I)
- It will conform to the focus group requirement that groups be homogeneous (participants are drawn from the same lifestyle area through "snowball" reference); yet that homogeneity will not be defined by one demographic variable alone, but rather by a richer, more realistic aggregate of variables that can determine or influence consumer and humanistic values regarding health services. Although the focus groups may be homogeneous in lifestyle, the data collection method will allow for identification of responses from specific individuals and groups by the common descriptors of age, race, sex, income, and geographic area. (Stage II)

Number of Groups

Focus group research has shown that more groups do not mean more information. Typically, the first two groups of a particular population segment provide "a considerable amount of new information, but by the third or fourth session, a fair amount may have already been covered."[25(p.84)] The suggested rule of thumb is to plan for four groups with similar composition; only add more groups if new information is still being generated.

Group Size

Ideally, a focus group is comprised of 7 to 10 people with similar backgrounds. "Focus groups with more than twelve participants are not recommended: they limit each person's opportunity to share insights and observations. In addition, group dynamics change when participants are not able to describe their experiences."[26(p.87)] The smaller number will also reduce the amount of time necessary for identifying willing participants through "snowball" reference.

Focus Group Settings

The location of group discussion is an important part of focus group methodology. To avert the possibility that a health care environment may bias the responses of the focus group participants, health departments, hospitals, or voluntary health organizations should not be used as settings for the sessions. Rather, schools, churches, businesses, or nonhealth community facilities should be selected by the local facilitator.

Facilitator Training

Facilitator training is a major aspect of finalizing the process for conducting the public forums. Selection of forum sites is but one aspect of moderator competence that must be accomplished if the focus group approach is to succeed. Additionally, consultants may help prepare facilitators by coaching them in the skills necessary for exercising the mild unobtrusive control required of focus group processes. These skills include tape recording oral discussion, brief notetaking, introduction of group discussion and maintenance of "ground rules," insertion of key questions, the use of "pause and probe," body language, and neutral response in encouraging full and open discussion, the maintenance of conversation flow, and conclusion of the session.

Data Collection and Analysis

Content analysis, a means of quantifying focus group response, is the most common method of data collection used in focus group discussion. As an analysis strategy, it can "make inferences by objectively and systematically identifying specified characteristics of messages."[27(p.12)] It accomplishes this by counting the number of times a word or theme is spoken or written. Content analysis is most successful in identifying beliefs, values, or ideologies if a deliberate effort is made to control very specific topics of discussion; this strategy is dependent on the skill of the facilitator in eliciting a spoken text that is a reliable indicator of the speaker's intent. This is a weakness of content analysis if it is the only analytical method used to make sense of the focus group discussions. Another related limitation is that this method often cannot account for context, use of negatives, meaningful inflections, or irony in spoken speech. To address these problems, Morgan, one of the two leading experts in focus group methodology, insists that an ethnographic interpretation of the oral recording be done as well.[28] Krueger, the other expert, strongly recommends that an assistant facilitator take written notes for this purpose; these notes complement the tape recording by identifying the speakers, noting switches in opinion or position, and providing general context and meaning to the comments—all of which content analysis cannot do.[29]

A comprehensive examination of the focus groups, which includes content analysis and ethnography, will therefore include several steps or components:

- tape recording of discussions
- note taking by the facilitator
- in-depth note taking by an ethnographic recorder or assistant facilitator
- typed transcription of tapes
- identification of key themes and ideas for quantification
- use of a computer software ("Ethnograph") in quantifying concepts using a content analysis dictionary (content analysis) and identifying values and beliefs in context (ethnographic analysis)

Analysis of an oral group discussion has advantages and disadvantages. The major ones are noted below:

- *Advantage:* The dynamic nature of group interaction when conducted in the presence of a skilled facilitator can produce the most reliable information regarding community opinion.
- *Disadvantage:* The process is extremely time-consuming if the number of groups is excessive. It is not unusual for one hour of discussion to require six to eight hours of typing time if the typist receives the tape "cold." Transcribers who attend the discussions usually require a full day of secretarial time to transcribe a two-hour focus group. Unless an attempt is made to limit the number of focus groups, the task can be "absolutely overwhelming."[30]

Alternative to Oral Content Analysis

An alternative to content analysis of oral discussion is content analysis of written text. The sessions may be conducted in much the same way as oral focus groups, the difference being that the major analysis is performed on written responses to questions that are posed through a process called "ideawriting."[31] In this method, each identified participant reacts in writing to a stimulus question and then places his or her pad in the center of the group. Each participant reacts, in writing, to what is written on each of the other pads. If the intent of the group is to prioritize or identify their most important ideas and values, this can be achieved through subsequent discussion.

Piloting the Methodology

Regardless of the type of content analysis performed, it is suggested that the methodology be piloted in several locations that have been identified as representative lifestyle clusters. This is to ensure that participant identification procedures are workable and to test the feasibility of focus group processes.

Scientific Considerations

Human feelings, values, or beliefs are not simple quantifiable descriptions of a community like income or occupation; therefore, any project that attempts to identify these "qualities" in a group of people must be able to defend its basic soundness. To achieve this, the proposed methodology and analysis must address the following questions:

- *Can the data collection method developed compile information about the values and beliefs that are truly representative of those beliefs?* That is, have the "right" questions been asked, have they been asked in the "right" way, and have the responses been recorded so that accurate data are produced?
- *How truthful are the findings or conclusions that have been interpreted from the data?* For example, if most of the population states that they do not believe in artificially extending life, can we conclude that most people will not support the cost of such medical intervention for their own family members?

These two questions refer to what is commonly called internal validity in quantitative studies. The methodologic approach must ensure the credibility of the data and findings; that is, the inquiry will be conducted in such a manner that the subject of health care values and beliefs is accurately identified and described.

- *How applicable are the findings to other settings or groups of people?* The study may reveal that some forums of elderly white groups hold values or express concerns very similar to some forums of elderly black groups; yet dissimilarity may be displayed by these groups in other forums. This is to be expected to a certain extent within the study because many factors additional to race and age may affect forum responses.
- *Would the data be replicated if the project were repeated using the same participants?* We want to know how consistent the data are; if the forum were held six months later, would the health care values of the population be different?

It is highly probable that the responses of some individuals would change if the study were replicated. Qualitative studies cannot display the "reliability" or replicability of quantitative studies because human beliefs are changeable. It is necessary, therefore, that the methodology must have strong dependability—it must be able to consistently extract a representative value system from the participants, although focus group members, settings, and facilitators may change.

Because of this expected variability that would appear to threaten the "external validity" or generalizability of a quantitative study, it is important that the sampling methodology used identify multiple data sources for each major demographic group. This approach will support the confirmability of a study. By drawing information from many elderly sessions, for instance, their responses can be compared to confirm the validity of generalized values and beliefs of this group.

- *How may results of the study be biased?* Whose beliefs are being represented?

Objectivity is essentially the same concept in all types of studies, quantitative or qualitative. The methodology used must ensure that the data collected are based on the beliefs of the participants, not the researchers or representatives of the health care system.

An example of results obtained from several focus groups using the process just described on the attitudes, beliefs, and values of Georgians about health care reform is shown in Exhibit 7–3. The process by which these results were obtained is outlined in Figure 7–4. Specifically, Georgia Health Decisions, a nonprofit group, was challenged to elicit public opinion on the health care reform debate. To accomplish this, focus groups were convened by PRIZM clusters (socialeconomic clusters) in the state. The flowchart (Figure 7–4) shows the process and the steps to arrive at a vision for health care reform in Georgia. As a result of this analysis, four super clusters and their beliefs were identified, which represented about 90 percent of Georgia's population.

BRAINSTORMING

Leebov and Ersoz have described brainstorming as "a quick, powerful, and energizing technique to elicit from a group (an improvement team, a community forum, a customer group, or a focus group) an outpouring or list of ideas, perceptions, problems, opportunities, questions, possible causes, dimensions of a problem, alternate solutions, and so forth. It is an extremely versatile tool. In fact, it is often used as one part of many other process improvement methods."[32(p.151)] Brainstorming may be used for identifying, collecting, and displaying data; it is quick, simple, and also very useful and important for making quality improvement decisions.

The purpose of brainstorming is to generate the information needed to proceed to other steps in the quality improvement process. Specifically, brainstorming helps a group to generate creative ideas in a relatively rapid time period, without criticisms or judgment, as well as without discussion along the way. The key to

Exhibit 7–3 An Analysis of Change Beliefs by Super Cluster, Georgia 1991: Change Beliefs "What Changes Do You Want in the Health Care System."

Polite Conservatives

% of Georgia Population: 19%

What Cluster Group Is Concerned About:
- Demand accountability
- Regulate the industry
- Emphasize preventive medicine
- Provide some means of access to the uninsured

Areas of Tension:
- Demand of the health care industry what they demand of their own businesses.
- They want regulation, but they see government as ineffective.
- Strain between the ideal of universal access and beliefs about high taxation and inferior quality of "socialized" system.

The Bottom Line:
- They want to modify the present system, but they don't want to eliminate the role of the private sector.

Transitional Hardliners

% of Georgia Population: 16.1%

What Cluster Group Is Concerned About:
- Regulation
- Control malpractice
- Increase access for special populations and the uninsured
- Consider a universal coverage model

Areas of Tension:
- May be losing out as compared to the more wealthy and the welfare beneficiaries.
- Moving cautiously, the super cluster considers the benefits of a universal system.

The Bottom Line:
- See what government leadership can do in regulation. Don't take any intransigent position on a changing health care system.

Needy Self Reliants

% of Georgia Population: 50.3%

What Cluster Group Is Concerned About:
- Regulation
- Prevention
- Control malpractice
- Reduce benefits of welfare programs
- Increase access
- Provide more services

Areas of Tension:
- Reduce the dominance of the powerful (regulate) and reduce or take away the benefits of non-contributors. Increase access and services to the needy. Suspicious of changes which may increase exploitation.

The Bottom Line:
- They argue for improving their position in the present system by competing against "welfare" and reducing the influence of controlling powers. Local control is very important.

Benefits Bunch

% of Georgia Population: 6.9%

What Cluster Group Is Concerned About:
- Regulation
- Prevention
- More access and facilities
- Adopt socialized medicine

Areas of Tension:
- Need a more humane face to delivery of public services. Adopt universal coverage, even if some don't contribute. HM can't understand why some (less productive) get services; working poor don't.

The Bottom Line:
- Maintain present public system but with improvements in pt/provider relationship and more opportunity for recipient autonomy. Or better, provide a universal health care system for all citizens.

Source: Reprinted with permission from G.E.A. Dever, "The Health Care Reform Effect in Rural America," *GAFP Journal*, Vol. 16, No. 4, p. 15, © 1994.

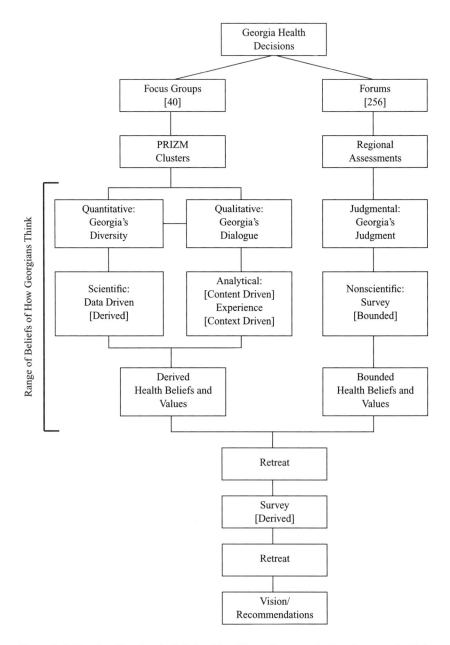

Figure 7–4 Flowchart Showing the Relationship of Focus Groups to the Development of a Vision and Recommendations for Making Health Decisions. *Source:* Adapted with permission from G.E.A. Dever, "The Health Care Reform Effect in Rural America," *GAFP Journal,* Vol. 16, No. 4, p. 14, © 1994.

successful brainstorming is that judgment or discussion is withheld. Thus, this technique becomes especially useful when all members of the group participate and no boundaries of thought are defined.

In typical large group discussions, people respond to one another's ideas with judgments; thus others become discouraged from speaking because they fear having their thoughts questioned or attacked.[33]

Brainstorming, when conducted appropriately, encourages people's thoughts to flow. Since judgments are not allowed, creativity is enhanced and people are most willing to participate because they have nothing to fear from other participants.

Conducting Brainstorming Sessions

Brassard has suggested that brainstorming be conducted in one of two ways:

1. *Structured*—In this method, every person in a group must give an idea as his or her turn arises in the rotation or pass until the next round. It often forces even shy individuals to participate but can also create a certain amount of pressure to contribute.
2. *Unstructured*—In this method, group members simply give ideas as they come to mind. It tends to create a more relaxed atmosphere but also risks domination by the most vocal members.[34]

In both methods, the general "rules of the road" are the same.

In fact, Leebov and Ersoz have suggested three phases for conducting brainstorming sessions: generation, clarification, and evaluation.[35]

Generation Phase

The rules of the brainstorming session are reviewed with group members, the question or purpose is clearly noted and written on a flipchart, and then responses are invited and recorded. This phase can be either structured or unstructured.

The rules for conducting a brainstorming session must be outlined in the generation phase, and they are

- Preparation for the session is as important as the session itself.
- All rules must be reviewed and understood before the session.
- Quantity of responses, not quality, is important.
- Discussion, judgment, and criticism are all suspended during the generation process.

- It is fine to build on ideas already presented.
- Practicality is unimportant; far-out ideas are welcome.
- Six- or seven-word maximum; otherwise, you will hear speeches.

Tips that may facilitate the generation phase of the process are noted:

- Record *every* idea in the speaker's own words.
- Minimize technical language in all comments.
- Follow the rules. One conversation at a time. Suggest a method to signal a violation of the rules. This avoids a verbal reprimand when someone has broken the rules. Utilizing a signal is especially important when the group is just learning how to brainstorm.
- Identify a scribe who takes direction from the facilitator or arbitrator only.
- The session arbitrator will make the final decision when a topic is hung and follow up with post-session decisions.
- A typical brainstorming session should move quickly; probably about 5 to 10 minutes is sufficient. A warning sign is appropriate before ending the session so any ideas left unsaid can be recorded.

Clarification Phase

After the list, which is usually numbered, is generated, the group reviews the list to clarify the meaning of all items. The generation phase has a "quantity, not quality" emphasis; therefore, some items may be expressed in vague terms. When this occurs, everybody is energized to determine the meaning of the terms or statements. Such clarification is important before ideas are judged so that in later discussion unclear ideas are not dismissed along with unworkable ideas.[36]

Evaluation Phase

The brainstormers now review the list and eliminate duplications, nonrelevant ideas, or ideas that are beyond the scope of the session. Combine items that seem similar, but only with the agreement of the group. As a next step, develop a matrix for decision making that would be useful in evaluating ideas according to a set of criteria specified by the group. Potential criteria may be the impact on the problem, cost, or ease of implementation. The Hanlon Method for setting priorities in public health practice could be utilized at this point to focus on a few of the more important problems that evaluate magnitude, effectiveness, cost, and amenability to improvement.[37] In other words, sort and narrow down the list of ideas to a few that may be utilized to focus a program.[38] This process may also be combined with nominal groups—multivoting or weighted voting techniques.

Uses of Brainstorming

The possibilities are many and the public health practitioner would be most wise to use this technique frequently. Brainstorming helps in establishing ownership in the process and it involves the people. Some possible uses of brainstorming include:

- Brainstorm ideas and alternative solutions to a problem that the group would like to solve.
- Brainstorm factors that allow one to search for root causes. For instance, brainstorm the possible causes of a problem on a cause-and-effect diagram or in a force-field analysis (see Chapter 8).
- Use brainstorming to identify alternative problem statements before agreeing to the specific program indicators that were targeted previously.
- Brainstorm outcomes to be evaluated for a public health program.
- Brainstorm ideas on how to improve the registration of vital record events.
- Brainstorm the approaches to use in public health practice for assessment.
- Brainstorm benefits of a publication for "marketing prevention."
- Brainstorm ideas about the development of a customer satisfaction survey in the community.[39]

NOMINAL GROUPS

This technique, a continuation of brainstorming, may be used to refine and narrow down a set of critical indicators or ideas after the brainstorming session. Once a list of ideas is generated, then the process of prioritizing or ranking of ideas begins. Ranking is accomplished by one of three popular methods: multiple voting, weighted voting, or simple ranking. A second list is generated, with the ideas ranked accordingly, and is presented for implementation in process improvement. This technique is especially helpful in condensing the number of ideas into a shorter, more manageable list of "best" ideas.[40]

Multiple Voting Technique

As a complementary technique to brainstorming, multiple voting is another way to shorten, evaluate, critique, and rank a long list of ideas.[41] Multiple voting is performed by the members of the group who generated the original list of ideas. Thus, multivoting may be used to refine and narrow down the critical indicators during a CQI session. It is a way to conduct a straw poll or to select the most important items from a list with limited discussion and difficulty. This is accomplished through a series of votes, each cutting the list in half—even a list of 30 to 50 items can be reduced to a workable number in four or five votes. Multivoting often follows a brainstorming session to identify the few items worthy of immediate attention. The steps involved are

1. First, generate a list of items and number each item.
2. If two or more items seem very similar, combine them, but only if the group agrees that they are the same.
3. If necessary, renumber all items.
4. Have all members choose several items they would like to discuss or address by writing down the number of choices equal to at least one-third of the total number of items on the list (48-item list = 16 choices; 37-item list = 13 choices).
5. After all the members have silently completed their selections, tally votes. You may let members vote by a show of hands as each item number is called out. If there is a need for secrecy, conduct the vote by ballot.
6. To reduce the list, eliminate those items with the fewest votes. Group size affects the results. A rule of thumb is, if it is a small group (five or fewer members), cross out items with only one or two votes. If it is a medium group (6 to 15 members), eliminate anything with three or fewer votes. If it is a large group (more than 15 members), eliminate items with four votes or fewer.
7. Repeat steps 3 through 6 on the remaining list with the choices reduced accordingly. Continue this until only a few items remain. If no clear favorite emerges by this point, have the group discuss which item should receive top priority. Or you may take one last vote.[42]

The new and final list of ideas is then presented for implementation in the processes involved.

Weighted Voting Technique

This technique, similar to multiple voting, is useful in preparing a final list containing the best ideas. As with multiple voting, each member is allowed to cast his or her vote to determine whether the full list of ideas or a short list will be submitted. Each group member is allowed a set number of votes. Members have the freedom to spread their votes across the ideas generated. A grid or a matrix is set up to record the voting pattern of the members and determine the total number of votes each idea receives.[43]

Nominal Group Techniques—An Example

In public health practice, there is a need to establish or determine which programs deserve priority for funding in the next legislative budget cycle. To devise this list, a CQI team (district health director and the state management team) must come to a consensus on the importance of what programs to support for funding. An appropriate approach to use to analyze this problem would be the nominal group technique. The participants generated a list of programs that were recorded on a board or flipchart. Duplicates were eliminated, and a final list of five programs was identified. The five programs listed by letter were

Letter	Program
A	Immunization
B	Hypertension
C	Environmental health
D	Vital records
E	Health assessment

Letters rather than numbers were used to identify each program so that team members did not get confused by the ranking process.

Each team member recorded the corresponding letters on a piece of paper and rank ordered the statements. For example, the health director from Atlanta ranked the programs as identified below:

Letter	Program	Rank
A	Immunization	5
B	Hypertension	4
C	Environmental health	3
D	Vital records	2
E	Health assessment	1

This example uses "5" as the most important ranking and "1" as the least important. Because individual rankings will later be combined, this "reverse order" minimizes the effect of team members leaving some statements blank. Therefore, a blank (value = 0) would not, in effect, increase its importance.[44]

For illustration purposes only, five district health directors recorded their responses, and they are noted below by the major city in the district.

Program	Atlanta	Albany	Savannah	Macon	Dalton		Total
A Immunization	5	5	4	2	4	=	20
B Hypertension	4	4	5	1	5	=	19
C Environmental health	3	1	3	4	1	=	12
D Vital records	2	2	1	5	2	=	12
E Health assessment	1	3	2	3	3	=	12

As a result of this process, the immunization program (A) would receive top priority. The team would work on this first and then move through the rest of the list as needed.

FLOWCHARTS

The easiest way to get a grip on a process is to draw a picture of it. Simply put, that is what a *flowchart* is—a picture of a process. Thus, when you need to identify the actual ideal paths that any program or service follows to identify deviations, use a flowchart.[45] Like a road map, a flowchart vividly portrays, sequentially and in picture form, every activity or step in a process intended to lead to an output. Typically, no one individual in a group knows the entire process. By mapping out the process, group members can gain a shared understanding of it and use their shared understanding to collect data, narrow down the problem, focus discussion of the process, and identify resources. Although it seems obvious that to improve and control a process you must first understand it, many managers and teams try to attack problems and make improvements without taking the critical first step of creating a flowchart to understand the existing situation.

Flowcharts range from the simple to the complex. A simple flowchart can be extremely powerful when you want to understand your current situation, pinpoint opportunities for improvement, revamp your process to reflect the improvements, and build on the changes to standardize the improvement. A flowchart, which is most helpful in group problem solving, includes symbols for activities, decisions, waits, stops-and-starts, arrows, and documentation (Figure 7–5). Using precise symbols, the group can specify the exact nature of an element in the process, whether it is a process, a decision, or a terminal.[46] For example, when you reach the analysis stage, you can look at all the wait symbols and ask whether and why they are necessary. Or you can look at the decision points and clarify the criteria for making the right decisions.[47] Banks has noted that "a standard flowchart diagram connects a series of different shapes. Each shape has a specific meaning [see Figure 7–5]. Although currently, there are no universally accepted rules for constructing flowcharts, methods and standards have been proposed."[48(p.112)] A

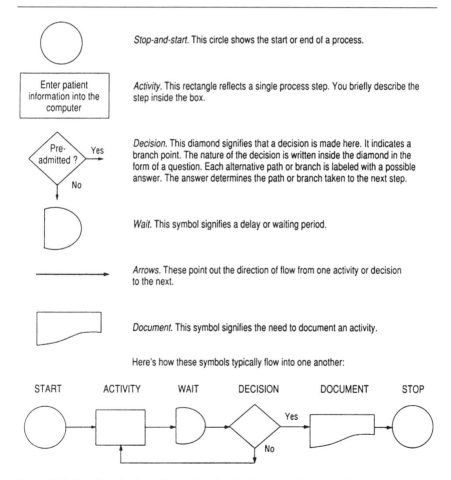

Stop-and-start. This circle shows the start or end of a process.

Enter patient information into the computer

Activity. This rectangle reflects a single process step. You briefly describe the step inside the box.

Pre-admitted ?   Yes   No

Decision. This diamond signifies that a decision is made here. It indicates a branch point. The nature of the decision is written inside the diamond in the form of a question. Each alternative path or branch is labeled with a possible answer. The answer determines the path or branch taken to the next step.

Wait. This symbol signifies a delay or waiting period.

Arrows. These point out the direction of flow from one activity or decision to the next.

Document. This symbol signifies the need to document an activity.

Here's how these symbols typically flow into one another:

START   ACTIVITY   WAIT   DECISION   DOCUMENT   STOP

Yes   No

Figure 7–5 Flowchart Symbols. *Source*: Reprinted with permission from *The Health Care Manager's Guide to Continuous Quality Improvement,* by Wendy Leebov, EdD, and Clara Jean Ersoz, MD, published by American Hospital Publishing, Inc., copyright 1991.

more benign flowchart that does not use the traditional symbols but yet does impart the message of investigating and controlling an epidemic is shown in Figure 7–6. In public health practice, this type of flowchart is very common. It offers a basic design and flow of an epidemiologic process, with branches suggesting decisions to be made concerning an epidemiologic analysis to determine if it is a disease investigation process versus a disease control approach. Further, a flowchart depicting patient flow in a public health clinic is shown in Figure 7–7.

Flowcharts may be used to (1) describe a process, (2) describe which problem will be addressed first, (3) identify a problem, (4) generate a process, (5) group similar processes, and (6) implement a new process. In constructing a flowchart, there is potential for committing some very common errors. Banks has outlined these possible errors and has suggested solutions to overcome these problems (Table 7–7). A flowchart may be used in conjunction with brainstorming, nominal group techniques, and focus groups.

CONCLUSION

Quality improvement methods used for problem identification in public health practice have been used very sparingly. It has been the intent of this chapter to explicitly outline six quality improvement tools for problem identification. They are surveys, checksheets/logs, focus groups, brainstorming, nominal groups, and flowcharts. The basic theme that links these methods is that when we use them we are generally working with ideas—a qualitative approach as opposed to working with numbers. Many readers will clearly recognize many of these methods and in many cases have used these tools. However, in public health practice most applications have been directed toward the efforts of describing data. A major purpose of this chapter was to demonstrate that these methods can also be used for analyzing, evaluating, and monitoring an improvement process (Table 7–1). Public health practitioners must use these quality improvement methods more often to support their decision-making process. As noted previously, many public health practice decisions are based on intuition, rhetoric, and anecdote; thus, these improvement methods are offered to provide public health practitioners specific methods to base decisions on evidence.

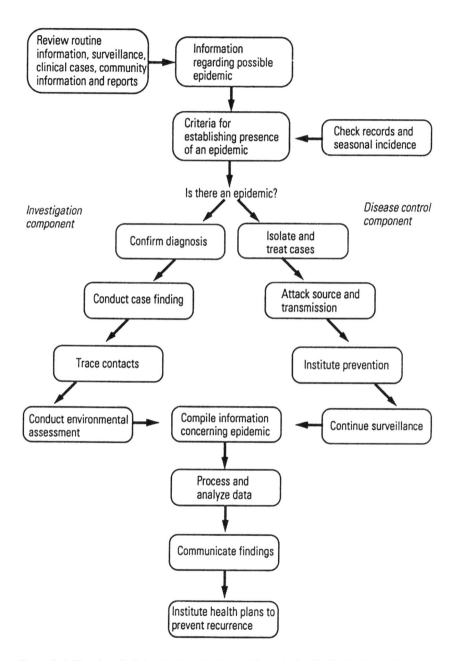

Figure 7–6 Flowchart Outlining the Investigation and Control of an Epidemic. *Source*: Reprinted with permission from J.P. Vaughan and R.H. Morrow, *Manual of Epidemiology for District Health Management,* p. 61, © 1989, World Health Organization.

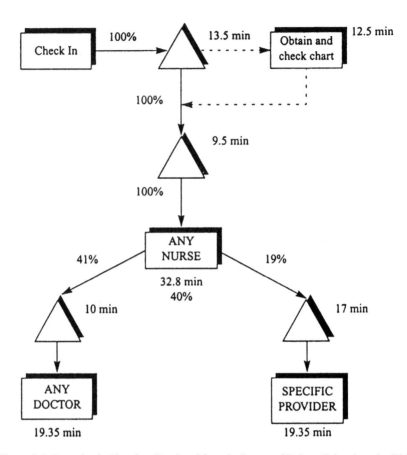

Figure 7–7 Example of a Flowchart Developed from the Process of Patients Going through a Walk-in Clinic (Average Times and Patient Volumes Are Noted on This Example). *Source*: Reprinted from S.P. Johnson and C.P. McLaughlin, "Measurement and Statistical Analysis in CQL," in *Continuous Quality Improvement in Health Care: Theory, Implementation, and Applications,* C.P. McLaughlin and A.D. Kaluzny, eds., p. 78, © 1994, Aspen Publishers, Inc.

Table 7–7 Common Errors and Solutions in Constructing Flowcharts

Flowchart Errors	*Flowchart Solutions*
Lack of consistency within the same flowchart in the direction of the arrows representing YES and NO	Reword text in decision nodes or rearrange subsequent decision and action nodes so that all the YES answers lead from the node in the same direction
Using a single flowchart to describe more than one algorithm—for example, one algorithm for both drug treatment decisions and drug inventory control process	Construct separate algorithms and indicate the entry from one to the other with connector shapes
Giving decision nodes more than two paths outward for multiple choices	Construct a series of yes-no decision nodes that cover all options
Giving decision nodes only one exit path, which assumes that there is no other option or no interest in another option	Provide alternate path, ending with the terminal shape for "stop"
Using the same shape for different meanings or different shapes for the same meaning	Review all meanings, and standardize the shapes used for each type
Looping arrows back or exiting to more than one subsequent series of steps, making sequencing hard to follow	Use connectors to show a loop or connection to other steps that are drawn separately
Ending a path with a process shape	Use a terminal shape to signal the end of each pathway
Writing questions or statements on the connecting arrows	Write all text within the appropriate shape

Source: Adapted from N.J. Banks, "Constructing Algorithm Flowcharts for Performance Measure Evaluation," *Using Clinical Practice Guidelines to Evaluate Quality of Care*, Vol. 2—Methods, p. 114, 1995, U.S. DHHS, PHS, Pub. No. 95-0046.

NOTES

1. W. Leebov and C.J. Ersoz, *The Health Care Manager's Guide to Continuous Quality Improvement* (Chicago: American Hospital Publishing, 1991).
2. P.E. Plsek and A. Onnias, *Juran Institute Quality Improvement Tools: Problem Solving/Glossary* (Wilton, CT: Juran Institute, 1989).
3. K. Ishikawa, *Guide to Quality Control* (Minato-Ku, Tokyo, Japan: Asian Productivity Organization, 1982).
4. T. Pyzdek, *Pyzdek's Guide to SPC: Volume One—Fundamentals* (Tucson, AZ: Quality Publishing, 1990).
5. E.J. Gaucher and R.J. Coffey, *Total Quality in Healthcare* (San Francisco: Jossey-Bass, Publishers, 1993).
6. C.P. McLaughlin and A.D. Kaluzny, *Continuous Quality Improvement in Health Care: Theory, Implementation, and Applications* (Gaithersburg, MD: Aspen Publishers, 1994).
7. Centers for Disease Control and Prevention, *The 1991 Behavioral Risk Factor Survey* (Atlanta, GA: CDC, 1991).
8. A.F. Al-Assaf and J.A. Schmele, eds., *The Textbook of Total Quality in Healthcare* (Delray Beach, FL: St. Lucie Press, 1993), 128.
9. Ibid., 129.
10. J.V. Peavy, "Surveys and Sampling," in *Field Epidemiology*, ed. M.B. Gregg (New York: Oxford University Press, 1996), 152–163.
11. Al-Assaf and Schmele, *Textbook of Total Quality in Healthcare*, 131.
12. Ibid.
13. Leebov and Ersoz, *Health Care Manager's Guide to Continuous Quality Improvement*, 109–110.
14. The Hospital Association of Pennsylvania (HAP), *A Guide for Assessing and Improving Health Status: Community... Planting the Seeds for Good Health* (Harrisburg, PA: 1993), 13.
15. Ibid., 14–15.
16. Ibid., 15.
17. *The Prevention Index: A Report Card on the Nation's Health,* 1995 Summary Report (Emmaus, PA: Rodale Press, 1995) (A project of *Prevention* Magazine).
18. Leebov and Ersoz, *Health Care Manager's Guide to Continuous Quality Improvement,* 117.
19. Ibid.
20. K. Ozeki and T. Asaka, eds., *Handbook of Quality Tools* (Cambridge, MA: Productivity Press, 1990), 163.
21. Al-Assaf and Schmele, *Textbook of Total Quality in Healthcare*, 133–134.
22. Leebov and Ersoz, *Health Care Manager's Guide to Continuous Quality Improvement,* 119.
23. Ibid., 105.
24. VNU Business Information Services, Inc. *Claritas PRIZM.* Arlington, VA.
25. R.A. Krueger, *Focus Groups: A Practical Guide for Applied Research* (Newbury Park, CA: Sage Publications, 1988).
26. Ibid., 87.
27. C. Marshall and G.B. Rossman, *Designing Qualitative Research* (Newbury Park, CA: Sage Publications, 1989), 12.
28. D.L. Morgan, *Focus Groups as Qualitative Research* (Newbury Park, CA: Sage Publications, 1988).

29. Krueger, *Focus Groups*.

30. H.R. Bernard, *Research Methods in Cultural Anthropology* (Newbury Park, CA: Sage Publications, 1988).

31. C.M. Moore, *Group Techniques for Idea Building*, Applied Social Science Series (Newbury Park, CA: Sage Publications, 1987).

32. Leebov and Ersoz, *Health Care Manager's Guide to Continuous Quality Improvement*, 151.

33. Ibid.

34. M. Brassard, *The Memory Jogger Plus+* (Methuen, MA: GOAL/QPC, 1989), 270–271.

35. Leebov and Ersoz, *Health Care Manager's Guide to Continuous Quality Improvement*, 151.

36. Ibid., 152.

37. G.F. Pickett and J.J. Hanlon, *Public Health Administration and Practice*, 9th ed. (St. Louis, MO: C.V. Mosby, 1990).

38. Leebov and Ersoz, *Health Care Manager's Guide to Continuous Quality Improvement*, 152.

39. Ibid., 152–153.

40. Al-Assaf and Schmele, *Textbook of Total Quality in Healthcare*, 137.

41. Ibid., 138–139.

42. Immunization CQI JAD Workbook (Workbook presented by the Texas Department of Health, Integrated Client Encounter System Project, Austin, TX, April 1993), 2–3.

43. Al-Assaf and Schmele, *Textbook of Total Quality in Healthcare*, 138–139.

44. M. Brassard and D. Ritter, *The Memory Jogger II* (Methuen, MA: GOAL/QPC, 1994), 92–93.

45. Brassard, *The Memory Jogger Plus+*, 267.

46. N.J. Banks, "Constructing Algorithm Flowcharts for Performance Measure Evaluation," in *Using Clinical Practice Guidelines to Evaluate Quality of Care*. Vol. 2—Methods (Rockville, MD: U.S. Department of Health and Human Services, Agency for Health Care Policy and Research, 1995). DHHS Pub. No. (PHS) 95-0046. GPO Stock No. 1995-380-940.

47. Leebov and Ersoz, *Health Care Manager's Guide to Continuous Quality Improvement*, 143–144.

48. Banks, "Constructing Algorithm Flowcharts for Performance Measure Evaluation," 112.

Chapter 8

Measurement for Quality Improvement in Public Health Practice—Problem Analysis

In Chapter 7, six basic quality improvement tools for identifying problems in public health practice were discussed. Many of those tools discussed were not new, and their use in public health practice has been extensive. The quality improvement tools (surveys, checksheets/logs, focus groups, brainstorming, nominal group techniques, and flowcharts) are important to the assessment process—one of the core public health functions. A review of Table 7–1 reveals the importance of each of the six problem identification tools in the quality improvement planning process. This chapter builds on the previous tools used for identifying problems and develops additional quality improvement tools for problem analysis. Specifically, the focus is on histograms, Pareto charts, cause-and-effect diagrams, run charts, stratification, scatter diagrams, control charts, and force-field analysis. Table 8–1 classifies these tools based on problem identification, problem analysis, or both and further classifies the tools according to working with ideas or working with numbers. In addition, for public health practitioners, Table 8–2 outlines the relationship of the continuous quality improvement (CQI) process including the Plan-Do-Check-Act (PDCA) cycle for building healthy communities to the tools for working with ideas (problem identification) and for working with numbers (problem analysis). Clearly, it is important to completely understand that the CQI process in public health practice may be applied to any one of the core functions of public health—assessment, policy development, and assurance. It just so happens that most public health practitioners will probably focus most on the assessment function as it relates to the CQI process and outcome measurement. No matter the situation or the focus, all quality improvement tools must be used appropriately and in correct situations. Thus, the purpose of this chapter is to outline the tools listed above and show applications in the public health arena.

Table 8–1 Quality Improvement Tools Classified by Problem Identification and Problem Analysis for Use in Public Health Practice

Quality Improvement Tools	Working with Ideas*	Working with Numbers*
Problem Identification		
Surveys		■
Checksheets/logs		■
Focus Groups	■	
Brainstorming	■	
Nominal group technique	■	
Flowcharts	■	
Problem Identification and Analysis		
Pareto charts		■
Cause-and-effect	■	
Run chart		■
Stratification		■
Problem Analysis		
Histogram		■
Scatter diagrams		■
Control chart		■
Force-field analysis	■	

*Brassard and Ritter in *Memory Jogger II* have classified these quality improvement tools by typical improvement situations such as working with ideas and working with numbers.

Source: Adapted with permission from *The Memory Jogger*™ *II*, Copyright 1994, by GOAL/QPC, 13 Branch Street, Methuen, Massachusetts, and from *The Memory Jogger*™, Copyright 1989 by GOAL/QPC, 13 Branch Street, Methuen, Massachusetts.

HISTOGRAMS

Histograms are not new to the public health practitioner; they have been used frequently and appropriately for describing data. However, they have been used very little for identifying and analyzing community health problems. To do this, we must understand how to use the histogram as part of the CQI process in working with numbers. A histogram is simply a statement of data collected and categorized by various groups to represent a picture of the situation that was investigated. When displayed, such information provides a description of that situation; however, when the structure of the data is examined according to a time sequence or the data are reexamined looking for possible causes or trends related to the distribution of the data, then the public health analyst is using the histogram to identify a problem or to analyze the problem based on the information gathered. In Chapter 6, frequency distributions (histograms) were discussed in some detail as to their shape and meaning as applied in public health. The pri-

Table 8-2 Relationship of the 12 Steps in the Quality Improvement Process to the Tools Used for Problem Analysis

Steps in the Continuous Quality Improvement Process

Problem Analysis Tools for Public Health Practice	Plan						Do		Check/Act			
	(1) Identify outputs, customer's expectations	(2) Describe current process	(3) Measure and analyze	(4) Focus on an improvement opportunity	(5) Identify root cause	(6) Generate and choose solutions	(7) Map out a trial run	(8) Implement a trial run	(9) Evaluate the results	(10) Draw conclusions	(11) Standardize the change	(12) Monitor; hold the gains
Histograms	◗		●		◗							○
Pareto charts		◗	●	●	●					●		
Cause-and-effect diagrams					●							
Run charts	◗		●	◗	●			●	●			●
Stratification	◗	◗	●		●				◗			●
Scatter diagrams	○	○	○	○	●	○						○
Control charts			●		●			●	●			●
Force-field analysis					●	◗	●	●	◗		●	

Legend: ● = often used; ◗ = used less often; ○ = used rarely.

Source: Adapted with permission from *The Health Care Manager's Guide to Continuous Quality Improvement*, by Wendy Leebov, EdD, and Clara Jean Ersoz, MD, published by American Hospital Publishing, Inc., copyright 1991 and adapted from *Quality Improvement Tools®: Problem Solving/Glossary* by P.E. Pisek and A. Onnias, © 1989 Juran Institute, Inc., p. 23.

mary focus was on the variation displayed in the histograms and what situations in a public health context each may represent. The intent in this section is to be more specific in the use, development, and application of the histogram in the CQI process for public health practice.

The histogram is a frequency distribution with vertical bars on an x-axis with a continuous scale (variable data), whereas the y-axis displays the frequency of the item being analyzed. A histogram provides a picture of the distribution of the data of the characteristics being measured. Some analysts confuse the frequency distribution with the bar chart. A bar chart displays on the x-axis a discrete value (attribute data) that usually shows separation of the bars.

How To Construct a Histogram

- Collect the data; count the total number of observations or data points.
- Arrange the data points in ascending order (i.e., rank the data).
- Determine the range of the data by subtracting the lowest value from the highest value.
- Calculate the number of columns for the histogram. A minimum of 5 and a maximum of 20 are recommended (Table 8–3).
- Calculate the width of the classes. Divide the range by the number of classes to establish the width of each class interval, for example,

$$Class\ interval\ width = \frac{range}{number\ of\ classes} \quad or \quad w = \frac{r}{k}$$

where w = class interval width
r = range
k = number of classes

- Write the class intervals along the horizontal or x-axis.
- Write the frequency scale (numbers or percentages) along the vertical or y-axis.

Table 8–3 Relationship of the Number of Observations to the Number of Classes

Number of Observations (n)	Number of Classes (k)
<50	5–6
50–100	7
101–200	8
201–500	9
501–1000	10
>1000	11–20

- For each class interval, draw the number of bars that reflect the number of data points in each interval.
- Label each axis and title the histogram.
- Identify and classify the pattern of variation (see Figure 6–5).

Infant Mortality—An Example

Infant deaths by day of occurrence are shown in Table 8–4. These infant deaths occurred in an urban county over a period of three years. On review of these data, it is difficult to tell how they are distributed. By inspecting the data, the lowest number in the table is 22 and the highest is 307. That is, an infant died on the 22nd day (the lowest value) and an infant died on day 307 (the highest value). Beyond that, however, there is not much to say about the data points by simply looking at them.

As suggested in the steps to construct a histogram, the data may be classified into equal intervals. Experts recommend between 5 and 20 intervals, as noted in Table 8–3. More than 20 intervals are difficult to manipulate and fewer than 5 may result in information being lost.

To decide on the actual number, it is appropriate to inspect the data. The data points in Table 8–4 range from 22 to 307. Subtracting 22 from 307 produces a range of 285. Many researchers arbitrarily divide the data into 10 intervals. If you were to divide these data into 10 intervals, the width of each would be 28.5 per interval. However, for infant mortality a 30-day or 1-month category is typical. The number of intervals, the width of each, and the upper and lower boundaries are many times selected arbitrarily, but they should be calculated to ensure interpretation of the information.

If the method outlined previously is applied to determine interval width, the result would be the range divided by the number of classes based on the number of observations. Therefore, the range (285) divided by 7 (because we had 79 observations) equals 40 days (i.e., $285 \div 7 = 40$ days). That is, the formula determination of interval width would be 40 days. In this example, 30 days is used

---

Table 8–4 Infant Deaths by Age in Days

271	174	164	225	130	96	102	148	130	81	80	46
226	64	20	65	187	117	42	51	116	28	38	66
77	120	79	176	108	117	96	85	61	87	80	65
299	134	181	65	150	88	108	95	25	108	60	80
53	57	90	138	76	99	28	67	22	113	110	114
199	34	104	47	90	151	80	92	115	23	165	87
65	77	45	42	32	44						

because this would be considered appropriate in public health practice. Actually, an interval of 28 days would be more appropriate because the 28-day interval equates to the neonatal mortality period. Table 8–5 displays the data grouped into 30-day intervals (months). The data grouped in this manner makes more sense than in Table 8–4. For example, many deaths occur between 61 and 90 days (two to three months), and very few deaths occur after 180 days (six months). As illustrated in Table 8–5, the data begin to provide a meaningful pattern. A graphic display will make the patterns, variations, and characteristics even more evident. Figure 8–1 shows the histogram for the infant deaths by age in days. This graphic presents a clear picture of the possible problems or the components of the problem. For example, this histogram reflects a skewed or isolated peak-type pattern (see Figure 6–5 for an analysis of histograms patterns).

Histogram Evaluation

If this is a true skewed distribution (Figure 8–1) (skewed distributions are not inherently bad), then the pattern observed suggests a distinct pattern of rare occurrences that are concentrated at the beginning of the process, and it diminishes gradually to the extent no events extend beyond a certain point. It would be prudent to investigate the events at the far right of the distribution to distinguish the differences in the events that occur rarely compared with those that appear more frequently. As noted, this pattern also represents an isolated peak-type of distribution. It is recommended to evaluate critically the conditions surrounding the data in the small peak to see if one can isolate a particular time, procedure, environment, family type, health status, etc. Small isolated peaks could represent errors in measurement or possibly two separate isolated events occurring.

To help evaluate the histogram, one could consider the following issues: (1) what are the consequences of this variation? and (2) what clues does this pat-

Table 8–5 Frequency Distribution of Infant Deaths by Age in Days

Age Interval (Days)	Number of Deaths
<30	6
31–60	13
61–90	23
91–120	18
121–150	7
151–180	5
181–210	3
211–240	1
241–270	0
>270	2

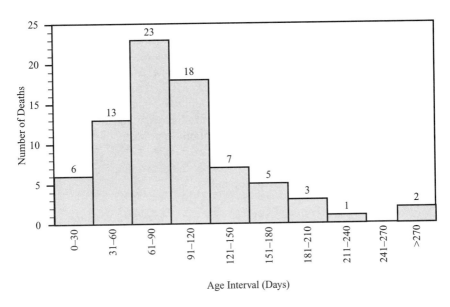

Figure 8–1 Histogram of Infant Deaths by Age in Days

tern of variation give about the scope and nature of the infant death problem? What questions does it raise that need to be investigated? What hypotheses need to be tested further?

Consequently, histograms are used to understand the variability of a process and to help generate *alternative* theories about the dynamics of processes and causes of problems, theories that then need to be confirmed or discarded through additional observations or analysis. In Chapter 6 (Figure 6–5), several types of histograms were presented, and the corresponding variation in patterns was evaluated as to the potential reasons for those shapes (i.e., causes, problems, etc.). Thus, to evaluate the pattern in the histogram and shed light on possible causes for that pattern, use Figure 6–5 as your guide.

Histograms—Summing Up

Leebov and Ersoz have noted that "All repeated events or processes vary in the results they produce over time. The degree and nature of this variation help to generate theories about problems in the process, the conditions under which the problem is most severe, and how to focus efforts on improving the process. A histogram visually communicates information about variation in a process in a way that helps to generate questions and focus improvement efforts. After creating the histogram, revisit the process to answer questions the histogram raises."[1(p.125)]

It is important to push for alternative explanations of the variation instead of accepting the first explanation that seems reasonable. Many may be misled by sticking to their first hunch about what might explain a pattern when, in fact, an explanation should be verified by gathering additional information.

The example of the distribution of infant deaths by day illustrates that a histogram is critical to revealing a pattern or variation—a powerful tool for descriptive epidemiology analysis in public health practice.

Juran has identified four key concepts about the data and use of histograms in problem identification and problem solving.

1. *Values in a set of data almost always show variation.* Variation is everywhere. It is inevitable in the output of any process—registration of vital events, health services, or administrative. It is impossible to keep all factors in a constant state all the time.
2. *Variation displays a pattern.* Different phenomena will have different variation, but there is always some pattern to the variation. These patterns of variation in data are called "distributions." For our purposes, it is enough to know that there are usually discernible patterns in the variation, and these patterns often tell us a great deal about the cause of a problem. Identifying and interpreting these patterns are the point to evaluating histograms.
3. *Patterns of variation are difficult to see in simple tables of numbers.*
4. *Patterns of variation are easier to see when the data are summarized pictorially in a histogram.*[2]

PARETO CHARTS

A Pareto chart is a specialized form of a bar graph that shows the relative frequency of events in descending order. The charts display the importance of the problems or causes that have been identified in the investigation of a problem. Although the chart was first developed by Vilfredo Pareto (1897), the more popular use in CQI was advanced by Juran.[3] Juran applied the principle of "a few people hold most of the money," and this principle was advanced by Pareto to problems of quality in which the focus is on the "vital few" as opposed to the "trivial many." This concept became known as the 80-20 rule—where 80 percent of the effect is a result of 20 percent of the causes. In public health practice, this could be applied by suggesting that (1) 80 percent of the coding errors in vital statistics could be attributed to 20 percent of the staff, (2) 80 percent of the customers complaining can be attributed to 20 percent of the problems, (3) 80 percent of the district health plans are completed by 20 percent of the staff, (4) 80 percent of the incomplete clinical records are due to 20 percent of the staff, and (5) 80 percent of the resistance to quality improvement in public health is due to 20 percent of the staff. The resulting notion or principle is that most of the problems result from a relatively small number of causes. Therefore, in the interest of time and the fact that one cannot focus on all problems or root causes at once, it is imperative to select a problem or root cause that will maximize returns and minimize the time.

Pareto Charts—How To Do It!

The basic concept of making a Pareto chart is quite easy. The following steps are suggested:

1. Identify a public health problem to be studied (e.g., behavioral risk factors in a community health assessment).
2. Determine a time period for data collection and design an approach to collect the data (e.g., survey, brainstorming, existing data).
3. Summarize the data by categorizing the information in descending order of percentage responses.
4. Calculate the frequency and make a chart that ranks the results in descending order from left to right (i.e., the largest first, the second largest second, and so on).
5. Label the vertical axis—counts or frequency. Some charts may label the left vertical axis with counts, whereas the right vertical axis could be percentages (0 to 100 percent).
6. Label the horizontal axis—categories, problems, or causes.
7. Add the percentage values of each bar and calculate the cumulative total for each bar. For clarification, the actual percentage for each bar may be placed on the bar.
8. Construct the bar chart.
9. If necessary, a line graph may be plotted showing the cumulative percentages to assess the 80-20 rule (Pareto curve).
10. Title the graph (i.e., add all necessary labels, sources, etc.).

Pareto Charts—Uses

Ozeki has outlined several ways in which Pareto charts may be used in CQI.[4] Some examples include the following:

- to focus on the major aspect of a problem (i.e., focus attention on the "vital few" instead of the "trivial many" problems or processes needing attention)

- to decide which problems to pursue for making improvements—the major cause may not always be the cause to pursue—need to evaluate what is practically important versus statistically important
- to evaluate the causes related to a problem (e.g., determining the importance of risk factors to the overall health status of a community)
- to evaluate the effectiveness of the improvement using a pre- and post-Pareto chart (Figure 8–2)
- to identify improvements to make that are easy and act on them immediately even if they are low priority (i.e., on the far right of the horizontal axis)

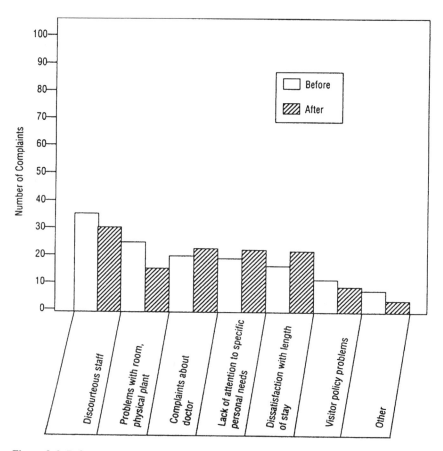

Figure 8–2 Before-and-After Pareto Chart. *Source:* Reprinted with permission from *The Health Care Manager's Guide to Continuous Quality Improvement,* by Wendy Leebov, EdD, and Clara Jean Ersoz, MD, published by American Hospital Publishing, Inc., copyright 1991.

- to make graphic explanations and presentations about the relative importance or severity of a problem
- to provide a diagnostic and monitoring device that can be used to identify
and monitor progress made after improvement measures are implemented[5]

Leebov and Ersoz have illustrated some of the uses noted above,[6] specifically
the use in selecting an improvement opportunity (second item above) and identifying a powerful cause (third item above).

The Pareto chart in Figure 8–3 was based on patient survey results and was
used to help a nursing team determine which three problems to work on. "Listen-
ing" to the chart, the team decided to work on (1) communicating more effectively about what the patient can expect, (2) answering calls more rapidly, and

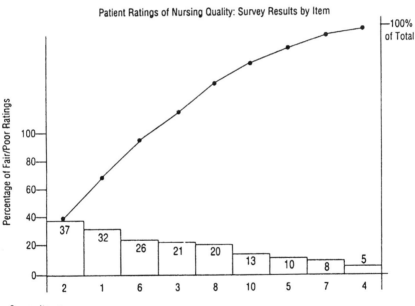

Figure 8–3 Pareto Chart Used To Determine Which Problems To Target for Improvement. *Source:*
Reprinted with permission from *The Health Care Manager's Guide to Continuous Quality Improvement,* by Wendy Leebov, EdD, and Clara Jean Ersoz, MD, published by American Hospital Publishing, Inc., copyright 1991.

(3) improving friendliness.[7] Thus, the group was able to decide on which improvement opportunity to select for solving.

Further, to identify a powerful cause, an improvement team may use a Pareto chart to compare the relative length of delays at each step in the process for patients entering the public health clinic (Figure 8–4). This type of chart suggests that delays based on administrative issues (completing forms) and block appointments were the two steps in the process that consumed the most unnecessary time. If these causes of delays could be alleviated, the overall delay would be significantly reduced.

Pareto charts, obviously, can be very useful; however, there are many cases in which simple line charts, bar charts, or pie charts may be used instead of or in addition to Pareto analysis.

Pareto Pointers

There are some basic elements or points to be aware of when utilizing these charts in quality improvement for public health practice.

- Always separate that which is of practical importance versus statistical importance. The Pareto chart assumes quality is important; however, one quality issue may easily override any quantity value. One complaint about an abusive practitioner is certainly more important than 10 complaints of poor carpeting.
- Beware of the "flat" Pareto chart with several categories. When all causes attain the same or near the same value, then the chart has little to contribute

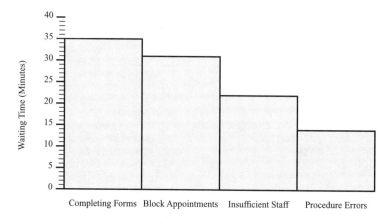

Figure 8–4 Pareto Chart Showing Reasons for Waiting Times at a Public Health Clinic

to define a specific problem for improvement. In this event, it is better to group or collapse categories if possible. If not possible, this situation could very well indicate overall significant quality problems and potential collapse of a program.

- Pareto charts should be considered based on causes and/or costs. Cause one may be one-tenth of the cost of cause four. Prioritize based on cost if appropriate.

CAUSE-AND-EFFECT DIAGRAMS

In public health practice, most analysts use sophisticated statistical methodologies and observational and experimental research designs to determine cause-and-effect relationships. Obviously, these types of tools may be used in the CQI process, but a beginning step that may be input to these approaches could be cause-and-effect diagrams. A cause-and-effect diagram is a visual display of the suggested causal relationship between a quality character (e.g., health status profile), the effect and the variables (e.g., demographics, health status indicators), and the cause. The purpose is to suggest possible theories about root causes and note relationships among them so one can select those causes deemed important for further analysis. The cause-and-effect diagram was developed by Kaoru Ishikawa that has become known as a "fishbone" diagram.[8] A generic cause-and-effect diagram is displayed in Figure 8–5. On the far right side of the chart is the effect or problem to be evaluated (the quality characteristic), and the left side of the chart contains the major categories potentially contributing to the effect. These become the causes. Specifically, there is a backbone, spine, or trunk that connects to the quality characteristic, and the remaining "branches" or "bones" reflect various levels of causes that may contribute to the effect. The central construction of such a chart must identify the quality characteristic, the trunk line, then add the headers or major categories and draw lines to connect to the trunk line, and then finally add contributing causes or the "branches" or "bones" attached to the categories or header line. The result is a design similar to Figure 8–6, which shows, among other variables, that prenatal care related to infant mortality is a quality characteristic (the effect) to be analyzed.

The Hospital Association of Pennsylvania has developed a cause-and-effect diagram (Fishbone Summary) to analyze a potential area for improvement (the cause) and the variables (the effect). Examples of the categories investigated include demographics, health status indicators, capacity/utilization, and small area analysis (Figure 8–7). This figure also gives the reader a basis for interpreting the information related to the cause-and-effect diagram. In Figure 8–8, the specific causes linked to the categories and subsequently linked to the effect are detailed. In public health practice, the assessment of a problem in a particular

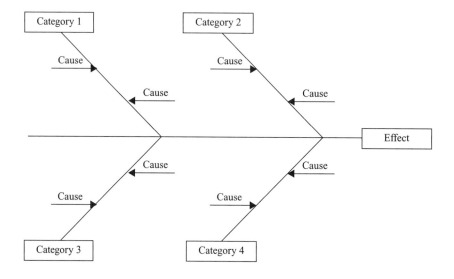

Figure 8–5 Generic Cause-and-Effect Diagram

geographic area provides the potential categories and causes that may be related to a particular effect. For instance, to understand the effect (teenage pregnancy) there must be an understanding of the causes (demographics, utilization, health status, and small area variation). The specific cause related to each category is then listed and noted as "branches" on the cause-and-effect graph. Thus, a possible theory could be that teenage pregnancy is related to the demographics of an area that is influenced by the educational attainment of the population. Each theory is listed as possible, thereby linking it to the effect. A good cause-and-effect design will have many theories, smaller branches, or "twigs"; if it does not, then it demonstrates that the understanding of the problem is superficial. Most times, the causes generated for a cause-and-effect design are a result of a brainstorming session or even from a flowchart or other quality improvement tools that use creative and critical thinking processes.

Developing Cause-and-Effect Diagrams

In public health practice, the reliance on the basic sciences of epidemiology, biostatistics, critical appraisal of the medical literature, research design, and behavioral sciences becomes the cornerstone for creative, critical, and divergent thinking necessary to foster theory about a problem being investigated. In public health practice, as in CQI, the same steps would be used to develop the process,

STEP ONE: Identify the Problem (Spine of Diagram)

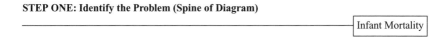

STEP TWO: Label Categories (Branches)

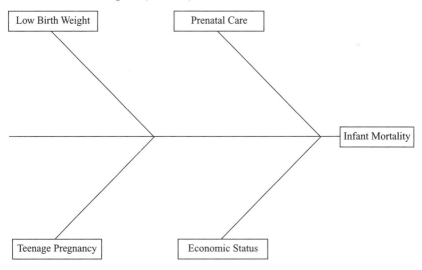

STEP THREE: Brainstorm for Causes of the Problem (Additional Branches)

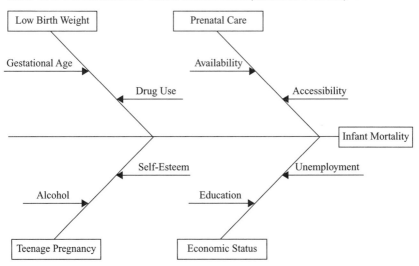

Figure 8–6 Construction of a Cause-and-Effect Diagram

COUNTY HEALTH PROFILE—"FISHBONE SUMMARY"

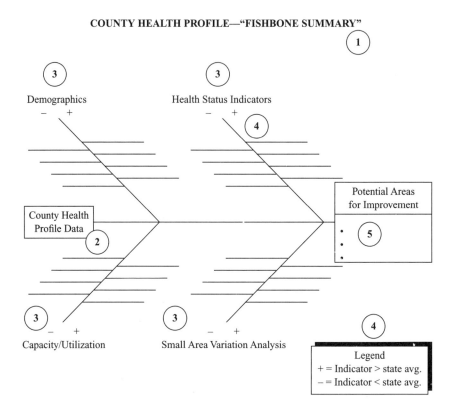

(1) The "cause-and-effect" diagram is used to illustrate the relationships between "potential areas for improvement" that could be identified from all the possible "causes." In this case, the cause-and-effect diagram links significant information from sections of the *County Health Profile* with areas in which the community might want to focus their attention.

(2) Source of the data is the *County Health Profile*.

(3) Identifies the major sections of information presented in the *County Health Profile*.

(4) Deviations from statewide values are indicated by placing that factor on the "+" side if the county value is higher than the state value, and on the "–" side if the county value is lower than the statewide figure. Statistical significance, when available, is reported in the *County Health Profile*.

(5) As a result of analyzing the trends reflected by those factors that are either higher or lower, there may be some initial problems or opportunities that emerge for further evaluation targets for improvement.[9]

Figure 8–7 How To Read a Cause-and-Effect Diagram. *Source:* Reprinted with permission from *A Guide for Assessing and Improving Health Status: Community...Planting the Seeds for Good Health,* p. B-7, © 1993, The Hospital Association of Pennsylvania.

COUNTY HEALTH PROFILE—"FISHBONE SUMMARY"

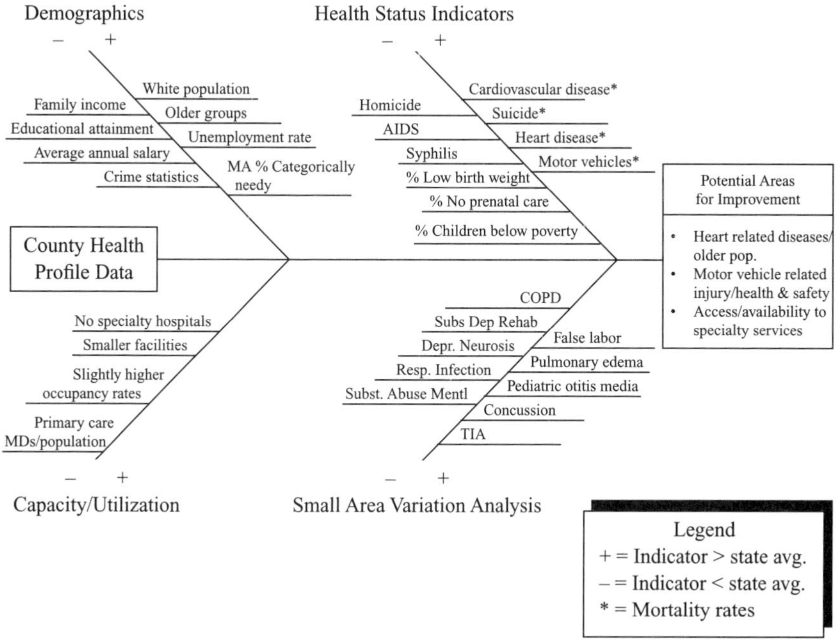

Figure 8–8 County Health Profiles—Cause-and-Effect Diagram. *Source:* Reprinted with permission from *A Guide for Assessing and Improving Health Status: Community...Planting the Seeds for Good Health,* p. 12, © 1993, The Hospital Association of Pennsylvania.

but in addition for public health practice, the focus must be on the use of the basic medical/public health sciences. Thus, to construct a cause-and-effect diagram, the following steps are observed.

1. Specifically define the effect to be analyzed. Place the effect statement in the effect box of your diagram (e.g., teenage pregnancy).
2. Determine headers. These are the broad categories to spark the thinking process about possible causes. Header boxes are connected to the main trunk of the diagram (e.g., demographic, health status, utilization).
3. Use brainstorming to develop potential headers and the elements of each broad category to be considered as possible causes related to the effect (e.g., unemployment, educational attainment, family function).
4. Develop headers and elements related to the headers using sound epidemiologic principles based on the concept of person, place, and time, including focusing on the who, what, where, when, how, and why of the effect. These

become the primary issues or causes, and then the team would take each primary cause and theorize as to secondary causes and deem their relevance in the process. For example, if the focus was on "who" or "person," the header might be demographics or population.

5. Add causes related to each main header identified in step 4 until your chart reflects what is believed as the root cause for each branch. Because most times brainstorming was used to get to this point and notably not all branches would be pertinent, it is appropriate to evaluate and determine the validity of some of the connections or links (i.e., check the logical validity of your graph).

6. Focus on the theories. The team may use nominal group techniques, focus groups, critical appraisal of the literature, evidence-based medicine, clinical practice guidelines, or any method that allows an independent consensus that may be summed to decide where to focus initial efforts.

7. Rule out causes or effects that are believed not amenable to change.

8. Focus on the basic themes of the final cause-and-effect diagram (the manageable significant few not the trivial many) by collecting data to test the theory.

Uses of Cause-and-Effect Diagram

- *to formulate theories*—it is a diagrammatic tool to identify the primary root cause or causes, the primary level of prevention for having an effect on a public health problem
- *to address resistance to change*—specifically to expand into alternative solutions and to focus on doing the right things right and avoid the "tunnel behavior" of doing the wrong things right
- *to provide a graphic output of a detailed brainstorming session* by organizing thought into categories (headers) and basic causes related to the effect
- *to identify solutions to problems* and ways to focus on a goal or a Year 2000 objective (i.e., map out a strategy of how to achieve an infant mortality rate of 7 infant deaths per 1,000 live births by the year 2000)

RUN CHARTS

In public health practice, run charts may be used for a preliminary analysis of any data measured on a continuous scale that can be organized in a time sequence.

Run chart candidates include such things in public health practice as the analysis of low birth weight (percentage) over time in a community or of changes in a clinical outcome for an individual or as an aggregate statistic for the program or clinic over time, weight changes over time in nutritional supplement programs, or infant mortality patterns in a community over time. In all cases, the intent is to monitor the process and determine whether the long-range process was in control (i.e., within acceptable standards) or whether it is changing. Therefore, when the need is to display trends for a variable over a specified period of time, a run chart is a beginning first step.

Pyzdek has defined run charts as "plots of data arranged in time sequence. Analysis of run charts is performed to determine if the patterns can be attributed to common causes* of variation, or if special causes* of variation were present."[10(p.71)]

In epidemiology, the cornerstone of public health practice, surveillance of public health problems, depends on the collection, analysis, and interpretation of data critical to the assessment, planning, implementation, and evaluation of public health programs. The monitoring of these surveillance functions uses line graphs to understand the time sequence of events. A run chart, a form of line graph, is a valuable tool and asset to analyze the data obtained from the surveillance process. The specific uses of run charts with surveillance data are to (1) understand the natural history of disease, (2) test hypotheses, (3) identify and evaluate the impact of intervention programs, (4) monitor changes, (5) detect changes in health practices (small area variation), and (6) plan activities to aid in the management of public health programs.[11] Obviously, a run chart is not a panacea to analyzing surveillance data for detecting patterns attributed to common causes of variation or to determining if special causes of variation are present. However, it is a simple line chart of continuous variable data, and the statistical analysis is "non-parametric" (i.e., no assumptions are made regarding the underlying distribution of data reflecting the process). This is an important point because in public health practice there are many instances where we are faced with data that are not normally distributed, and on many occasions our data values are too few or small to be evaluated statistically. A run chart allows a first and simple step to discuss variation in the process being analyzed. Unlike the other tools presented, the run chart displays the nature of the process over a period of time. A run chart is a forerunner to the more sophisticated tools for problem analysis, namely control charts.

---

*These terms are used frequently in evaluating outcomes in the quality improvement process as demonstrated with run charts and control charts. There are two types of variation that when combined account for all variation in a process that is uncontrollable. *Common cause* variation is the result of change that occurs in the everyday operations of a program or the variation inherent in the process. *Special cause* variation is the result of change that can be attributed to a particular source or event, the variation that is controllable and readily identifiable. It is the special causes that run charts and control charts were designed to detect.

How To Construct a Run Chart

1. Develop a chart with the vertical axis (y) being the variable of interest (e.g., low birth weight).
2. Define the horizontal axis (x) as the data representing a time sequence (months, years).
3. Connect the data points on the graph with a line.
4. Find the median of the data. This may be done statistically as noted in Chapter 6 or more simply, graphically. When the data are plotted on the graph, place a straightedge on the graph parallel to the x-axis and lower the straightedge until half of the data points are above that line and half below. At this point, draw a line horizontally across the chart—this is the "median" line or $\tilde{X}$.
5. Remember that if there is an odd number of data points, the horizontal line will run though the one odd data point (i.e., one value will be exactly on the median).
6. Evaluate the run chart.

Figure 8–9 shows the results of applying these steps to determine the "median" line of the run chart. The chart displays 22 points; therefore, there should be 11

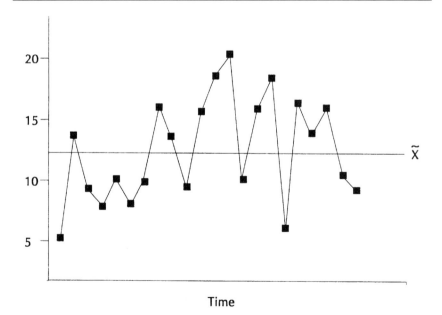

Figure 8–9 Sample Run Chart

points below the median and 11 points above the median. Once the median line is determined, the run chart is evaluated for run length, number of runs, and trends (increases or decreases). Statistical tests can be applied to these runs to determine if there is a special cause of variation to be investigated.

Run Length

A run length is the number of consecutive points that fall on the same side of the median line. The run length is determined by counting the number of consecutive points on the same side of the median (Figure 8–10). If more than one point falls on the median, then allocate the value to one side of the median or the other so that 50 percent falls on one side and 50 percent on the other. Usually, a long series of consecutive points will not fall on the same side of the median, unless the process is being influenced by special causes.[12] Therefore, by checking run length one is able to evaluate the process for special cause of variation. Thus, we determine the longest run and compare the length of the longest run to the values in Table 8–6. If the longest run is longer than the maximum allowed, then the process was probably (approximately a 95 percent probability) influenced by a special cause of variation.[13]

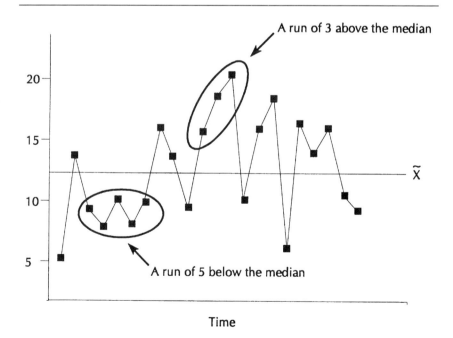

Figure 8–10 Example Run Chart Demonstrating Run Length

Table 8–6 Maximum Run Length

Number of Values	Maximum Run Length*
10	5
15	6
20	7
30	8
40	9
50	10

*Critical values based on alpha level 0.05. Actually, unless the cost of investigating is very high, "borderline situations" are often worth investigating.

Source: Reprinted with permission from T. Pyzdek, *Pyzdek's Guide to SPC: Volume One—Fundamentals,* p. 74, © 1990, Quality Publishing, Inc.

Number of Runs

The number of runs expected from a controlled process can also be mathematically determined. A process that is not being influenced by special causes will not have either too many runs or too few runs. The number of runs is found by simple counting.[14] For example, a run is the number of points above the median line before the next value goes below the line (Figure 8–11). Thus alternating above and below the median line constitutes a new run. In other words, if one point is above the median line and the next point is below the line, then the first point is considered a run. Once the data point shifts above or below the line, no matter how many points are above or below the line, the shift constitutes a run.

Table 8–7 is used to evaluate the number of runs. If you have fewer runs than the smallest allowed or more runs than the largest allowed, then there is a high probability that a special cause is present.[15]

Trends

A trend is defined as a series of consecutive points moving in the same direction—up or down, regardless of whether it crosses the median. If a process is stable, a long trend would not be evident. To evaluate trends, consecutive increases or decreases are determined. The run chart should not have any unusually long series of consecutive increases or decreases. If it does, however, then a trend is indicated, and it is probably due to a special cause of variation. Compare the longest count of consecutive increases or decreases to the longest allowed shown in Table 8–8; if your count exceeds the table value, then there is a strong probability that a special cause of variation caused your process to drift up or down.[16]

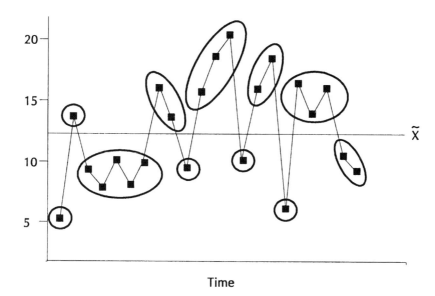

Figure 8–11 Example Run Chart Demonstrating the Number of Runs (11: 5 Above the Median and 6 Below the Median)

Pyzdek has specified the following pointers for using run charts.

- Run charts should not be used if too many of the numbers are the same. As a rule of thumb, do not use run charts if more than 30 percent of the values are the same. For example, in the data set 1, 3, 4, 4, 5, 9, 9, 13, 19, 24, the number 4 appears twice and the number 9 appears twice. Thus, 4 of the 10, or 40 percent of the values are the same.

- Run charts are preliminary analysis tools; if you have continuous data in time-order, always sketch a quick run chart before doing any more complex analysis.

- Run charts are one of the least sensitive quality improvement tools. They are especially insensitive to "freaks," single points dramatically different from the rest. Thus, run charts may fail to find a special cause even if a special cause was present. In statistical parlance, run charts tend to have large type II errors (i.e., they have a high probability of accepting the hypothesis of no special cause even when the special cause actually exists).

- Use run charts to aid in troubleshooting. The different run tests indicate different types of special causes.

  1. A long run on the same side of the median indicates a special cause that created a process *shift*.

Table 8–7 Limits on Number of Runs

Number of Values	Smallest Run Count*	Largest Run Count*
10	3	8
12	3	10
14	4	11
16	5	12
18	6	13
20	6	15
22	7	16
24	8	17
26	9	18
28	10	19
30	11	20
32	11	22
34	12	23
36	13	24
38	14	25
40	15	26
42	16	27
44	17	28
46	17	30
48	18	31
50	19	32

*Critical value based on alpha level 0.05.
Source: Reprinted with permission from T. Pyzdek, *Pyzdek's Guide to SPC: Volume One—Fundamentals*, p. 76, © 1990, Quality Publishing, Inc.

Table 8–8 Maximum Consecutive Increases or Decreases

Number of Values	Maximum Consecutive Increases or Decreases*
5–8	4
9–20	5
–21–100	6
–101+	7

*Critical values based on alpha level 0.05.
Source: Reprinted with permission from T. Pyzdek, *Pyzdek's Guide to SPC: Volume One—Fundamentals*, p. 77, © 1990, Quality Publishing, Inc.

2. A long series of consecutively increasing or decreasing values indicates a special cause that created a *trend*.

3. Too many runs often indicate *mixture* of several sources of variation in the sample.

4. Too few runs often occur in conjunction with a process shift or trend.

• Evaluate the distribution produced by the run chart. Figure 8–12 outlines five distribution patterns produced by a run chart. Each of these run patterns suggests special causes of variation that would be appropriate for investigation.

1. Chart A (*run length*) shows 7 points out of 11 on one side of the median, which is significant at the 0.05 level (Table 8–6). Given a distribution of 11 points, we would expect at most a run length of only 5. This would warrant further investigation (e.g., a decline in infant mortality with some recent increases).

2. Chart B shows occasional *freak values,* separated by periods of relative stability. This may be due to an error in recording the data, reacting to an out of specification condition, or over adjusting the previous process.[17] Also, investigate further to see if "small numbers" may be the culprit. Freak values are better evaluated using control charts, which are discussed in the next chapter.

3. *Trends,* as indicated by Chart C, are often caused by intentional program improvement or possibly reduction in resources causing increases in the outcome. Common examples are infant mortality, low birth weight, or trends in cardiovascular disease.

4. Chart D shows *sudden large shifts* followed by periods of relative stability. Try to find out what happened at the change points.[18] Were there policy changes or changes in risk behavior?

5. Chart E shows a *cyclical pattern.* A zigzag or periodicity of measurements is also abnormal and suggests special causes. Many epidemics follow this pattern. An epidemiologic delight!

Always evaluate the distribution pattern in the run chart and determine what special causes need to be investigated and what questions need to be asked.

Precautions should include the following:

• Changes made during the process in data collection could render your data misleading and maybe invalid. If this should occur, beware of your interpretation.

• You must remember to always look for the obvious causes before you think more serious factors are contributing to the variation. In medicine, you learn if you hear "hoof beats" to think of horses, not zebras.

• Other quality improvement tools should be used to investigate the special cause variation.

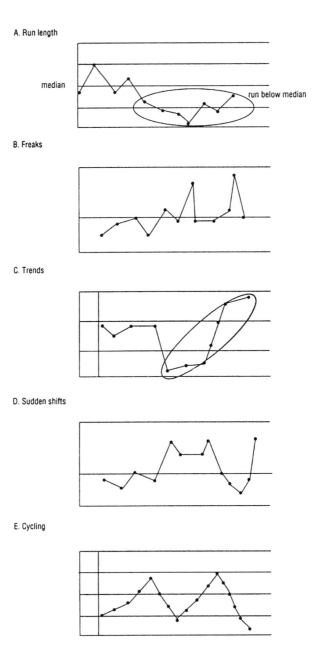

Figure 8–12 Run Charts with Different Distributions. *Source:* Reprinted with permission from *The Health Care Manager's Guide to Continuous Quality Improvement,* by Wendy Leebov, EdD, and Clara Jean Ersoz, MD, published by American Hospital Publishing, Inc., copyright 1991.

Infant Mortality—An Example

In a rural county, the infant mortality was evaluated using a run chart. The data for years 1971–1990 were plotted on a line graph to determine the distribution of the points by year. The median was determined using a straight edge (the graphical method), and the line was drawn on the graph showing 10 data points above the median line and 10 data points below the median line. Figures 8–13 through 8–16 show respectively the run chart (infant mortality rates for the years 1971–1990), the run chart for detecting run length, the run chart for detecting the number of runs, and the run chart detecting the trends. An analysis of the run length on Figure 8–14 shows we have a run of eight below the median where we would expect only a run of seven based on 20 observations (Table 8–6). Because this value is above expected, then the process is out of control and we must look for special causes that have created this variation. Figure 8–15 shows the chart based on the number of runs. This analysis produced seven runs (four above the median and three below the median). The process would be evaluated as being in control because the range for runs is 6 to 15 for 20 observations—our data on infant mortality had seven runs, which is within the range, however, close to the lower limit. Figure 8–16 evaluates the trend in the infant mortality data. Normally, based on 20 observations, we would expect five consecutive increases or decreases (Table 8–8); however, we had eight. Therefore, the process is out of control, and we must investigate for special causes. This example is not unusual; we see there is a decline in infant mortality during a seven-year period but yet increases occurred for five years after the decline. This is exactly the reason for doing a run chart, to evaluate the special causes that may have created the decline so the management can get the process back on track, because the last five years have increased. Of course, these last five years must be investigated to determine the causes for this change. Further, this method allows us to evaluate data or rates that may be based on small numbers because we are evaluating the length, the runs, and the trends and not the numbers themselves. *This certainly is a tool to be used in small-area analysis.*

STRATIFICATION

A technique called *stratification* is often used by epidemiologists in analyzing data to minimize confounding in epidemiologic investigations. In CQI, it is used to find improvement opportunities. Stratification helps analyze problems in which data actually mask the real facts. This often happens when the recorded data are from many sources but are treated as one number.[19] In public health practice, analysts regularly study data based on age, gender, race, and socioeconomic status. The major reason for stratification is to potentially eliminate the confounders

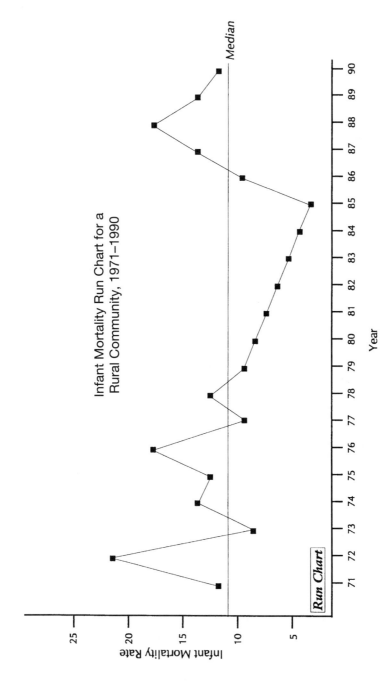

Figure 8–13 Run Chart

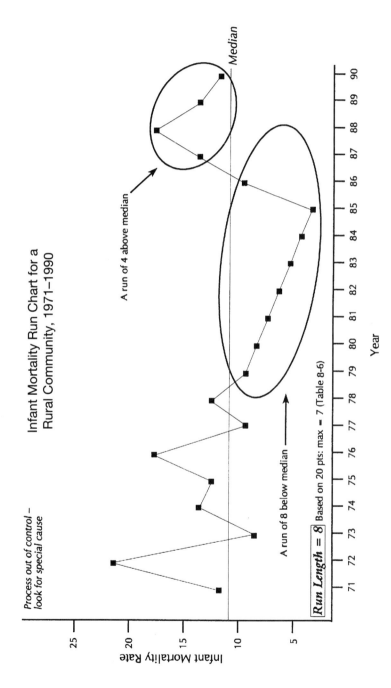

Figure 8-14 Run Length—Infant Mortality

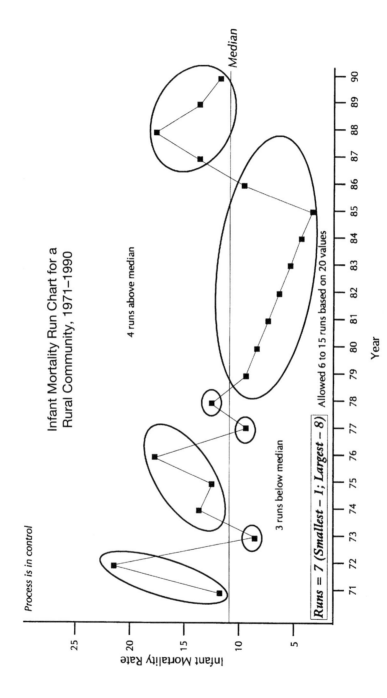

Figure 8–15 Number of Runs

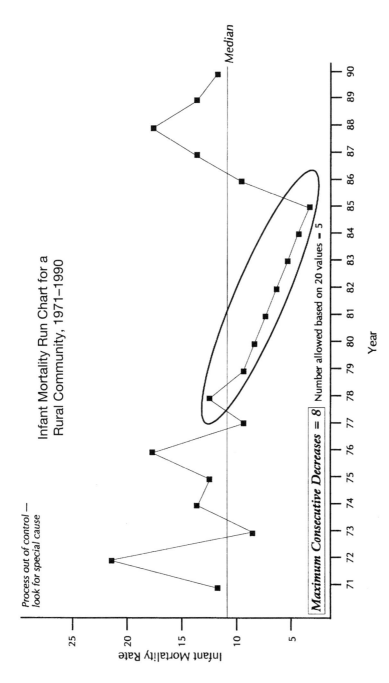

Figure 8–16 Consecutive Increases or Decreases

or variables that may be having an effect on the process. If we stratify by age group, then we have potentially eliminated age as a special cause in the process being evaluated or we find that age is the special cause creating the process.

For example, data on motor vehicle accidents in a county may be recorded as a single value either increasing or decreasing (Figure 8–17). But that number is actually the total of all motor vehicle accidents. If we study the accidents by the following categories, a different picture emerges:

- by environment: rain, clear, foggy
- by location: city, rural, highway
- by age: younger than 19, 20–44

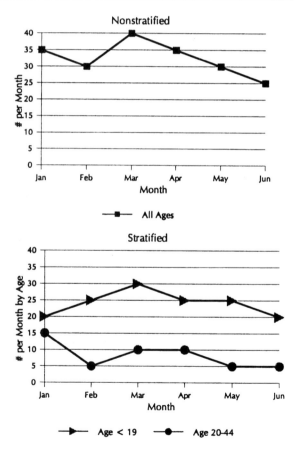

Figure 8–17 Comparison of Motor Vehicle Accidents between Stratified and Nonstratified Data Based on Age Groups

Clearly, stratification by age breaks down simple numbers into meaningful categories or classifications to focus action for correction. Notably, a public health practitioner would focus further efforts on the younger than 19 age group. Further stratification could evaluate the type of environment or the location for the age group younger than 19 to determine additional special causes.

SCATTER DIAGRAMS

A *scatter diagram* is a graph used when you need to display what happens to one variable when another variable changes to determine the relationship between the two variables. The scatter diagram may be used to test for possible *cause-and-effect* relationships. It cannot prove that one variable *causes* the other, but it does make it clear whether a relationship or association exists and the strength of that relationship or association.[20]

A scatter diagram, like most line graphs, has a horizontal axis (x-axis), to represent the measurement values of one variable, and a vertical axis (y-axis) to represent the measurements of the second variable.[21]

This technique is useful in displaying data obtained from two variables that may relate to (but not necessarily have an impact on) each other (e.g., low birth weight and teenage pregnancy). The data collected from the two variables are plotted on a graph, with one variable on the x-axis and the other on the y-axis. If a pattern is detected, then a positive or a negative relationship may be concluded. This technique is considered the easiest way of recording correlation analysis without actually quantifying the strength or the significance of the relationship between the variables. It is, however, simple to construct and is useful in showing data patterns and providing support data to construct a cause-and-effect diagram. Figure 8–18 gives examples of scatter diagrams between paired data.[22] Although scatter diagrams are sometimes used to plot pairs of discrete data (e.g., number of vital events), they are most useful when plotting continuous data (e.g., teenage pregnancy rates).

When two variables behave in the manner as shown for the numbers 1 through 5 (positive and negative correlation) in Figure 8–18, then it may be concluded that if we control x we will have a good chance of controlling y. For example, if we controlled teenage pregnancy, we would probably improve the low-birth-weight ratios.

Testing Correlation with Scatter Diagrams

Scatter diagrams can be used to determine whether there is a correlation between two sets of data. When correlation does exist, it is helpful to know the

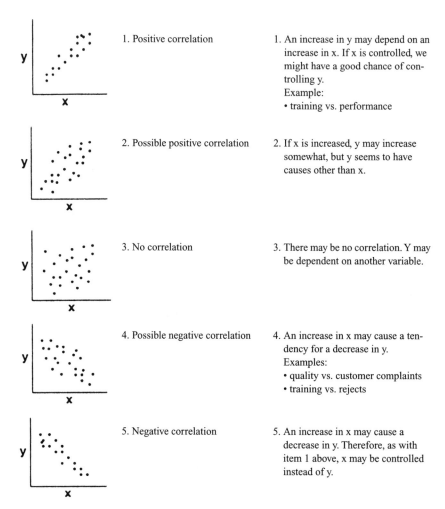

Figure 8–18 Various Patterns and Meanings of Scatter Diagrams. *Source:* Adapted with permission from *The Memory Jogger™,* Copyright 1989 by GOAL/QPC, 13 Branch Street, Methuen, Massachusetts.

extent of the correlation. Either of two methods can be used. One is to calculate the coefficient of correlation, and the other method (median) uses the binomial properties of the distribution. The most practical and the easiest one is presented—the so-called median method for analyzing correlations.[23] Ishikawa has outlined the following steps to test the correlation with scatter diagrams.[24] They are

1. Find the x median ($\tilde{x}$) and the y median ($\tilde{y}$). Use the straightedge method to draw both median lines on the scatter diagram (Figure 8–19).

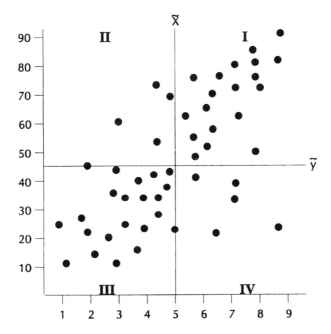

Figure 8–19 Drawing a Median Line

2. Mark the quadrants I, II, III, and IV made by the median lines, starting from the upper right and going counterclockwise. Count the points in each area (Figure 8–19) and display the points in a table (Table 8–9).
3. Find the number of points for II and IV and N (total number of data points minus number of points on the line). Number of points in II and IV is $4 + 5 = 9$, and $N = 50 - 2 = 48$. Number of points in I and III is $50 - 9 - 2 = 39$.
4. Compare the total number of points in II and IV with the "limit of number of points" column indicated in Table 8–10. If the number of points in the two areas is less than the limit as specified in Table 8–10, then a correlation exists.

   When $N = 48$, the limit is 16. As 16 is greater than 9, a positive correlation exists.[25] Alternately, if II and IV = 9 points, then I and III = 39 points (given two were on the line); therefore, because the number in I and III is greater than II and IV, a positive correlation exists.

Scatter Diagrams and Stratification

As noted previously, stratification may help to understand the variation and look for special causes. Therefore, stratification may be an important step to eval-

Table 8–9 Points in Each Area

Area	Points
(I)	19
(II)	4
(III)	20
(IV)	5
On the line	2
Total	50

Source: Reprinted with permission from K. Ishikawa, *Guide to Quality Control,* p. 92, ©1982, Asian Productivity Organization.

Table 8–10 Sign Test Table

N	Limit of Number of Points for II + IV	N	Limit of Number of Points for II + IV
20	5	42	14
21	5	44	15
22	5	46	15
23	6	48	16
24	6	50	17
25	7	52	18
26	7	54	19
27	7	56	20
28	8	58	21
29	8	60	21
30	9	62	22
32	9	64	23
34	10	66	24
36	11	68	25
38	12	70	26
40	13		

Note: Table 8–10 is part of a sign test table. This table is limited to $N = 20$ to 70 at a 5 percent level of significance.
Source: Reprinted with permission from K. Ishikawa, *Guide to Quality Control,* p. 93, ©1982, Asian Productivity Organization.

uate in using scatter diagrams. Figure 8–20 shows a hypothetical example of the relationship between birth weights for mothers aged 15 to 19 (x) and prenatal care (y). In the diagram at the top, the data were simply plotted, whereas the diagram at the bottom uses the same data—but the data were stratified (according to black and white) before plotting. This is an example of a situation in which, on the whole, there seems to be no correlation, but when the data are stratified, a correlation is seen to exist. The reverse can also be true—when the data are stratified, there seems to be no correlation, but when viewed as a whole, there really is.[26] Again, this becomes an important quality improvement tool to understand the problem, examine the variation, and look for special causes.

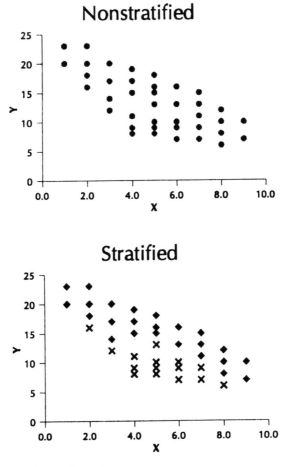

Figure 8–20 Stratification in a Scatter Diagram

CONTROL CHARTS

Control charts are used with statistical methods to detect the presence of special causes of variation in a process. A control chart is not a statistical test of hypotheses testing to determine if the process has changed.[27] Specifically, hypotheses tests are descriptive statistical methods that describe static populations or events, whereas control charts are analytical statistical tools that aid in understanding the dynamics of the process. Brassard has indicated that "a *Control Chart* is used when you need to discover how much variability in a process is due to random variation and how much is due to unique events/individual actions in order to determine whether a process is in statistical control."[28(p.288)] Further, he states that "a Control Chart is simply a run chart with statistically determined upper (Upper Control Limit) and possibly lower (Lower Control Limit) lines drawn on either side of the process average."[29(p.288)]

The fluctuations of the points within the limits result from variation built into the process. This results from *common causes* within the *system* (e.g., design, choice of program, preventive maintenance) and can only be affected by changing that system. However, points outside of the limits come from a *special cause* (e.g., people errors, unplanned events, freak occurrences), which is not part of the way that the process normally operates. These special causes must be eliminated before the control chart can be used as a monitoring tool. Once this is done, the process would be "in control," and samples can be taken at regular intervals to make sure that the process does not fundamentally change.[30]

Control charts are probably the most important quality improvement tools to be used in monitoring a process and evaluating outcomes to assess variation and identify special causes. The discussion on control charts in this chapter is purposefully brief because Chapter 9 is devoted to control charts for attribute data and Chapter 10 focuses on control charts for variable data. The primary functions of a control chart is to measure and analyze a problem, implement a trial run, evaluate the results (outcome measurement), and monitor the process to hold the gains (Table 8–2).

REMEMBER: "Control" does not necessarily mean that the product or service will meet your needs. It only means that the process is *consistent* (may be consistently bad).[31]

FORCE-FIELD ANALYSIS

In public health practice, many times we are faced with the status quo; we are stuck, and we need to move from the position we are in to a more favorable one and realize there may be another way to accomplish the task. To produce this improvement or move toward a goal, you have to challenge the status quo. You can do this in two ways: you can (1) strengthen the forces that are currently pushing performance upward (the driving forces) or (2) weaken or eliminate the forces that are impeding improved performance (the restraining forces). This is the logic that underlies force-field analysis.[32] Leebov and Ersoz say

> When you want to tackle a problem or goal, it helps to start by examining the forces that are contributing to the status quo, or the current situation. These include opposing forces that create a balance, a static force field or frozen condition. Change happens when one type of force overwhelms another. Performance *deteriorates* when restraining forces overpower driving forces, in other words, when restraining forces inhibit or block improvement or solutions. Performance *improves* when driving forces overpower restraining forces, in other words, when driving forces push toward, encourage, or support improvement or solutions.[33(p.165)]

Brassard gives us the following example:

> Consider the practical example of *"losing weight"* [in a preventive maintenance program provided by a public health clinic (Table 8–11)]: If the restraining forces are stronger than the driving forces, then the desired change will not happen. It stands to reason that some change (lost weight) will occur if the driving forces are more powerful than those on the restraining side of the ledger.[34(p.299)]

Table 8–11 Force-Field Analysis Driving and Restraining Forces—for Losing Weight

CURRENT PREFERENCE LEVEL

0% Satisfaction	*100% Satisfaction*
Driving Forces ⇒	⇐ *Restraining Forces*
Health threat	Lack of time
Cultural obsession with being thin	Genetic traits
Plenty of thin role models	Unsympathetic friends and family
Embarrassment	Lack of money for exercise
Negative self-image	Lack of interest
Positive attitude toward exercise	Bad advice
Lack of temptation	Years of bad eating habits
Clothes do not fit	Amount of sugar in any prepared food

Source: Adapted with permission from *The Memory Jogger*™, Copyright 1989 by GOAL/QPC, 13 Branch Street, Methuen, Massachusetts.

Brassard further notes that force-field analysis helps make changes happen because (1) it forces people to think together about all the facets of a desired change; it encourages creative thinking; (2) it encourages people to agree about the relative priority of factors on each side of the "balance sheet;" the team can use the nominal group technique to reach consensus quickly; and (3) it provides a starting point for action.[35]

How To Construct a Force-Field Analysis

Leebov and Ersoz have outlined the following basic steps in the construction of a force-field analysis.

1. Identify the improvement that is planned, and write down the goal statement so the group can continuously focus on it.
2. Prepare an initial worksheet by drawing across the top of a sheet of paper a horizontal line representing a continuum related to the outcome measure or performance goal.

    0% ———————————————— 100%

3. Represent the current status or performance level by a vertical line down the middle of the page.

    Current Performance Level

    0% ——————————|—————— 100%

4. Before analysis, brainstorm the driving forces first and then the restraining forces that affect performance level. List the driving forces on the left under an arrow pointing in the direction of the performance level. List the restraining forces on the right under an arrow pointing backward, illustrating that the performance level is being held back.

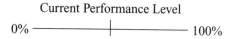

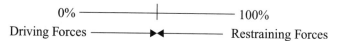

5. Reduce the lists to reflect only those forces that indicate the best potential for reaching the stated objective. From the final list select a few driving forces that can realistically strengthen the performance level and select an equal number of restraining forces that can be weakened (see Table 8–11 for a practical example related to losing weight).[36]

Leebov and Ersoz have noted at least four uses of force-field analysis. They are (1) to identify improvement opportunities, (2) to identify key causes that, if altered, would have a positive impact on a solution to a problem, (3) to evaluate the likelihood that a new program or proposed improvement would actually reap the intended benefits, and (4) to help think through a realistic implementation plan that includes countermeasures designed to diminish restraining forces or barriers, as well as strategies to capitalize on driving forces.[37]

CONCLUSION

In public health practice, analyzing problems is critical to the core public health function of assessment, policy development, and assurance. In this chapter, the quality improvement tools were detailed that may be used for analyzing public health problems, although four of the tools (Pareto charts, run charts, cause-and-effect diagrams, and stratification) may be used for identifying and analyzing problems. The remainder of the tools (histograms, scatter diagrams, force-field analysis, and control charts) are to be used for analyzing problems only. As noted in Table 8–1, most of the tools discussed in this chapter require that the practitioners work with numbers as opposed to just working with ideas. The use and application of these tools to public health problems will enhance the practice of public health and promote an "active" analysis of problems by continuously monitoring the process and by identifying special cause variation to ensure that the gains that are made are held. This change from the "passive" analysis of collecting data and producing a "static" document to an "active" analysis of collecting data and monitoring the situation producing a "dynamic" process is the future of public health practice.

NOTES

1. W. Leebov and C.J. Ersoz, *The Health Care Manager's Guide to Continuous Quality Improvement* (Chicago: American Hospital Publishing, 1991), 125.

2. P.E. Plsek and A. Onnias, *Juran Institute Quality Improvement Tools: Histograms* (Wilton, CT: Juran Institute, 1989), 4–7.

3. J.M. Juran and F.M. Gryna, eds., *Juran's Quality Control Handbook*, 4th ed. (New York: McGraw-Hill, 1988).

4. K. Ozeki and T. Asaka, eds., *Handbook of Quality Tools* (Cambridge, MA: Productivity Press, 1990), 144–146.

5. Ibid.

6. Leebov and Ersoz, *Health Care Manager's Guide to Continuous Quality Improvement,* 129–130.

7. Ibid., 129.

8. K. Ishikawa, *Guide to Quality Control* (Minato-Ku, Tokyo, Japan: Asian Productivity Organization, 1982).

9. The Hospital Association of Pennsylvania (HAP), *A Guide for Assessing and Improving Health Status: Community…Planting the Seeds for Good Health* (Harrisburg, PA: 1993), B-7.

10. T. Pyzdek, *Pyzdek's Guide to SPC: Volume One—Fundamentals* (Tucson, AZ: Quality Publishing, 1990), 71.

11. S.B. Thacker, "Surveillance," in *Field Epidemiology,* ed. M.B. Gregg (New York: Oxford University Press, 1996), 28–30.

12. Pyzdek, *Volume One—Fundamentals,* 72–74.

13. Ibid., 74.

14. Ibid.

15. Ibid., 74–75.

16. Ibid., 75–76.

17. Ibid., 79.

18. Ibid.

19. M. Brassard, *The Memory Jogger Plus+* (Methuen, MA: GOAL/QPC, 1989), 301.

20. Ibid., 285.

21. Ibid.

22. A.F. Al-Assaf and J.A. Schmele, eds, *The Textbook of Total Quality in Healthcare* (Delray Beach, FL: St. Lucie Press, 1993), 136.

23. Ishikawa, *Guide to Quality Control,* 92.

24. Ibid., 92–93.

25. Ibid.

26. Ibid., 93–94.

27. Pyzdek, *Volume One—Fundamentals,* 90.

28. Brassard, *Memory Jogger Plus+,* 288.

29. Ibid.

30. Ibid., 288–289.

31. Ibid., 289.

32. Leebov and Ersoz, *Health Care Manager's Guide to Continuous Quality Improvement,* 165.

33. Ibid.

34. Brassard, *The Memory Jogger Plus+,* 299.

35. Ibid.

36. Leebov and Ersoz, *Health Care Manager's Guide to Continuous Quality Improvement,* 166–167.

37. Ibid., 168.

Chapter 9

Public Health Practice—
Quality Improvement Control
Charts for Counts

Control charts take the practice of public health from passive, static, enumerative, statistical methods to describe populations to active, dynamic, analytical statistical methods to understand and monitor processes. Certainly, public health practice uses sophisticated statistical methods and advanced research designs to understand the nature of the disease process and the practice and performance of clinical medicine. However, as mentioned previously, this latter aspect of serving individuals in clinics is diminishing as a major public health practice. A main purpose to this book has been to bring to the practice of public health the quality improvement methods and tools to be used and applied to public health problems focusing on outcome measurement. Additionally, it is hoped that the understanding of these methods and tools becomes part of the training and education of the public health scientist. To further both of these objectives, a basic understanding of control charts is essential. There are basically two types of control charts: attribute control charts and variables control charts. In this chapter, the use, application, and interpretation of attribute control charts in public health practice are explored. In the next chapter, variables control charts are discussed.

CONTROL CHART CONCEPTS

Control charts were first introduced by W.A. Shewhart in 1924 with the intent of eliminating abnormal variation by distinguishing variations due to assignable (special) causes from those due to random or chance (common) causes. Table 9–1 shows the distinction between the two types of causes based on the description and interpretation of the causes. In the analysis of a public health problem,

Table 9–1 Distinction between Random (Common) and Assignable (Special) Causes of Variation

Random (Common) Causes	Assignable (Special) Causes
Description	
Consists of many individual causes	Consists of one or just a few individual causes
Any one random cause results in a minute amount of variation (but many random causes act together to yield a substantial total)	Any one assignable cause can result in a large amount of variation
Interpretation	
Random variation cannot economically be eliminated from a process	Assignable variation can be detected; action to eliminate the causes is usually economically justified
An observation within the control limits of random variation means the process should not be adjusted	An observation beyond control limits means the process should be investigated and corrected
With only random variation, the process is sufficiently stable to use sampling procedures to predict the outcome of interest	With assignable variation present, the process is not sufficiently stable to use sampling procedures for prediction

Source: Adapted with permission from J.M. Juran and F.M. Gryna, *Quality Planning and Analysis*, 3rd ed., p. 110, © 1993, McGraw-Hill, Inc.

whether it be infant mortality, motor vehicle accidents, patient satisfaction, or waiting times in clinics, it is important to understand the variation and whether it may be due to common or special causes.

The intent of using the control chart is to determine which causes are special as opposed to those that are not. A control chart consists of a central line (an average, median, proportion, etc.), control limits—upper and lower, and the data values plotted on the chart that represent the state of the process (problem) being investigated. An example of a generic control chart is shown in Figure 9–1. When these values (central line and control limits) are isolated and placed on the chart, they divide the vertical scale of the chart into two regions: one is associated with special causes and one with chance (common) causes. The plotted values that fall outside (above or below) the control limits are interpreted as signals of possible special causes, whereas data points that fall within the control limits are usually (not always) considered to be absent of special causes. Thus, the control charts may be used, for example, to (1) monitor the low birth weights of infants in hospitals in a health district or for various counties in a health district, (2) determine

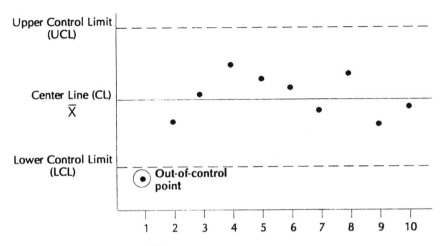

Figure 9–1 Generic Format of a $\overline{X}$ Control Chart

if a process over time or in space is in control, (3) improve process performance (patient-customer satisfaction of picking up birth certificates in a vital records unit), (4) evaluate statistical significance (comparing the infant mortality rate with a standard—Year 2000 objective), and (5) provide an early warning system of problems that could have economic/social significance (changes in teenage pregnancy). Thus, by using the control chart, the approach is to improve the process performance over time by studying variation and potentially identifying the root cause, that special cause.

Specifically, the control chart provides the public health organization with the following:

- focuses attention on detecting and monitoring process variation over time
- distinguishes special from common causes of variation, as a guide to community or management action
- serves as a tool for the ongoing monitoring of a process
- helps improve a process to perform consistently and predictably for higher quality, lower mortality/morbidity, and improved effective outcomes
- provides a common language for discussing process performance[1]

TYPES OF CONTROL CHARTS

There are two basic types of control charts so classified based on the type of data unique to the calculations required for each type of chart. The type of data is considered either to be attribute data (discrete or countable) or variable data (continuous or measurement). Thus, control charts are considered to be attribute- or variable-type charts. Attribute data examples include number of births, deaths, teenage pregnancies, prenatal care visits, and motor vehicle accidents, whereas variable data examples include age, height, infant mortality rates, cancer death rates, and teenage pregnancy rates. Clearly, when items are simply classified as occurring or not occurring, we are dealing with two categories or discrete counts —mainly attribute data. However, if characteristics are measured on a continuous scale, then we have variable data. Thus, based on the type of data (attribute or variable) and further based on sample size, the appropriate chart may be selected for the particular problem being investigated. Figure 9–2 provides a flow diagram for selecting the most appropriate control chart based on data type and sample size. It is apparent that there is considerable variability in the sample size required for the proper application of each of the control charts.

INTERPRETING CONTROL CHARTS—RULES FOR DETECTING SPECIAL CAUSE

Most of the control charts may be interpreted in the same manner with the same rules, providing certain criteria are met. A typical control chart format is displayed in Figure 9–3, which consists of a center line, an upper control limit, and lower control limit. The center line definition is dependent on the type of control chart; in our example, a generic format is presented.

There are many types of patterns in a control chart that may signal a possible or probable existence of special causes. Figure 9–4 shows a control chart divided into three zones, which represent one, two, and three standard deviation limits based on a calculation of a center line for a chart. These zones are important to the evaluation of the process and the pattern of points displayed on a chart. There are rules to evaluate patterns based on the fact that points on the chart fall within and/or beyond the three standard deviation control limits, and there are rules that are based on the examination of the pattern of points that occur without regard to the control limits. Figure 9–5 illustrates graphically the two types of rules resulting in eight tests. Additionally, Table 9–2 provides a list of points to be considered when evaluating the eight tests. The evaluation of the pattern of points based on a runs chart without reference to control limits was detailed in Chapter 8. With run charts, we assumed nothing about the distribution, and our tests were, therefore, less sensitive to changes than charts in which the distribution is assumed to be normal or when the points are assessed to be randomly scattered about the center line. To evaluate the attribute control chart's pattern within the control limits, use the rules as defined in Figure 9–5. Nonrandom patterns of any kind signal the possible presence of special causes.

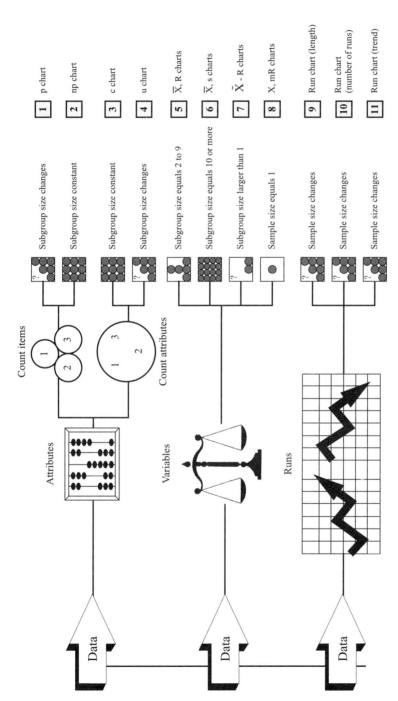

Figure 9–2 Guide for Selecting the Appropriate Type of Control Chart. Source: Adapted from and reprinted with permission from *SPC: Control Charts* software. (This text's author added the bottom branch to CCC's decision tree.) Copyright © 1994 Computer Curriculum Corporation. All rights reserved. For information about *SPC: Control Charts*, contact Quality America, Inc. (CCC's distributor) at (800) 722-6154. Computer Curriculum Corporation (CCC) is a leading provider of educational software and services.

+ 3σ   Upper Control Limit

$\overline{X}$ Center Line

− 3σ   Lower Control Limit

Figure 9–3 Typical Format of a Control Chart

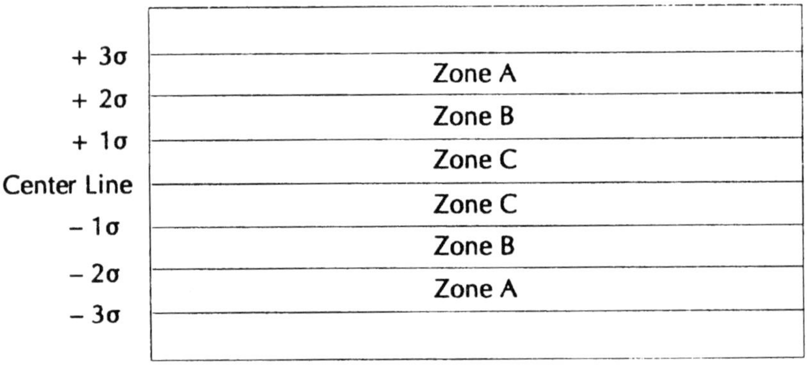

+ 3σ
+ 2σ   Zone A
+ 1σ   Zone B
Center Line   Zone C
− 1σ   Zone C
− 2σ   Zone B
− 3σ   Zone A

Figure 9–4 Control Chart Divided into Sigma Zones

Typically, control charts based on the three standard deviation limits assume that the distribution or statistic follows a normal distribution. Given the three standard deviations, one is able to estimate that 0.27 percent of the time a point may fall outside the control limits even when no special cause is present. Thus by using the 0.27 percent limit, the control chart establishes a standard for a false alarm. Naturally, the wider the control limits, the less chance of detecting special causes. In public health practice, a usual practice is to use two standard deviations as the control limits for detecting special causes; thus 5 percent of the time a point may fall outside the limit even when no special cause is present (i.e., 2.5 percent above the limit and 2.5 percent below the limit). To follow this procedure, we would substitute in the formulas we have been given 1.96 (the 95 percent control limit) as opposed to 2.57 (the 99 percent control limit).

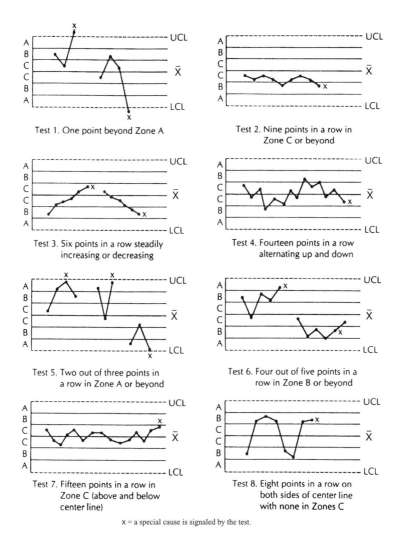

Test 1. One point beyond Zone A

Test 2. Nine points in a row in Zone C or beyond

Test 3. Six points in a row steadily increasing or decreasing

Test 4. Fourteen points in a row alternating up and down

Test 5. Two out of three points in a row in Zone A or beyond

Test 6. Four out of five points in a row in Zone B or beyond

Test 7. Fifteen points in a row in Zone C (above and below center line)

Test 8. Eight points in a row on both sides of center line with none in Zones C

x = a special cause is signaled by the test.

Figure 9–5 Illustrations of Eight Rules for Detecting Special Causes in Control Charts. *Source:* © 1996, American Society for Quality Control. Reprinted with permission.

Thus, points that fall outside either the two or three standard deviation limits may signal special causes. Again, in the case of two standard deviations, a 2.5 percent value is set above and below the control limit, whereas for three standard deviations, a 0.27 percent value is set (i.e., 0.135 percent above and below the control limit). The basic idea associated with detecting special causes is that a stable process should produce only a random pattern of points on the control

Table 9–2 Criteria for Evaluating the Eight Rules for Detecting Special Causes (Figure 9–5)

1. These tests are applicable to average (X̄) charts and to individuals (X) charts. However, for p charts (charts for evaluating a process using percentages abnormal) if lower control limit is greater than 0 and upper control limit is less than *n,* then these rules apply. A normal distribution is assumed. Tests 1, 2, 5, and 6 are to be applied to the upper and lower halves of the chart separately. Tests 3, 4, 7, and 8 are to be applied to the whole chart.

2. The upper control limit and the lower control limit are set at three standard deviations above the center line and three standard deviations below the center line. For the purpose of applying the tests, the control chart is equally divided into six zones, each zone being one standard deviation wide. The upper half of the chart is referred to as A (outer third), B (middle third), and C (inner third). The lower half is taken as the mirror image. In public health, outcomes may be evaluated using two standard deviations.

3. When a process is in a state of statistical control, the chance of (incorrectly) getting a signal for the presence of a special cause is less than 5 in 1,000 for each of these tests.

4. It is suggested that tests 1, 2, 3, and 4 be applied routinely. The overall probability of getting a false signal from one or more of these is about 1 in 100.

5. It is suggested that the first four tests be augmented by tests 5 and 6 when it becomes economically desirable to have earlier warning. This will raise the probability of a false signal to about 2 in 100.

6. Tests 7 and 8 are diagnostic tests for stratification. They are very useful in setting up a control chart. These tests show when the observations in a subgroup have been taken from two (or more) sources with different means. Test 7 reacts when the observations in the subgroup always come from both sources. Test 8 reacts when the subgroups are taken from one source at a time.

7. Whenever the existence of a special cause is signaled by a test, this should be indicated by placing an (x) just above the last point if that point lies above the center line, or just below it if it lies below the center line.

8. Points can contribute to more than one test. However, no point is ever marked with more than one (x).

9. The presence of an (x) indicates that the process is not in statistical control. It means that the point is the last one of a sequence of points (a single point is test 1) that is very unlikely to occur if the process is in statistical control.

10. Although this can be taken as a basic set of tests, analysts should be alert to any patterns of points that might indicate the influences of special causes in their process.

Source: © 1996, American Society for Quality Control. Reprinted with permission.

chart. Any nonrandom pattern signals the possibility of special causes. To detect these nonrandom patterns, Farnum has suggested that five of those rules noted in Figure 9–5 are the most frequently used. They are

1. one point outside the (three standard deviations) control limits (rule 1)

2. six successive points that increase (or decrease) (rule 3)
3. two out of three points that are on the same side of the center line, both at a distance exceeding two or three standard deviations from the center line (rule 5)
4. four out of five points that are on the same side of the center line, all four at a distance exceeding one standard deviation from the center line (rule 6)
5. eight successive points on the same side of the center line (rule 8)[2]

As Farnum notes, "There are additional rules (e.g., some…replace 'eight' by 'seven' in rule 8 above), but these five are probably the most frequently used…. The rules in the list are designed to be comparable in the sense that each has approximately the *same* probability of giving a false signal."[3(p.172)] The probability for each is 0.27 percent if three standard deviations or 5 percent if two standard deviations. Finally, for most of the problems encountered in public health practice, it is sufficient to use the tests outlined in Figure 9–5. If one thinks that special tests are essential to fit a particular situation using any of the control charts—especially the attribute charts, which may not meet the criterion for a normal distribution—the reader should check the *Statistical Quality Control Handbook.*[4]

ATTRIBUTE CHARTS

Attribute control charts are charts that use attribute data that measure the performance of a process by counting. Typically in nonhealth industries, the "things" being counted are "flaws," "nonconformities," or "defects." For instance, the number of errors on invoices in a purchasing department or the number of cars that do not pass inspection are examples of industry-type problems that may be analyzed using attribute control charts. In public health practice, there is more concern about events (births, death, disease) being measured and being counted as "abnormal," "above or below a standard," or "too few or too many cases." For instance, the number of infant deaths occurring in a rural community or the number of establishments that did not pass inspection by the public health officials is an example that may be analyzed by using attribute control charts.

Four basic types of attribute control charts may be applied to public health practice problems. They are:

1. "p" chart for percentage abnormal
2. "np" chart for number abnormal
3. "c" chart for number of occurrences for equal sample size
4. "u" chart for number of occurrences for variable sample size

As noted in Figure 9–2, the algorithm for selecting the appropriate attribute control chart is dependent on (1) whether we are using discrete events (coding errors on death certificates, percentage of babies who are low birth weight, number of nurses who are absent from the clinic) or (2) whether the data are measuring an "abnormal" event that may be classified as abnormal based on having multiple problems (attributes) or measuring an "abnormal" event that is classified as abnormal based on having not met the accepted criteria or standard for being normal. For example, a baby born with multiple problems—low birth weight, congenital malformations, respiratory distress syndrome, and fetal alcohol syndrome—would be considered abnormal because any one of these conditions represents an abnormal baby; therefore, this event would be classified abnormal (attribute data) and we would use a c or u chart depending on subgroup size, i.e., constant or not constant. If another baby is born with low birth weight, then this birth would also be considered abnormal. Thus, the number of birth-related problems are being counted for each baby delivered. In this example, there were four problems for the first infant and one problem for the second infant. In other words, the outcome of the event is either good (live birth = acceptable = normal) or bad (one or more multiple problems/birth defects = unacceptable = abnormal), no matter whether the birth has one abnormality or more than one, it would be classified as abnormal. Obviously, there will be many times when there are births with no abnormalities. To analyze this type of problem, a c or u chart is used.

If, however, the number of infant deaths occurring within the first year of life is measured as a percentage of all births, the birth is being defined as alive or dead, normal or abnormal. In other words, the outcome of this event is either good, which is normal (live birth = acceptable), or bad (infant death = unacceptable), which is abnormal. To analyze these types of problems, p and np charts are used. Thus, given either of these two situations for classifying events as abnormal or normal, "abnormal" may be used in the continuous quality improvement (CQI) process for using attribute control charts as a way to describe an event (birth, death, morbidity, etc.) as a defect.

To be more specific, attribute control charts base their control limit calculations on either the binomial or the Poisson distribution (these are elaborated in the discussion on small area analysis in a later chapter). These distributions are appropriate because both the binomial and Poisson random variables *count* the number of occurrences of an event.

The binomial distribution is used for the control limits for the p and np charts, which evaluate "nonconforming," "defective units," or from a public health perspective, abnormal events. That is, an event (birth, death, or outcome) is either normal or it is not normal. For example, a pregnancy may result in a live birth (normal event) or in an infant death (abnormal event). Thus, to describe the number of occurrences of these types of events (normal, not normal), the binomial distribution is the most appropriate.

The Poisson distribution provides the control limits for c and u charts, which evaluate "nonconformities," or "defects," which count the multiple possibilities or opportunities for a defect in a given unit or "area of opportunity" (i.e., a population group, time period, etc.). In public health practice, as suggested previously, if a high risk pregnancy program was evaluated and the pregnancies were monitored as to outcomes, any one of the following events (low birth weight, respiratory distress syndrome, fetal alcohol syndrome, congenital malformations) would be considered as abnormal but would not make the pregnancy a complete failure—but the program would still attempt to limit or eliminate the number of abnormal multiple outcomes. Thus, when there are several or multiple possibilities related to one event or area of opportunity and more than one outcome is possible, then a c or u chart is used. However, when an event is discrete and a single problem (death) makes the event abnormal, then a p or np chart is used. The description and application of these charts in subsequent sections should aid the reader in making this distinction.

p Chart—for Percentage Abnormal

When a public health agency needs to monitor a nonmeasurable characteristic (i.e., a count) in a program, a p, np, c, or u chart is used. Specifically, the p chart helps to monitor and evaluate the percentage of abnormal events over time or among communities. The use of a control chart for determining differences among communities is appropriate; however, in public health practice, rates, confidence intervals, and statistical analysis can be used to accomplish a similar result. The chapter on small area analysis provides the detail using rates, confidence intervals, and statistical analysis. Thus, to monitor the percentage of abnormals, diseased, or those who died over a period of time, use a p chart. The *p* in p chart stands for *percentage*.

The p chart is based on counts or the number of times an event is observed; therefore, they can be applied to any variable in which the outcome measure is a count. The p chart and likewise the np chart are based on the binomial distribution. To this end, there are certain conditions that must be satisfied to characterize the behavior of the counts on a control chart. These conditions are

- *Binomial condition 1:* The samples to be evaluated for the count must consist of *n* distinct items.
- *Binomial condition 2:* Each of the *n* distinct items must be classified as abnormal (not having) or normal (having) the outcome. This outcome is usually some type of abnormality based on a standard.
- *Binomial condition 3:* Let *p* denote the probability that an event has the outcome being counted. The value of *p* must be the same for all *n* items in any

one sample. Although the chart will check if *p* changes from sample to sample, the value of *p* must be constant *within each sample*.

• *Binomial condition 4:* The likelihood of an event possessing the outcome will not be affected by whether the preceding event possessed the outcome. (Abnormal events do not naturally occur together in clusters, and counts are independent of each other.)[5]

When these conditions are met, the p chart and the np chart may be used based on the binomial probability model. These charts can then be based on the relationship of the mean and standard deviations of the binomial distribution. This relationship allows chart limits to be based on the one statistic—the average proportion abnormal. This relationship further makes the control limits less susceptible to sampling variation. However, some count data and percentages do not satisfy the conditions stated and, therefore, should not be calculated using a p or np chart. Obviously, percentages based on measurement data as opposed to discrete data should not be charted on a p chart. It may be true that the percentage defines a proportion, but if it is not discrete, then a p chart is not appropriate. In this case, an average and range chart or more generally variables control charts would be appropriate. This is discussed in Chapter 10.

Constructing p Charts

The following formulas are used for constructing p charts. The calculation of a p chart may be based on a standard (i.e., Year 2000 objectives) or based on the process that the data create during measurement (i.e., over time or among communities).

The formulas are

• based on a standard

$$CL_p = P_o$$

$$UCL_p = P_o + 3\sqrt{\frac{P_o(1 - P_o)}{\bar{n}}}$$

$$LCL_p = P_o - 3\sqrt{\frac{P_o(1 - P_o)}{\bar{n}}}$$

• based on process data

$$CL_p = \bar{p}$$

$$UCL_p = \bar{p} + 3\sqrt{\frac{\bar{p}(1-\bar{p})}{\bar{n}}}$$

$$LCL_p = \bar{p} - 3\sqrt{\frac{\bar{p}(1-\bar{p})}{\bar{n}}}$$

where

   p = the number abnormal (%)
   P_o = the standard or target considered (Year 2000 objective)
   n = sample size
   $\bar{n}$ = average sample size
   $\bar{p}$ = the average number abnormal (%) based on the number of time periods
      or communities selected (i.e., the center line for the p chart)
   CL_p = center line of the chart
   UCL_p = upper control limit of the chart
   LCL_p = lower control limit of the chart

To calculate the limits for two and one standard deviations, substitute the value 2 or 1 in the above equation for the value 3. This calculation will define the boundary for two standard deviations and one standard deviation, respectively. Thus for p charts we calculate the percentage abnormal in the following way. If we reviewed 100 birth records and noted we had two infant deaths (abnormals), we would define the percentage abnormal as

$$p = 2 \div 100 \times 100 = 2\%$$

This calculation for percentage abnormal is determined for all time periods or communities over time.

p Chart—Low-Birth-Weight Example

The data displayed in Table 9–3 show a sample of 25 months in a health district where the number of births was reviewed to determine the number of low-birth-weight babies. In the 25 months, there were 36,060 births, and 2,103 were low-birth-weight babies.

Therefore, the average number or percentage of low-birth-weight babies is

$$\bar{p} = \frac{\Sigma p}{\Sigma n}$$

$$\bar{p} = \frac{2,103}{36,060}$$

$$\bar{p} = 0.0583 \text{ or } 5.83\%$$

where

$\bar{p}$ = average number of abnormal births (low-birth-weight)

p = total number of low-birth-weight births

n = total number of births

Σ = summation

Also, the average number of births reviewed in the 25 months is[*6]

$$\bar{n} = \frac{n}{k}$$

$$\bar{n} = \frac{36,060}{25 \text{ (number of months)}}$$

$$\bar{n} = 1,442 \text{ live births/months}$$

where

$\bar{n}$ = average number of live births per subgroup

n = total number of births

k = number of subgroups (months)

Thus, to construct a p chart for low birth weights, the following steps are followed:

- Collect or obtain a set of data that gives the number of births and the number of low-birth-weight births in a 25-month period. The month subgroup sample size should be greater than 50. (See Table 9–3.)[†7]
- Compute the average number of low-birth-weight births and convert to a percentage. This is the center p line of the chart.

$$\bar{p} = \frac{2,103}{36,060}$$

$$\bar{p} = 0.0583 \text{ or } 5.83\%$$

---

[*]If the samples to be used for a p chart are not of the same size, it is permissible to use the *average sample size* for the series in calculating the control limits. The largest sample in the series should not be more than twice the average sample size, and the smallest sample in the series should not be less than half the average sample size.

If the individual samples vary more than this, either separate or combine samples to make them of suitable size or calculate control limits separately for the samples that are too large or too small.

P charts are most useful when this problem is avoided by keeping the sample size constant (Western Electric Company, 1956). However, it is not necessary to have constant sample sizes.

- Calculate the average ($\bar{n}$) number of births in the 25 sampled months.

$$\bar{n} = \frac{36,060}{25}$$

$$\bar{n} = 1,442 \text{ live births/month}$$

- Compute the control limits.
  1. center line (CL)

$$CL = \bar{p}$$

$$CL = \frac{2,103}{36,060}$$

$$CL = 5.83\% \text{ (rounded to 6\%)}$$

  2. upper control limit (UCL)

$$UCL = \bar{p} + 3\sqrt{\frac{\bar{p}(1 - \bar{p})}{\bar{n}}}$$

---

†Before we construct a p chart, it is good to have an estimate of the appropriate subgroup size to use. Setting the subgroup size requires that a reasonable estimate of p be available. When p is small, larger subgroup sizes are necessary to accurately estimate the subgroup proportions. For larger values of p, smaller subgroups can be used. The overriding concern is that the subgroup be large enough to find some abnormals. With too small a subgroup, the proportions (p) can easily be 0 (even if p is not 0), which may lead to $\bar{p} = 0$ and control limits of 0, rendering the chart useless.

One approach to setting the sample size when p is small relies on the fact that a binomial variable X can be approximated by a Poisson random variable with parameter $\gamma = np$, where n is the subgroup size and p is the underlying proportion of abnormal events. To ensure that some abnormalities are found in a subgroup, one specifies that the probability, γ, of finding at least one such item should be fairly high (e.g., about 0.90 or 0.95).

Thus,

$$n = -\frac{\ln(1 - \gamma)}{p}$$

where ln denotes the natural logarithm (log base e). This formula is easy to apply, but when $\lambda = 0.95$, it is especially simple because $\ln(1 - 0.95) = -2.996$. Rounding this result to -3 and substituting into the formula yields the simple formula

$$n = \frac{3}{p} \qquad (\gamma) = 0.095$$

To illustrate, if one had specified $\gamma = 0.95$ and if p (the proportion abnormal) was estimated to be about 0.05, then using the above formula suggests that subgroup sizes of about $3/0.05 = 60$ would be sufficient for the p chart. Thus, to develop an effective p chart for a process with $p = 0.05$, subgroups should not be allowed to be smaller than 60 (Farnum, 1994).

Table 9–3 Low Birth Weights during a 25-Month Period in a Health District

Month (k)	(1) Number of Births (n)	(2) Number of LBW[1] Babies (p)	(3) % of Births LBW (p ÷ n)	(4) Above (+) or Below (–) Control Limits[2]
1	1,524	70	4.59	0
2	1,275	53	4.16	0
3	1,821	132	7.25	0
4	1,496	91	6.08	0
5	1,213	32	2.64	–
6	1,371	55	4.01	0
7	1,248	69	5.53	0
8	1,123	67	5.97	0
9	1,517	159	10.48	+
10	1,488	94	6.32	0
11	2,052	105	5.12	0
12	1,696	37	2.18	–
13	1,427	58	4.06	0
14	1,277	75	5.87	0
15	1,613	73	4.53	0
16	1,987	145	7.30	0
17	1,360	41	3.01	–
18	1,439	50	3.47	–
19	1,723	118	6.85	0
20	2,035	169	8.30	+
21	1,314	88	6.70	0
22	215	24	11.16	+
23	1,384	77	5.56	0
24	1,995	185	9.27	+
25	467	36	7.71	0
TOTAL	36,060	2,103		

[1]LBW = Low birth weight—a low-birth-weight baby is defined as less than 2,500 g or 5.5 lb.
[2] + = above calculated control limits; – = below calculated control limits; 0 = within calculated control limits.

$$UCL = 0.0583 + 3 \sqrt{\frac{(0.0583)(0.942)}{1,442}}$$

$$UCL = 0.0583 + 0.0185$$

$$UCL = 0.0768 = 7.680\%$$

3. lower control limit (LCL)

$$LCL = \bar{p} - 3 \sqrt{\frac{\bar{p}(1-\bar{p})}{\bar{n}}}$$

$$LCL = 0.0583 - \sqrt{\frac{(0.0583)(0.942)}{1,442}}$$

$$LCL = 0.0583 - 0.0185$$

$$LCL = 0.0398 = 3.980\%$$

- Using the CL, UCL, and LCL, create a p chart by plotting the individual values on the graph (Figure 9–6).[*]

$$CL = 5.83\%$$

$$UCL = 7.68\%$$

$$LCL = 3.98\%$$

- Evaluate the pattern.
  1. There are 5 months above the UCL (test 1—Figure 9–5).
  2. There are 4 months below the LCL (test 1—Figure 9–5).
  3. There are 2 out of 3 months in a row above or below the UCL and LCL (test 5—Figure 9–5).
  4. There are 16 months within the UCL and LCL.
- Apply the rules for detecting special causes.
  1. Interpret the p chart pattern.

---

[*]The control limits in Figure 9–6 were calculated using an average value of $\bar{n}$ (1,442). It is possible given unequal sample size to calculate control limits for each point on the p chart using the individual values of *n* (Table 9–3). Following the procedure, an irregular or stairstep effect is created (Figure 9–7). Small sample sizes create wide control limits, whereas large sample sizes create small control limits. This stairstep type of chart is more difficult to interpret and should be used minimally. However, if we do not meet the criteria for computing an average sample size ($\bar{n}$) for all communities or time periods sampled (see previous footnote), then individual limits may be calculated for only those samples not meeting the criteria. In our example, the 22nd and 25th month do not meet the criteria.

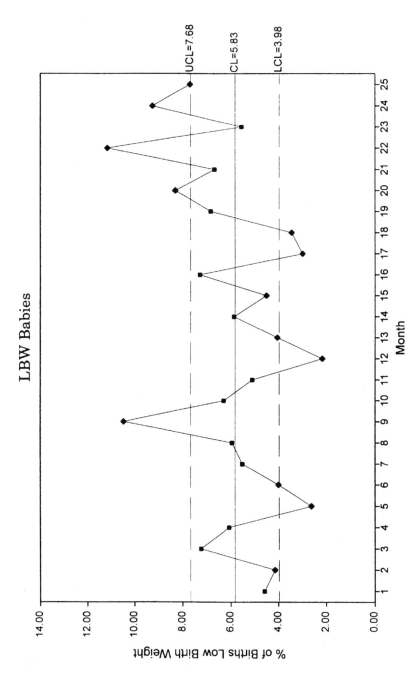

Figure 9–6 Low-Birth-Weight p Chart Using Average n ($\bar{n}$)

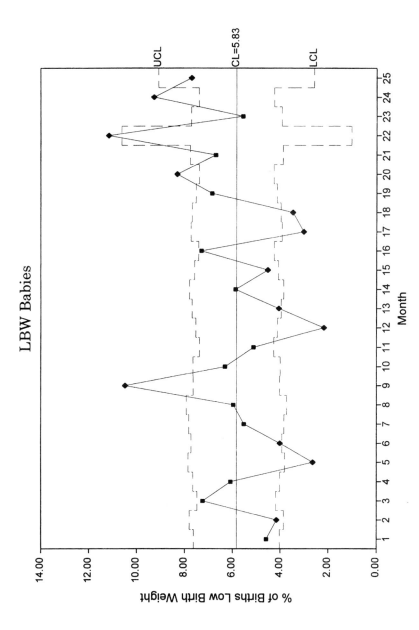

Figure 9–7 Low-Birth-Weight p Chart Using Individual Values: A Stairstep Pattern Develops Given the Variable Limits Based on Each Individual *n*

- For a p chart, if the LCL is greater than zero and the UCL is less than *n*, one may use the same tests for detecting a run as used for average (variables control charts) charts. If the LCL is less than zero, then the LCL is set at zero. As noted in the previous step, there are several situations that meet the test rules for detecting special causes.

Given, this example was attempting to determine if any of the months based on the low-birth-weight average of all the months were in control or produced a pattern that was expected. Clearly, several months were detected as "special cause situations"—they were outside the control limits or met one of the test rules for detecting special causes based on an evaluation of the pattern within the control limits (run length, number of runs, and trend—maximum consecutive increases or decreases). Thus, the cause for not having low-birth-weight births in control can be attributed to months 5, 9, 12, 17, 18, 20, 22, 24, and 25 (test rule one— one or more points outside the UCL or LCL). In addition, according to test rule five, there could be additional months, notably months 6 and 13. To improve this outcome of reducing the percentage of low-birth-weight babies (i.e., the process) by using the CQI approach, the above numbered months must be examined critically. The public health scientist now has target months to examine and develop a plan (i.e., the Plan-Do-Check-Act [PDCA] cycle) to improve the outcome and continue to monitor this health district in the months ahead using the p chart to measure the progress, obviously hold the gains, and continuously improve the quality of the program.

np Chart—for Number Abnormal

A variation of the p control chart is the np chart, in which the actual numbers of abnormal events or defects are analyzed instead of the proportion or percentage abnormal. The np stands for the number of abnormal events or parts. In public health practice, it may be more suitable many times to use a control chart that plots the number instead of the percentage of events that are abnormal in the sample. A major difference between the p chart and the np chart is that for the np chart, the size of each sample must be the same or constant. Therefore, for each time period, community, or clinic, an identical number of records must be sampled each time. This chart and others are based on a sample and do not include the universe. In the practice of public health, there must be a greater emphasis on the concept of sampling versus attempting to analyze the universe of elements.

The p chart and the np chart are interchangeable if subgroup sizes are constant; the only difference would be the sample of values on the vertical axis: number versus percentage. As with the p chart, the categorization of data into classes (normal versus abnormal) suggests a binomial process.

Constructing np Charts

The following formula is used for constructing np charts. The calculation of an np chart may also be based on a standard (i.e., Year 2000 objectives) or on the process being measured for the characteristic investigated.

The formulas are:

- based on a standard

$$CL_{np} = {}_nP_o$$

$$UCL_{np} = nP_o + 3\sqrt{{}_nP_o(1 - P_o)}$$

$$LCL_{np} = nP_o - 3\sqrt{{}_nP_o(1 - P_o)}$$

- based on process data

$$CL_{np} = n\bar{p}$$

$$UCL_{np} = n\bar{p} + 3\sqrt{n\bar{p}(1 - \bar{p}_o)}$$

$$LCL_{np} = n\bar{p} - 3\sqrt{n\bar{p}(1 - \bar{p}_o)}$$

where
    np = number of abnormal events
    P_o = the standard or targeted process number for abnormal events
    n = sample size (constant)
    $\bar{p}$ = the average number abnormal (fraction) based on the number of time
        periods or communities selected (i.e., the center line for the np chart)
  CL_{np} = center line of the chart
UCL_{np} = upper control limit of the chart
LCL_{np} = lower control limit of the chart

To calculate the control limits based on one or two standard deviations, substitute in the above formula a 1 or 2 in place of the 3. The result produces control limits based on one or two standard deviations.

Thus for np charts, the fraction abnormal or the number abnormal is determined from the sample selected. Remember the sample size is constant for np charts. If 150 records were reviewed (the sample size) and 5 were abnormal, the number or fraction abnormal (np) would be determined as

$$np = 5 \div 150$$

$$np = 0.033$$

The fraction abnormal is evaluated for all time periods or communities for the time period investigated.

np Chart—Teenage Pregnancy Example

The data displayed in Table 9–4 show a sample of 20 months of 150 records (constant) in a health district that were reviewed to determine the number of teenage pregnancies (ages 10 to 17).[8] During the 20 months, there were 3,000 records sampled, and 87 teenage pregnancies were recorded.

Table 9–4 Teenage Pregnancies in a Health District during a 20-Month Period

Month	Number of Births Sampled (n)	Number of Teenage Pregnancies (x)	Fraction of Teenage Pregnancies (p)*
1	150	4	0.027
2	150	2	0.013
3	150	4	0.027
4	150	4	0.027
5	150	8	0.053
6	150	4	0.027
7	150	4	0.027
8	150	3	0.020
9	150	5	0.033
10	150	3	0.020
11	150	5	0.033
12	150	2	0.013
13	150	3	0.020
14	150	5	0.033
15	150	2	0.013
16	150	8	0.053
17	150	4	0.027
18	150	3	0.020
19	150	8	0.053
20	150	6	0.040
TOTAL	3,000	87	$\bar{p} = 0.029$

*p is the fraction or proportion abnormal (in this example, the proportion of teenage pregnancies in the sample).

The average number of "abnormals" or "defects" (i.e., teenage pregnancies) is

$$\bar{p} = \frac{\Sigma p}{\Sigma n}$$

$$\bar{p} = \frac{87}{3,000}$$

$$\bar{p} = 0.029$$

where
    $\bar{p}$ = average number of teenage pregnancies (fraction)
    p = number of teenage pregnancies
    n = sample size
    Σ = summation

To determine if the number of teenage pregnancies during the 20-month period is in control (normal) or needs correction (improvement), an np chart is constructed. To do this, the following steps are recommended:

- Collect or obtain a sample set of data that provides the number of births and the number of births there were to teenagers (aged 10 to 17) for a 20-month period. The subgroup size (k), in this instance, months, should be about 20 to 25.
- Compute the average number of teenage pregnancies as a fraction. This is used to calculate the center line of the np chart.

$$\bar{p} = \frac{87}{3,000}$$

$$\bar{p} = 0.029$$

- Compute the control limits.
  1. center line (CL)

$$\mathrm{CL}_{np} = n\bar{p}$$

$$\mathrm{CL}_{np} = 150\,(0.029)$$

$$\mathrm{CL}_{np} = 4.35$$

  2. upper control limit (UCL)

$$\mathrm{UCL}_{np} = n\bar{p} + 3\sqrt{n\bar{p}(1-\bar{p})}$$

$$UCL_{np} = 4.35 + 3\sqrt{(4.35)(0.971)}$$

$$UCL_{np} = 4.35 + 3(2.0552)$$

$$UCL_{np} = 10.52 \text{ (or 11 rounded)}$$

3. lower control limit (LCL)

$$LCL_{np} = n\bar{p} - 3\sqrt{n\bar{p}(1-\bar{p})}$$

$$LCL_{np} = 4.35 - 3\sqrt{(4.35)(0.971)}$$

$$LCL_{np} = 4.35 - 3\,(2.0552)$$

$$LCL_{np} = -1.8156 \text{ (or zero)}$$

- Using the CL, UCL, and LCL, create an np chart by plotting the individual values on the graph (Figure 9–8).

$$CL = 4.35$$

$$UCL = 10.52 \text{ or 11 rounded}$$

$$LCL = -1.8 \text{ (or zero)}$$

When a negative LCL is obtained, one may set the LCL to equal zero because negative events are not possible (i.e., negative teenage pregnancies).
- Evaluate the pattern.
  1. All numbers of abnormal events (teenage pregnancies) for this time period are within the control limits.
- Interpret the np chart pattern.
  1. Apply the rules for detecting special causes.
  2. The same rules as noted for p charts also apply for np charts. However, if the LCL is less than zero and UCL is less than n (sample size), then special tests are used.[*]

In this example, none of the months examined are considered out of control, so the process is in control, or variation in the number of teenage pregnancies during the 20 months does not exhibit any special causes and the outcome (teenage preg-

---

[*]See the *Statistical Quality Control Handbook* by the Western Electric Company. 1956. Indianapolis, IN: AT&T., pp. 180–183.

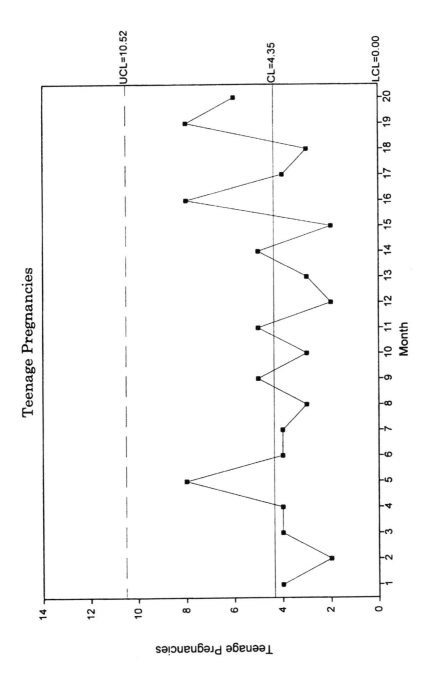

Figure 9–8 Teenage Pregnancy np Chart

nancies) has not changed. The process is performing as expected (i.e., there are no notable changes in the number of events that have occurred over the 20-month period). This is important to know, because if the public health agency does not have a teenage pregnancy prevention program in this area, then you would not have any reason to expect change; however, if a program had been implemented and the process performed as shown in this example, then the program has had no impact on the process or trend (i.e., no reduction in teenage pregnancies).

Further, this approach is especially useful for evaluating small numbers that may be associated with small areas. As can be seen in Figure 9–8, there is considerable variation; however, the peaks at months 5, 16, and 19 are not indicative of an increasing trend in teenage pregnancies because they are within the control limits. Further, there is no apparent pattern within the control limits. Apparently, from viewing this chart there has been no change in the number of teenage pregnancies over the past 20 months (no increases, no decreases). A public health practitioner would target this district to determine why there has been no improvement in the process. An alternative analysis would be to apply a standard number abnormal or defective (Year 2000 objective) to evaluate the process. The results of this might be considerably different if one indicated the standard abnormal (Year 2000 objective) is 0.012 instead of the 0.029 obtained from the 20-month process. By substituting in the formula based on a standard, the result would be UCL = 5.8 and LCL = 0. By reviewing Table 9–4, it is still apparent that none of the months exceed these limits, although the 5th, 16th, and 19th months show 0.053. Finally, if the analyst thought that the evaluation of the process should be based on two standard deviations versus the three that were presented here, then the interpretation of the control chart might indicate an out-of-control process. This decision is made programmatically or by the analyst who might calculate both the two and three standard deviation limits.

c Chart—for Number of Occurrences for Equal Sample Size

The c chart is a special type of attribute control chart that uses the number of abnormals or "defects" per item or event evaluated instead of the number of items abnormal or "defective." If n distinct items (births, disease) are classified as good (normal) or bad (abnormal), then p or np charts are used. However, if the number of problems related to each n distinct item are counted instead of the items themselves, c or u charts are used. In other words, if the number of peaches that are considered to be rotten in a box are counted, then a p and np chart would be used to analyze the process. However, if the number of blemishes on each peach in a box are counted, then a c or u chart would be used. Thus, with c charts, the question "Has a special cause of variation caused the process to produce an abnormally large or small number of occurrences over the time period observed?" is answered. Examples of questions to ask would be (1) the number of patient complaints in the clinic per 100 patients surveyed (duplicated count), (2) the number of customers served per week (duplicated count), (3) the number of patients visiting an outpatient clinic per month (duplicated count), and (4) the number of congenital malformations per birth during the past month. Each of these examples presents constant "areas of opportunity" (i.e., per 100 patients, served per hour, per week, and per month). In public health practice, these problems are usually handled by converting to rates if possible so that the area of opportunity is standardized for purposes of comparison. Obviously, however, if the area of opportunity for the event to occur is constant, then it is possible to make use of the counts instead of the rates. Further, the events for analysis in c charts should be relatively rare and be independent of each other.

When we are interested in counting the number of occurrences per time period (i.e., the interval) or area of opportunity (observations) the Poisson distribution is used as the basis for charting. The area of observation or opportunity is a finite region of space, time, or product. As you may recall, when analyzing data using the p and np charts, the binomial distribution was the basis for charting, and there was concern about the number of discrete events in which the result was 0 or 1 (i.e., normal or abnormal). A simple way to distinguish between binomial count data and Poisson count data is that binomial count data counts either the number normal or the number abnormal, whereas the Poisson count data can only count the abnormals—it will be impossible to count the nonabnormals. The Poisson distribution (discrete distribution) is applicable because the outcome is the number of times an event occurs as opposed to the binomial distribution (discrete distribution), which is applicable when the outcome is dichotomous (i.e., yes and no, positive and negative, or normal and abnormal). There are four conditions for using the Poisson distribution to characterize counts:

1. The counts are counts of discrete events.
2. The discrete events occur within some well-defined, finite region of space or time or program. This finite region is the area of opportunity.
3. The events occur independently of each other.
4. The events are rare.[9]

Small Average Counts

Another aspect of the c chart concerns the fact that the Poisson distribution is severely skewed when the average is small. This skewness changes the chances of getting a false alarm (false-positives or false-negatives). For average counts that are less than one per sample, there is an approximate chance of 3 to 4 percent that a point will exceed the upper three standard deviations. For average counts between one and three, the chance of a false alarm is about 2 percent, and for averages between three and seven, the chance of a false alarm is about 1 percent. When the average count is between 7 and 12, the chance of a false alarm drops to about 0.5 percent. At the same time, the formulas for the three standard deviations do not produce a lower control limit until the average count per sample exceeds nine. This makes it difficult to detect improvements when the average count drops below about 10.[10]

These problems with the usual three standard deviations are not overwhelming. The regular limits are sufficiently conservative to be useful in practice. However, because the assumptions justifying the use of a c chart also justify the use of the Poisson distribution, there is an easy way to remedy both of the shortcomings of three standard deviations for Poisson counts. This may be done by using the 0.005 LCL_c and the 0.995 UCL_c probability limits shown in Table 9–5. Although the 0.995 UCL_c is sometimes larger and sometimes smaller than the upper three standard deviations, the probability of a point falling above the 0.995 UCL_c is never greater than 0.005 when the process is in control. Likewise, although the 0.005 LCL_c is always greater than the lower three standard deviations, the probability of a point falling below the 0.005 LCL_c is never greater than 0.005 when the process is in control. Thus, these limits provide a balance between sensitivity to process improvements and process deterioration, while minimizing the chance of a false alarm. They are a reasonable alternative to the three standard deviations for a c chart and also effectively deal with small counts.

For average count values in excess of 20, one may use the following approximations for the 0.005 and 0.995 probability limits (LCL_c and UCL_c) for a c chart:[11]

$$0.005\ LCL_c \approx \bar{c} - 2.47\sqrt{\bar{c}} \qquad\qquad 0.995\ UCL_c \approx \bar{c} + 2.85\sqrt{\bar{c}}$$

Constructing c Charts

The following formulas are used for constructing c charts. As noted for p and np charts, a c chart may be based on a standard (average) or based on the process data, in which case the average must be estimated. The c chart must use a constant area of observation, and the average sample size should be greater than five. The reason for this is that this is approximately the cut-off point where the LCL will be greater than zero. An average value less than five produces an LCL of zero. Obviously, an average of five or more produces an LCL that can be evaluated from a practical perspective based on the problem investigated. However, if this is not critical, an average value of five or less may be evaluated quite easily from Table 9–5.

Table 9–5 Fixed Control Chart Limits for a c chart When Counts Are Less Than 20

Process Average Count	LCL*	UCL	Process Average Count	LCL*	UCL
0.00 to 0.10	0.0	1.5	9.65 to 10.36	2.5	19.5
0.10 to 0.33	0.0	2.5	10.36 to 10.97	2.5	20.5
0.33 to 0.67	0.0	3.5	10.97 to 11.08	3.5	20.5
0.67 to 1.07	0.0	4.5	11.08 to 11.81	3.5	21.5
1.07 to 1.53	0.0	5.5	11.81 to 12.54	3.5	22.5
1.53 to 2.04	0.0	6.5	12.54 to 12.59	3.5	23.5
2.04 to 2.57	0.0	7.5	12.59 to 13.28	4.5	23.5
2.57 to 3.13	0.0	8.5	13.28 to 14.02	4.5	24.5
3.13 to 3.71	0.0	9.5	14.02 to 14.14	4.5	25.5
3.71 to 4.32	0.0	10.5	14.14 to 14.77	5.5	25.5
4.32 to 4.94	0.0	11.5	14.77 to 15.53	5.5	26.5
4.94 to 5.30	0.0	12.5	15.53 to 15.66	5.5	27.5
5.30 to 5.58	0.5	12.5	15.66 to 16.28	6.5	27.5
5.58 to 6.23	0.5	13.5	16.28 to 17.05	6.5	28.5
6.23 to 6.89	0.5	14.5	17.05 to 17.13	6.5	29.5
6.89 to 7.57	0.5	15.5	17.13 to 17.82	7.5	29.5
7.57 to 8.25	0.5	16.5	17.82 to 18.57	7.5	30.5
8.25 to 8.43	0.5	17.5	18.57 to 18.59	8.5	30.5
8.43 to 8.95	1.5	17.5	18.59 to 19.36	8.5	31.5
8.95 to 9.27	1.5	18.5	19.36 to 20.00	8.5	32.5
9.27 to 9.65	1.5	18.5			

*Represents the 0.005 and 0.995 probability limits for c charts.
Source: Adapted with permission from D.J. Wheeler and D.S. Chambers, *Understanding Statistical Process Control*, 2nd ed., p. 274, © 1992, SPC Press, Inc.

The formulas are

- based on a standard

$$CL_c = \mu_0$$

$$UCL_c = \mu_0 + 3\sigma_c$$

$$= \mu_0 + 3\sqrt{\mu_0}$$

$$LCL_c = \mu_0 - 3\sigma_c$$

$$= \mu_0 - 3\sqrt{\mu_0}$$

- based on process data

$$CL_c = \bar{c}$$

$$UCL_c = \bar{c} + 3\sqrt{\bar{c}}$$

$$LCL_c = \bar{c} - 3\sqrt{\bar{c}}$$

where

c = the number of abnormal events in a sample

μ_0 = standard average number of abnormal events (population average or standard)

$\bar{c}$ = average number of abnormals in several samples

CL_c = center line of the chart

UCL_c = upper control limit of the chart

LCL_c = lower control limit of the chart

To calculate the limits for one or two standard deviations, substitute the value of 1 or 2 in the above equations for the value of 3. This procedure would define the limits—upper and lower—for one or two standard deviations.

For c charts, the estimated average of abnormal events is calculated by using the following formula:

$$\bar{c} = \frac{\Sigma c}{k}$$

where

$\bar{c}$ = average number of abnormals for the samples

c = the number of abnormal events in a sample

k = the number of samples

c Chart—Congenital Malformations in Infants

The data shown in Table 9–6 represent a sample of 20 births that were evaluated to determine the number of congenital malformations per birth. These samples were retrospectively selected over the past week. During the week, there were 23 malformations.

The average number of malformations is given by

$$\bar{c} = \frac{\Sigma c}{k}$$

$$\bar{c} = \frac{23}{20}$$

$$\bar{c} = 1.15$$

Table 9–6 Number of Congenital Malformations per Birth

Birth Number* (k)	Number of Malformations (c)
1	4
2	2
3	0
4	0
5	1
6	2
7	0
8	3
9	0
10	0
11	0
12	0
13	1
14	0
15	2
16	0
17	4
18	1
19	3
20	0

*Each sample birth certificate was reviewed to determine the number of congenital malformations.

To construct a c chart for determining if there is an unusual number of congenital malformations among the 20 births, the following steps are appropriate.

- Collect or obtain a sample of data that gives the number of malformations over a constant area of observation, specifically, individual birth certificates. It is recommended the average sample count be five or more.
- Compute the average number (count) of malformations. This also is the center line of the c chart.

$$\bar{c} = \frac{23}{20}$$

$$\bar{c} = 1.15$$

- Compute the control limits.
  1. center line (CL)

$$CL_c = \bar{c}$$

$$CL_c = 1.15$$

  2. upper control limit (UCL)

$$UCL_c = \bar{c} + 3\sqrt{\bar{c}}$$

$$UCL_c = 1.15 + 3\sqrt{1.15}$$

$$UCL_c = 1.15 + 3(1.07)$$

$$UCL_c = 1.15 + 3.22$$

$$UCL_c = 4.37 \text{ (or rounded to 4.4)}$$

  3. lower control limit (LCL)

$$LCL_c = \bar{c} - 3\sqrt{\bar{c}}$$

$$LCL_c = 1.15 - 3\sqrt{1.15}$$

$$LCL_c = 1.15 - 3(1.07)$$

$$LCL_c = 1.15 - 3.22$$

$$LCL_c = -2.07 \text{ (or zero)}$$

Because the number of malformations cannot be negative, the lower limit is set to zero.
- Using the CL, UCL, and LCL, create a c chart by plotting the individual counts of congenital malformation values on the graph (Figure 9–9). If one used Table 9–5 (determining the exact probability limits for the c chart based on the Poisson distribution) to determine the limits, the LCL would also be zero and the UCL would have been 5.5 as opposed to the calculated 4.4.
- Evaluate the pattern.
  1. Four out of five points beyond one standard deviation; therefore, the process is out of control (rule 6—Figure 9–5)

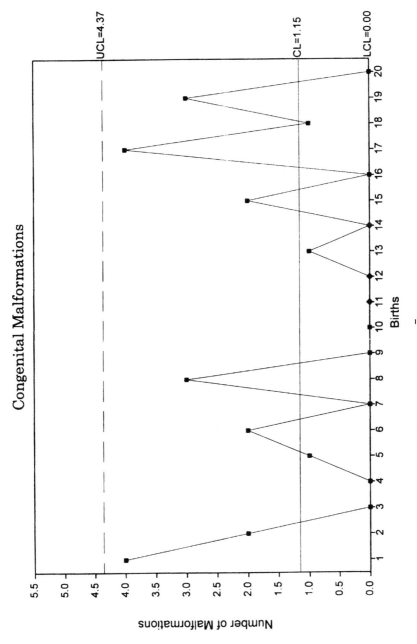

Figure 9–9 c Chart: Congenital Malformations by Birth—Using Average c $(\bar{c})$

- Interpret the c chart pattern.

    Apply the rules for detecting special causes. c charts are interpreted in the same way as p charts.

    The pattern exhibited in Figure 9–9 results in a process that is out of control. Specifically, statistically based on the fact that four of the five points (births 10, 11, 12, 13, 14) are beyond one standard deviation, the pattern is out of control. From a public health practice perspective, the counts can be evaluated based on small numbers to determine if there is any statistical significance to the variation. Of course, in this example it appears that there has been a substantial number of births (counts) that do not have any malformations. Finding this type of result indicates that it appears a reduction in the number of events (small numbers) over a recent period has occurred. This result at this point is also confirmed statistically based on the nonrandomness of the pattern by applying the Poisson distribution probability limits. The ultimate effort here is to have zero malformations. Obviously, a review of the 20 births suggests that there are still some significant problems. However, the test rule 6 indicating that the process is out of control suggests that from a practical point of view this is the pattern we wish to eliminate or find on inspection of 20 births for another time period.

u Chart—for Number of Occurrences for Variable Sample Size

The last attribute control chart to consider for application in public health practice for use in CQI to manage a process, analyze a process, or determine if the process is in control based on a standard is a u chart. Obviously all the charts discussed thus far provide the identical evaluation of a process. A u chart is similar to a c chart except the "area of opportunity" or the observations that occur within some well-defined, finite region of space or time or product varies from sample to sample, and therefore, the counts cannot be directly compared. As noted previously using the c chart, the area of opportunity was constant as in the congenital malformation example in which each birth certificate was reviewed during the past week to determine if the number of occurrences of congenital malformations was declining (i.e., improving). With u charts, before the counts can be charted or analyzed, they must be changed into rates. If the data satisfy the Poisson probabilities, then the appropriate rate to calculate is the number of abnormal events per the area of opportunity (i.e., region, space, time, or product) observed.

Constructing u Charts

In contrast to c charts, the area of opportunity for u charts changes from sample to sample, whereas the c chart is based on a constant from sample to sample. This fundamental difference establishes control limits based on variable sample sizes as opposed to constant sample sizes. The formulas for calculating u charts based on variable sample sizes are

- center line (CL)

$$CL_u = \bar{u}$$

- upper control limit (UCL)

$$UCL_u = \bar{u} + 3\sqrt{\frac{\bar{u}}{n}}$$

Note: We use n for detecting variable control limits (a control limit for each sampled observation) and $\bar{n}$ for determining standard control limits. In this example, variable control limits are presented.

- lower control limit (LCL)

$$LCL_u = \bar{u} - 3\sqrt{\frac{\bar{u}}{n}}$$

where

u = the number of abnormals per event in a sample
n = the number of observations
$\bar{u}$ = average number of abnormals

As with the other attribute charts, the control limits for one or two standard deviations is determined by substituting 1 or 2 in the above equation for the value of 3.

For u charts to calculate the estimated average number of abnormal events observed, we use

$$\bar{u} = \frac{\Sigma x}{\Sigma n}$$

$$\bar{u} = \frac{\text{total number of occurrences (events)}}{\text{total number of observations (sample)}}$$

where

$\bar{u}$ = average number of abnormals
x = number of occurrences (deaths, complaints, etc.)
n = number of observations (populations, patients)—population-at-risk
Σ = summation

u Chart—Complaints at a Public Health Clinic Example

The information in Table 9–7 represents 20 consecutive days (20 samples) of patients attending an afternoon public health clinic in a rural county. A u chart is

Table 9–7 Control Chart Calculations for a u Chart Based on Patient Complaints in a Public Health Clinic with Variable Subgroups

Days Sampled	Number of Patients (n)	Number of Complaints (x)	Number of Complaints per Patient (u)	$3\sqrt{\frac{\bar{u}}{n}}$	LCL_U	UCL_U
M	10	1	0.1	0.620	0.00	1.05
T	20	8	0.4	0.438	0.01	0.87
W	15	9	0.6	0.506	0.00	0.93
T	10	9	0.9	0.620	0.00	1.05
F	30	12	0.4	0.358	0.07	0.78
M	20	4	0.2	0.438	0.01	0.87
T	10	7	0.7	0.620	0.00	1.05
W	10	8	0.8	0.620	0.00	1.05
T	10	7	0.7	0.620	0.00	1.05
F	20	4	0.2	0.438	0.01	0.87
M	30	24	0.8	0.358	0.07	0.78
T	10	2	0.2	0.620	0.00	1.05
W	40	12	0.3	0.310	0.12	0.74
T	40	8	0.2	0.310	0.12	0.74
F	10	5	0.5	0.620	0.00	1.05
M	30	15	0.5	0.358	0.07	0.78
T	20	6	0.3	0.438	0.01	0.87
W	20	16	0.8	0.438	0.01	0.87
T	10	8	0.8	0.620	0.00	1.05
F	40	8	0.2	0.310	0.12	0.74
TOTAL	405	173	—			
MEAN	$\bar{n} = 20.3$		$\bar{u} = 0.43$			

used to determine, in this instance, whether there is an unusual number of patient complaints over the time period observed. To answer this question, the average must be calculated. Therefore,

$$\bar{u} = \frac{\Sigma x}{\Sigma n}$$

$$\bar{u} = \frac{173}{405}$$

$$\bar{u} = 0.43$$

To construct a u chart for patient complaints, the following is recommended:

• Collect the survey data from the patients who attended the afternoon public health clinics during the 20-day period. As noted in Table 9–7, the subgroup size (i.e., the number of patients surveyed) is variable. For example, on the first Monday only 10 patients were sampled, and on the first Tuesday 20 patients were sampled. It is recommended that, although the sample size n varies for each sample, as long as the variation falls within ±50 percent of $\bar{n}$ (the average sample size), you can use $\bar{n}$ and the method outlined here to determine control limits. In our example, n varies between a minimum of 10 and a maximum of 40. Because $\bar{n} = 405/20 = 20.3$, the variation does fall within the ±50 percent (10 to 30) of $\bar{n}$. Therefore, individual limits were calculated for each sample (Table 9–7).

• Compute the average number of patient complaints per patient. This is also the center line (CL) of the chart.

$$\bar{u} = \frac{173}{405}$$

$$\bar{u} = 0.43$$

• Compute the control limits.
  1. center line (CL)

  $$CL_u = \bar{u}$$

  $$CL_u = 0.43$$

  2. upper control limit (UCL)

  $$UCL_u = \bar{u} + 3\sqrt{\frac{\bar{u}}{\bar{n}}}$$

  $$UCL_u = 0.43 + 3\sqrt{\frac{0.43}{20.3}}$$

  $$UCL_u = 0.43 + 3\sqrt{0.0212}$$

  $$UCL_u = 0.43 + 3(0.1455)$$

  $$UCL_u = 0.43 + 0.4366$$

  $$UCL_u = 0.87$$

Note: The UCL and LCL calculations used $\bar{n}$ to show how the standard control limits are determined because the individual UCL and LCLs are presented in Table 9–7.

3. lower control limit (LCL)

$$LCL_u = \bar{u} - 3\sqrt{\frac{\bar{u}}{n}}$$

$$LCL_u = 0.43 - 3\sqrt{\frac{0.43}{20.3}}$$

$$LCL_u = 0.43 - 3\sqrt{0.0212}$$

$$LCL_u = 0.43 - 3(0.1455)$$

$$LCL_u = 0.43 - 0.4366$$

$$LCL_u = -0.007 \text{ (or zero)}$$

Because the number of patient complaints cannot be negative, the lower limit would be set to zero. Additionally, to calculate the control limits for each subgroup of patients by day, you replace $\bar{n}$ (average sample size) in the above formulas with n (subgroup sample size). This produces the UCL and LCL for each day sampled (Table 9–7).

- Using the CL, UCL, and LCL for the individual day sample size, a u chart is created by plotting the individual values for patient complaints on the graph, plus the average value ($\bar{u} = 0.43$) for the number of patient complaints is shown (Figure 9–10). The figure produced resembles a city skyline due to the individual calculations of the control limits for each subgroup.
- Evaluate the pattern.
  1. Day 11—a Monday (using the variable sample size, one point is outside the three standard deviation limit).
  2. Using the average sample size UCL, day 11 is inside the limit.
  3. Using the average sample size UCL, day 4 is outside the limit.
- Interpret the u chart pattern.

  As with all control charts, a special cause is probably present if there are any points beyond the UCL or LCL. However, an analysis of patterns between the control limits becomes complicated by two facts: (1) the distribution of the number of abnormal events follows the Poisson distribution, not the normal distribution; and (2) the control limits change as the subgroup of patients change. Because of this, run tests are not generally used to determine an out-of-control process. Also, remember that the variable control limits must be used if the variables from the average sample size are ±50 percent of $\bar{n}$.

  The pattern exhibited in Figure 9–10 shows a point in and out of control, depending on whether the UCL and LCL was based on average sample size

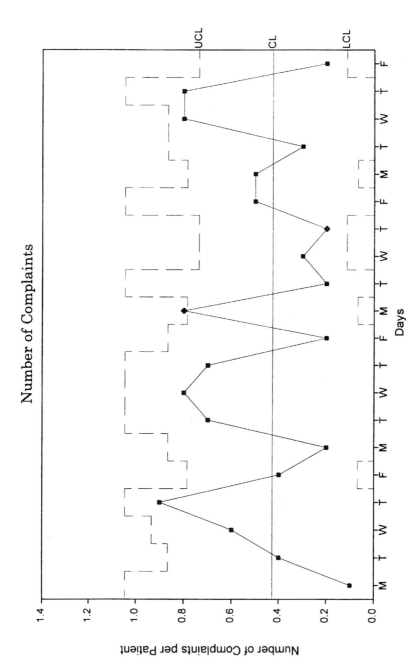

Figure 9–10 u Chart Patient Complaints in a Public Health Clinic Using Varying Sample Size

($\bar{n}$) or individual sample size (n), also known as "moving control limits." Because one point is outside the limit in either situation, then the process is out of control. However, a more intuitive interpretation tells us we should have as our improvement goal zero complaints. A further analysis would be to analyze (stratify) this data by day of the week to determine the cause of this pattern. If this revealed no clue to a cause, we could analyze by staff member or by shift to see if complaints can be targeted more specifically. To meet a targeted objective of 2 complaints per 10 patients as opposed to the average number of complaints of 4.2 per 10 patients, we would substitute the value 2 in the formula of $\bar{u} = \Sigma x / \Sigma n$. If we used the value 2, then $\bar{u} = 2$. This approach may be more relevant to implementing a process for improving the patient complaint issue. Obviously, by applying this chart to the PDCA cycle we are able to monitor the process and further hold the gains and continually improve the quality of the clinics by assessing patient satisfaction.

CONCLUSION

Attribute control charts that are based on counts can be broadly classified into two groups: (1) p charts and np charts, which are based on a binomial model of probability for counts, and (2) c charts and u charts, which are based on a Poisson model of probability for counts. When the conditions of use of the binomial and Poisson models are satisfied, then one may use the p and np charts and the c and u charts, respectively, for charting attribute data. Table 9–8 provides a summary of the attribute control charts and their formulas and sample sizes required for calculating the center line, the upper control limit, and the lower control limit. If the sample size is constant, then an np chart (binomial) and a c chart (Poisson) are appropriate; however, when the sample size, or area of opportunity, is variable, the counts must be converted into rates before using the p chart (binomial) or the u chart (Poisson). All four of these attribute charts, by satisfying the conditions of the binomial or Poisson model, assume that the variation is a function of the average and control limits accordingly. Obviously, if all these conditions are not met, then the application of these charts in public health practice would be inappropriate.

The specific use of these charts is also based on the count or the count converted to a rate or proportion. For example,

- A p chart may be used to help stabilize a process by indicating a lack of statistical control in the characteristic being measured as a *rate or proportion*. Sample sizes are variable.
- An np chart is mathematically equivalent to a p chart, but the *number*—not the *proportion or rate* with the characteristic—is charted. Sample sizes are constant.

Table 9-8 Summary—Attribute Control Charts for Public Health Practice

Type	Center Line	Upper Control Limit*	Lower Control Limit*	Sample Size	Model for Statistical Evaluation
p chart	$\bar{p}$	$UCL_p = \bar{p} + 3\sqrt{\dfrac{\bar{p}(1 - \bar{p})}{n}}$	$LCL_p = \bar{p} - 3\sqrt{\dfrac{\bar{p}(1 - \bar{p})}{n}}$	≥ 50 (variable)	Binomial
np chart	$n\bar{p}$	$UCL_{np} = n\bar{p} + 3\sqrt{n\bar{p}(1 - \bar{p})}$	$LCL_{np} = n\bar{p} - 3\sqrt{n\bar{p}(1 - \bar{p})}$	≥ 50 (constant)	Binomial
c chart	$\bar{c}$	$UCL_c = \bar{c} + 3\sqrt{\bar{c}}$	$LCL_c = \bar{c} - 3\sqrt{\bar{c}}$	$\bar{c} > 5$ (constant)	Poisson
u chart	$\bar{u}$	$UCL_u = \bar{u} + 3\sqrt{\dfrac{\bar{u}}{\bar{n}}}$	$LCL_u = \bar{u} - 3\sqrt{\dfrac{\bar{u}}{\bar{n}}}$	variable	Poisson

*To calculate control limits for one or two standard deviations, substitute 1 or 2 for the value of 3 in the above equations.

- A c chart is used when a single sample may have multiple events, such as the *number* of abnormals in a population. This chart helps to evaluate the process and stabilize the *number of events* when the sample size, or area of opportunity, is the same.
- A u chart is used when counts of the number of events are to be charted, but the count must be *converted to a rate* for appropriate comparison because the sample size varies from subgroup to subgroup.

Finally, a basic difference between the p/np charts and the c/u charts for deciding which chart to use is based on two decisions: (1) are items classified as normal or abnormal? (if so, use a p or np chart) and (2) are the number of abnormal events counted per the area of opportunity that is defined as a finite region of space, time, or product? (if so, use a c or u chart). It is the responsibility of the public health practitioner to ensure that the conditions are validated for appropriate application of each of these charts. Although it is true that attribute charts help identify special cause variation, they are only some of the analytical tools for quality improvement. To further analyze public health data and monitor the process and improve the outcome, variables control charts must be used. This is the subject of the next chapter.

NOTES

1. M. Brassard and D. Ritter, *The Memory Jogger II* (Methuen, MA: GOAL/QPC, 1994), 36.
2. N.R. Farnum, *Modern Statistical Quality Control and Improvement* (Belmont, CA: Duxbury Press, 1994), 171.
3. Ibid., 172.
4. Western Electric Company, *Statistical Quality Control Handbook* (Indianapolis, IN: AT&T, 1956), 180–183.
5. D.J. Wheeler and D.S. Chambers, *Understanding Statistical Process Control*, 2d ed. (Knoxville, TN: SPC Press, 1992), 260.
6. Western Electric Company, *Statistical Quality Control Handbook*, 18.
7. Farnum, *Modern Statistical Quality Control and Improvement*, 243–244.
8. R. Gulezian, *Process Control: Statistical Principles and Tools* (New York: Quality Alert Institute, 1991), 250–252.
9. Wheeler and Chambers, *Understanding Statistical Process Control*, 272.
10. Ibid., 274.
11. Ibid., 275.

Chapter 10

Public Health Practice— Quality Improvement Control Charts for Continuous Measurement

In the previous chapter, we outlined quality improvement control charts for counts or discrete data that are called attribute control charts. These charts were based on the binomial (p and np charts) and Poisson (c and u charts) probability models. The type of chart used depends on constant or varying sample sizes and whether the events being evaluated were classified as normal or abnormal (the number defective) or based on counts of the number of abnormalities or defects. This chapter presents control charts for application in public health practice that rely on continuous measurement data for assessing outcomes. These charts are usually referred to as variables control charts by quality control experts. The difference between discrete data or counts (attribute control charts) and continuous data measurement (variables control charts) may be determined by the following criterion—if it is possible to improve the accuracy of the measurement by using more sensitive methods or devices, then the characteristic being measured is continuous (variables control charts) or otherwise it is discrete (attribute control charts).[1]

Many practitioners have made the observation that a control chart resembles a heart monitoring device of one's heartbeat or pulse. In quality improvement, the use of the chart is intended to monitor for signals that are exhibited by a process related to the customer, community, or program, and it further offers a method for determining if the signal may be evidence of a problem related to the outcome indicator being investigated. Evaluating these problems may require further analysis of the process.[2]

The variables control charts for continuous measurement discussed in this chapter are

- $\overline{X}$ and R (average and range)
- $\overline{X}$ and s (average and standard deviation)
- $\tilde{X}$ and R (median and range)
- X and mR (individual and moving range).

Each of these charts is used in an ongoing cycle of process improvement. Public health practitioners must begin to institutionalize the quality improvement tools for improving and attaining the desired outcomes to create healthy communities. In public health, we are guided by the Year 2000 objectives but we must also be encouraged to review the process (i.e., the program, community, customer, etc.) that is creating the improved outcomes.

Typically, charts are used to analyze the process and maintain the process; however, for improving the process, especially if the variation now stems from common causes, more sophisticated methods and tools are appropriate, which are not discussed in this book.[3] If the variation found results only from common causes (remember the use of control charts is to identify special causes) when apparently special causes have been eliminated, then efforts to reduce this variation must focus on changes in the process itself. For example, if an analysis of teenage pregnancies (outcome variable) revealed from using control charts that there were no special causes (i.e., control chart was in control) but the management realized there were still too many teenage pregnancies, then a potential action would be a program review to understand the common causes for altering the process and policies relating to this program.

CONTROL CHARTS FOR MEASUREMENT

Control charts for measurement data (variables control charts) are important quality improvement tools that are used when we have measurements from a process. In public health, examples would be the mortality rate, the time to provide an immunization, or percentage of women who had adequate prenatal care. Thus, control charts for variables are useful in public health practice for several reasons:

1. In public health, many processes and their outputs have characteristics that are measurable.
2. A quantitative value (e.g., the infant mortality rate is 1 per 1,000 live births) contains more information than a single normal/abnormal statistic (e.g., the baby is alive or dead).

3. With variable data, the analysis of a process and levels of improvement related to the outcome can be quantified. Even if no out-of-control points exist, this is significant to advance to the ongoing analysis of the improvement process.

Control charts for measurement explain process data in terms of both spread (observation-to-observation variability) and location (process average). Consequently, control charts for variables are usually prepared in pairs—a chart for location ($\overline{X}$ chart) and a chart for dispersion (R charts and s charts). A flowchart for selecting the appropriate variables control chart was presented in Chapter 9 (Figure 9–2).

$\overline{X}$ AND R CHART (AVERAGE AND RANGE)

$\overline{X}$ (read x bar or average) and R (read range) control charts are based on variable data in which the sample size is usually small: from three to five observations. The statistical model that is used for the application is the normal distribution. We are basically concerned with the process average ($\overline{X}$) and the process variation (R). Any instability in these measures is an indication of process problems. An alternate to this $\overline{X}$ and R control chart is the $\overline{X}$ and s chart, which is used if the sample size is larger, usually 10 or more. This type of chart ($\overline{X}$ and s) is discussed later. Average charts answer the question—has a special cause of variation caused the central tendency of the process to change over time? However, range (R) or standard deviation (s) charts determine if a special cause of variation causes the process distribution (the spread or dispersion) to become erratic. In public health, much of the information is based on continuous measurement; therefore, these charts have wide applicability for assessing community health status, for monitoring change, and for continuously improving outcomes. As with all charts discussed, the systematic use and application must be implemented if benefits are to occur.

Constructing $\overline{X}$ and R Charts

The following formulas are used for constructing $\overline{X}$ and R charts. As was the case with attribute control charts, $\overline{X}$ and R charts may also be based on a standard (i.e., Year 2000 objectives) or based on the process of the observed data during measurement (i.e., over time or among communities).

The formulas are

• based on a standard or target ($\overline{X}$)

$$\text{Center line, } CL_{\bar{x}} = \mu$$

$$\text{Upper control limit, } UCL_{\bar{x}} = \mu + A\sigma$$

$$\text{Lower control limit, } LCL_{\bar{x}} = \mu - A\sigma$$

- based on sample data ($\bar{X}$)

$$\text{Center line, } CL_{\bar{x}} = \bar{\bar{X}}$$

$$\text{Upper control limit, } UCL_{\bar{x}} = \bar{\bar{X}} + A_2\bar{R}$$

$$\text{Lower control limit, } LCL_{\bar{x}} = \bar{\bar{X}} - A_2\bar{R}$$

where
   μ = a target (2000 objective) or specified mean
   σ = a target (2000 objective) or specified standard deviation
   $\bar{\bar{X}}$ = mean of the sample means
   $\bar{R}$ = mean of the sample ranges
   A = tabulated factor used to calculate control limits based on target μ and σ
   A_2 = tabulated factor used to calculate control limits based on process ranges

In addition to the formulas for calculating control limits for the $\bar{X}$ chart, we also need to define the formula for a R chart because the two charts are both used to determine if special causes are determined in the process. Therefore, the formulas for the R chart are

- based on a standard or target (R)

$$\text{Center line, } CL_R = d_2\sigma$$

$$\text{Upper control limit, } UCL_R = D_2\sigma$$

$$\text{Lower control limit, } LCL_R = D_1\sigma$$

- based on sample data (R)

$$\text{Center line, } CL_R = \bar{R}$$

$$\text{Upper control limit, } UCL_R = D_4\bar{R}$$

$$\text{Lower control limit, } LCL_R = D_3\bar{R}$$

where

$\overline{R}$ = mean of the sample ranges

d_2 = tabulated bias adjusted factor for the sample range as an estimate of σ

σ = a target (2000 objective) or specified standard deviation

D_1 = factor to calculate LCL for a range chart based on σ

D_2 = factor to calculate UCL for a range chart based on σ

D_3 = factor to calculate LCL for a range chart based on sample data

D_4 = factor to calculate UCL for a range chart based on sample data

To make use of these charts there are a series of constants or coefficients to be used as indicated by the symbols A, A_2, d_2, D_1, D_2, D_3, and D_4. These tabulated values are presented in an abridged form in Table 10–1 for sample sizes from 2 to 25. The chart does not provide the values for A, D_1, or D_2, which are constants to be used if the calculated control limits are to be based on targets of the μ and σ. Although in public health practice it is likely targets may be used, the reader is referred to a more elaborate display of these values.[4] Further, for the public health practitioner who would like to know where these control chart constants come from, see Wheeler and Chambers.[5]

$\overline{X}$ and R Chart—Average Times for an Immunization Visit

The data displayed in Table 10–2 represent a sample of times for five clinics providing an immunization service in 25 rural public health clinics. There has always been concern about the average time it takes to give an immunization injection because of the cost and, therefore, the amount to be reimbursed from the Medicaid program. In each of the 25 clinics, five nurses were sampled to see how long it took them to provide the immunization services. Another approach could have been to evaluate the times for the same nurse and sample five different patients. The steps included to analyze this process are:

- Collect the data at the 25 rural health clinics for the five nurses and display as in Table 10–2. The sample size for this type of chart is usually small—three to five observations.

- Calculate the average ($\overline{X}$) time for each subgroup (county health clinic).

$$\overline{X} = \frac{X_1 + X_2 + X_3 + \ldots X_n}{n}$$

where

n = sample size (in this example, it is 5)

Table 10–1 Table of Constants and Formulas for Control Charts

$\bar{X}$ and R Charts

Subgroup Size	Chart for Averages ($\bar{X}$) Factors for Control Limits	Chart for Ranges (R)		
		Divisors for Estimate of Standard Deviation	Factors for Control Limits	
n	A_2	d_2	D_3	D_4
2	1.880	1.128	—	3.267
3	1.023	1.693	—	2.574
4	0.729	2.059	—	2.282
5	0.577	2.326	—	2.114
6	0.483	2.534	—	2.004
7	0.419	2.704	0.076	1.924
8	0.373	2.847	0.136	1.864
9	0.337	2.970	0.184	1.816
10	0.308	3.078	0.223	1.777
11	0.285	3.173	0.256	1.744
12	0.266	3.258	0.283	1.717
13	0.249	3.336	0.307	1.693
14	0.235	3.407	0.328	1.672
15	0.223	3.472	0.347	1.653
16	0.212	3.532	0.363	1.637
17	0.203	3.588	0.378	1.622
18	0.194	3.640	0.391	1.608
19	0.187	3.689	0.403	1.597
20	0.180	3.735	0.415	1.585
21	0.173	3.778	0.425	1.575
22	0.167	3.819	0.434	1.566
23	0.162	3.858	0.443	1.557
24	0.157	3.895	0.451	1.548
25	0.153	3.931	0.459	1.541
>25	$3/\sqrt{n}$			

$$\text{UCL}_{\bar{x}}, \text{LCL}_{\bar{x}} = \bar{\bar{X}} \pm A_2 \bar{R}$$

$$\text{UCL}_R = D_4 \bar{R}$$

$$\text{LCL}_R = D_3 \bar{R}$$

$$\sigma = \frac{\bar{R}}{d_2}$$

Source: Copyright ASTM. Reprinted with permission.

Table 10–2 Clinic Times $\bar{X}$-R Chart—Time To Provide an Immunization Visit in 25 Public Health Clinics

Rural Public Health Clinic (k)	Nurse 1 (X₁)	Nurse 2 (X₂)	Nurse 3 (X₃)	Nurse 4 (X₄)	Nurse 5 (X₅)	ΣX	$\bar{X}$	R
1	47	32	44	35	20	178	35.6	27
2	19	37	31	25	34	146	29.2	18
3	19	11	16	11	44	101	20.2	33
4	29	29	42	59	38	197	39.4	30
5	28	12	45	36	25	146	29.2	33
6	40	35	11	38	33	157	31.4	29
7	15	30	12	33	26	116	23.2	21
8	35	44	32	11	38	160	32.0	33
9	27	37	26	20	35	145	29.0	17
10	23	45	26	37	32	163	32.6	22
11	28	44	40	31	18	161	32.2	26
12	31	25	24	32	22	134	26.8	10
13	22	37	19	47	14	139	27.8	33
14	37	32	12	38	30	149	29.8	26
15	25	40	24	50	19	158	31.6	31
16	7	31	23	18	32	111	22.2	25
17	38	1	41	40	37	157	31.4	40
18	35	12	29	48	20	144	28.8	36
19	31	20	35	24	47	157	31.4	27
20	12	27	38	40	31	148	29.6	28
21	52	42	52	24	25	195	39.0	28
22	20	31	15	3	28	97	19.4	28
23	29	47	41	32	22	171	34.2	25
24	28	27	22	32	54	163	32.6	32
25	42	34	15	29	21	141	28.2	27
TOTAL							746.8	685
AVERAGE							$\bar{\bar{X}}$ = 29.87	$\bar{R}$ = 27.44

The calculation for the first health clinic is

$$\overline{X} = \frac{47 + 32 + 44 + 35 + 20}{5}$$

$$\overline{X} = 35.6 \text{ (average time)}$$

- Calculate the range (R) for each subgroup.

$$R = \text{maximum value} - \text{minimum value}$$

The calculation for the first health clinic is

$$R = 47 - 20$$

$$R = 27$$

- Calculate the mean of the sample means ($\overline{\overline{X}}$).

$$\overline{\overline{X}} = \frac{\overline{X}_1 + \overline{X}_2 + \overline{X}_3 + \ldots \overline{X}_k}{k}$$

where
  k = number of subgroups (rural health clinics) (25 in this example)

Thus,

$$\overline{\overline{X}} = \frac{(35.6 + 29.2 + 20.2 + \ldots 28.2)}{25}$$

$$\overline{\overline{X}} = 29.9 \text{ (rounded)}$$

- Calculate the mean of the sample ranges ($\overline{R}$).

$$\overline{R} = \frac{R_1 + R_2 + R_3 + \ldots R_k}{k}$$

Therefore,

$$\overline{R} = \frac{(27 + 18 + 33 \ldots 27)}{25}$$

$$\overline{R} = 27.4 \text{ (rounded)}$$

- Calculate the control limits.
  1. $\overline{X}$ chart
     Central line

$$CL_{\bar{x}} = \overline{\overline{X}}$$

$$CL_{\bar{x}} = 29.9$$

Upper control limit

$$UCL_{\bar{x}} = \overline{\overline{X}} + A_2\overline{R}$$

$$UCL_{\bar{x}} = 29.9 + (0.577)(27.4)$$

$$UCL_{\bar{x}} = 29.9 + 15.8$$

$$UCL_{\bar{x}} = 45.7$$

Lower control limit

$$LCL_{\bar{x}} = \overline{\overline{X}} - A_2\overline{R}$$

$$LCL_{\bar{x}} = 29.9 - (0.577)(27.4)$$

$$LCL_{\bar{x}} = 29.9 - 15.8$$

$$LCL_{\bar{x}} = 14.1$$

  2. R chart
     Central line

$$CL_R = \overline{R}$$

$$CL_R = 27.4$$

Upper control limit

$$UCL_R = D_4\overline{R}$$

$$UCL_R = (2.114)(27.4)$$

$$UCL_R = 57.9$$

Lower control limit

$$LCL_R = D_3\bar{R}$$

$$LCL_R = (0)(27.4) \text{—not considered}$$

The LCL is not considered when n for D_3 is smaller than 6 (Table 10–1). As stated previously, A_2, D_3, and D_4 are constants and are determined by the size of the subgroup (Table 10–1).

- Using the CL, UCL, and LCL for the $\bar{X}$ and R, create the control charts by plotting the values (samples) and the limits on the chart (Figure 10–1).

  Therefore,

$\bar{X}$ (Average)	R (Range)
$CL_{\bar{x}} = 29.9$	$CL_R = 27.4$
$UCL_{\bar{x}} = 45.7$	$UCL_R = 57.9$
$LCL_{\bar{x}} = 14.1$	$LCL_R = \text{not considered}$

- Evaluate the pattern.
  1. no points out of control
- Apply the rules for detecting special causes.

The rules for detecting special causes were detailed in Chapter 9 when attribute control charts were discussed. The rules outlined previously also apply to the variables control charts discussed in this chapter. However, a brief review is in order so the reader is able to realize that the evaluation of the process of variables control charts is the same.

There are four basic interpretations of control charts to consider. They are

1. Points beyond the control limits
   The presence of one or more points beyond the control limit is evidence of a process out of control. Because points rarely are beyond the limits, it is assessed to be a special cause if it is beyond the limit.
   - points above the upper control limit may be a sign of
     - a miscalculation
     - worsened variability of the distribution—at a point in time or is part of a trend
     - change in the system of measurement

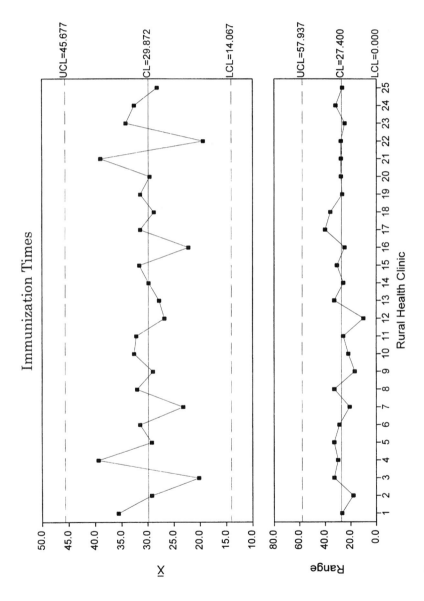

Figure 10–1 $\bar{X}$-R Chart

−an ineffective system of measurement for discriminating differences
  • points below the lower control limit may be a sign of
  −error in calculating center line
  −decreased spread of the distribution (i.e., become better)
  −change in measurement system
2. Patterns or trends within the control limits
  • Unusual patterns or trends could be a first warning of unfavorable conditions.
  • Certain patterns or trends could be favorable and should be studied for potential permanent improvement of the process.
3. Runs
  This was discussed in detail in Chapter 8. However, note when the sample size (n) is less than five, the possibility of runs below $\bar{R}$ increases, so a run length of eight or more may be necessary to signal a change in the process.
4. Nonrandom patterns
  • obvious trends even though they did not satisfy the runs tests
  • cycles
  −freaks
  −grouping or bunching
  −mixtures
  −natural pattern
  −stratification
  −tendency of one chart to follow another
Other nonrandom patterns, including those listed here, are illustrated elsewhere.[6]

The interpretations of the $\bar{X}$ and R charts are completed separately, but comparison of patterns between the two charts may give some added insight into special causes contributing to the process.

$\bar{X}$ AND s CHART (AVERAGE AND STANDARD DEVIATION)

In calculating the $\bar{X}$ for use with the s chart, the formulas are quite similar to those detailed in the discussion on the $\bar{X}$ and R chart. $\bar{X}$ and s charts, as $\bar{X}$ and R charts, are developed for data generated by the process and are always used as a pair. The s chart provides essentially the same information as range charts because they answer the question: Has a special cause of variation caused the process distribution to become more unstable? However, range charts were developed because of the ease of calculations, and they are rather efficient for small samples per subgroup of about three to five but definitely not more than above 10. s charts, however, are statistically more efficient than range charts because an increase in the process spread is more apt to be detected using sigma (standard deviation) charts than range charts for given sample sizes. In fact, as the sample size increases, the s chart is more appropriate for sample sizes per subgroup of more than 10. It is true that s charts are more complex to calculate and usually less sensitive in detecting special causes of variation based on the rule of a single value beyond the upper and/or lower control limits. Thus, when faced with a large sample size of 10 or more, use the $\overline{X}$ and s chart for assessing outcomes.

Constructing $\overline{X}$ and s Charts

The formula for determining the $\overline{X}$ of a chart was defined under the discussion of $\overline{X}$ and R charts. However, because there is one change in the formula, there is a need to present it again based on the constant A_3 (Table 10–3), which is substituted for the constant A_2 when the s chart is used. A_3 is the factor used to calculate control limits on a mean chart based on process data when the s chart is used with the $\overline{X}$ chart. Therefore, the formula for the $\overline{X}$ chart when using an s chart is

$$CL_{\bar{x}} = \overline{\overline{X}}$$

$$UCL_{\bar{x}} = \overline{\overline{X}} + A_3\overline{S}$$

$$LCL_{\bar{x}} = \overline{\overline{X}} - A_3\overline{S}$$

where
A_3 = tabulated factor used to calculate control limits on a mean chart based on process data (s).

However, as noted, this chart ($\overline{X}$ and s) includes the standard deviation; therefore, the formula for a chart based on s (standard deviation) will be detailed. The formulas are

• based on a standard or target (s)

$$\text{Center line, } CL_s = \sigma$$

$$CL_s = c_4\sigma$$

$$\text{Upper control limit, } UCL_s = B_6\sigma$$

$$\text{Lower control limit, } LCL_s = B_5\sigma$$

Table 10–3 Table of Constants and Formulas for Control Charts

	$\bar{X}$ and S Charts*			
	Chart for Averages ($\bar{X}$)	Charts for Standard Deviation (S)		
Subgroup Size	Factors for Control Limits	Divisors for Estimate of Standard Deviation	Factors for Control Limits	
n	A_3	c_4	B_3	B_4
2	2.659	0.7979	—	3.267
3	1.954	0.8862	—	2.568
4	1.628	0.9213	—	2.266
5	1.427	0.9400	—	2.089
6	1.287	0.9515	0.030	1.970
7	1.182	0.9594	0.118	1.882
8	1.099	0.9650	0.185	1.815
9	1.032	0.9693	0.239	1.761
10	0.975	0.9727	0.284	1.716
11	0.927	0.9754	0.321	1.679
12	0.886	0.9776	0.354	1.646
13	0.850	0.9794	0.382	1.618
14	0.817	0.9810	0.406	1.594
15	0.789	0.9823	0.428	1.572
16	0.763	0.9835	0.448	1.552
17	0.739	0.9845	0.466	1.534
18	0.718	0.9854	0.482	1.518
19	0.698	0.9862	0.497	1.503
20	0.680	0.9869	0.510	1.490
21	0.663	0.9876	0.523	1.477
22	0.647	0.9882	0.534	1.466
23	0.633	0.9887	0.545	1.455
24	0.619	0.9892	0.555	1.445
25	0.606	0.9896	0.565	1.435
>25			$1 - 3/(\sqrt{2n})$	$1 + 3/(\sqrt{2n})$

$$\text{UCL}_{\bar{x}}, \text{LCL}_{\bar{x}} = \bar{\bar{X}} \pm A_3 \bar{S}$$

$$\text{UCL}_s = B_4 \bar{S}$$

$$\text{LCL}_s = B_3 \bar{S}$$

$$\sigma = \frac{\bar{S}}{c_4}$$

*From *Manual on the Presentation of Data and Control Chart Analysis.* ASTM publication STP-15D. 1976. Philadelphia: ASTM, pp. 134–136.
Source: Copyright ASTM. Reprinted with permission.

• based on sample data (s)

$$\text{Center line, CL}_s = \bar{S}$$

$$\text{Upper control limit, UCL}_s = B_4\bar{S}$$

$$\text{Lower control limit, LCL}_s = B_3\bar{S}$$

where
σ = a target or specified standard deviation
$\bar{S}$ = the mean of the sample standard deviations
c_4 = tabulated bias adjusted factor for the sample standard deviation as an estimate of σ
B_3 = factor used to calculate LCL based on sample data
B_4 = factor used to calculate UCL based on sample data
B_5 = factor used to calculate LCL based on a target σ
B_6 = factor used to calculate UCL based on a target σ

To make use of the $\bar{X}$ and s charts, there is a series of constants or coefficients to be used as indicated by the symbols c_4, B_3, B_4, B_5, and B_6. These tabulated values are noted in an abridged Table 10–3 for sample sizes 2 to 25. The chart does not include the values for B_5 or B_6, which are coefficients to be used if the calculated control limits are to be based on targets of the σ. For derivation of the coefficients for the $\bar{X}$ and R chart and the $\bar{X}$ and s chart, see Gitlow et al.[7] It is sufficient for most public health analysts to be able to apply the charts in the most appropriate situations and not to be overwhelmed by the derivation of the coefficients. In any event, the coefficients are based on normally distributed processes, and in the use of the $\bar{X}$ and R chart, the assumption of normality is not required for interpretation.

$\bar{X}$ and s Chart—Prenatal Care Visits Example

One of the major outcome indicators to be assessed in rural areas or census tracts in urban areas is the risk of infant mortality. Many experts believe adequate prenatal care is a risk factor in reducing infant mortality. Public health analysts usually use the Year 2000 objectives as outcome indicators to determine if the communities are at risk. In continuous quality improvement (CQI) measurement, the data may be analyzed using an $\bar{X}$ and s chart to determine the variation among the areas and determine if there is an identified special cause that may be creating the variation. In this instance, the special cause could be a community that is not in control (i.e., outside the process limits) and, therefore, is labeled as a special cause. The data displayed in Table 10–4 represent 20 rural communities where for 10 consecutive months 100 birth records were sampled, and the average number of prenatal care visits was determined.

The steps required to analyze this problem are

- Collect the data for the 20 communities in the health district for the 10-month period; each month 100 birth records are sampled. The sample size for an $\overline{X}$ and s chart is usually large (i.e.,10 or more).
- Calculate the average ($\overline{X}$) for each subgroup.

Table 10–4 Prenatal Care Visits Based on 100 Births for 10 Consecutive Months in 20 Rural Counties

County (k)	Months (Measurements) 1 (x_1)	2 (x_2)	3 (x_3)	4 (x_4)	5 (x_5)	6 (x_6)	7 (x_7)	8 (x_8)	9 (x_9)	10 (x_{10})	Average ($\overline{X}$)	Standard Deviation (s)
1	13.0	11.0	12.0	12.5	10.5	9.5	11.0	11.6	13.7	9.8	11.5	1.36
2	10.1	11.0	11.5	9.7	12.5	11.2	11.0	9.0	10.4	10.8	10.7	0.98
3	12.2	10.5	9.3	10.8	11.5	12.7	9.5	11.1	11.2	11.0	11.0	1.06
4	10.8	11.2	11.1	12.8	10.0	9.5	11.5	11.4	12.8	13.1	11.4	1.20
5	9.8	13.0	13.1	11.2	10.8	11.0	11.5	13.5	11.2	12.6	11.8	1.21
6	11.2	13.0	10.1	12.0	11.1	9.3	10.2	12.5	10.5	11.0	11.1	1.15
7	9.2	11.0	11.3	10.2	9.3	11.7	12.4	9.8	13.4	11.2	11.0	1.36
8	10.4	11.4	11.8	11.2	10.0	10.2	10.5	13.4	11.2	10.5	11.1	1.01
9	10.8	9.2	11.4	12.0	10.2	10.4	9.4	10.5	11.2	10.6	10.6	0.86
10	12.0	11.3	11.9	11.6	10.3	12.5	12.0	12.4	11.0	10.3	11.5	0.79
11	12.5	9.1	9.6	10.4	9.3	10.8	12.9	14.2	11.0	10.0	11.0	1.70
12	12.4	13.4	14.0	12.6	11.3	11.5	10.8	10.2	10.5	11.8	11.9	1.25
13	11.3	11.6	11.2	12.2	11.2	10.7	10.4	12.8	11.2	11.0	11.4	0.70
14	10.8	13.1	11.2	11.8	11.5	11.7	9.8	10.5	10.0	12.6	11.3	1.07
15	10.8	12.6	11.3	9.4	13.0	11.5	10.7	10.2	12.2	11.8	11.4	1.11
16	11.4	10.2	11.4	9.4	13.0	10.8	9.4	11.2	11.5	13.6	11.2	1.37
17	10.6	11.2	9.8	11.2	12.0	10.2	11.9	10.3	10.2	10.9	10.8	0.74
18	11.4	12.2	11.8	12.7	11.7	12.6	11.5	10.7	10.2	13.6	11.8	0.99
19	10.7	10.5	9.7	10.5	11.6	10.2	10.2	11.4	10.7	10.0	10.6	0.59
20	11.3	9.0	11.2	10.4	14.0	11.2	11.5	10.1	13.0	11.4	11.3	1.41

$$\overline{X} = \frac{x_1 + x_2 + x_3 \ldots x_n}{n}$$

where

n = sample size (usually 10 or more)

The calculation for the first county in the health district is

$$\overline{X} = \frac{13.0 + 11.0 + 12.0 + 12.5 + \ldots 9.8}{10}$$

$$\overline{X} = 11.5 \text{ (prenatal care visits)}$$

Each $\overline{X}$ for the county in the health district is calculated in this manner. The results are displayed in Table 10–4.

• Calculate the s for each subgroup (rural county) using the following formula:

$$s = \sqrt{\frac{\sum_{i=1}^{i=n} (x_i - \bar{x})^2}{n - 1}}$$

The results of using this formula are also displayed in Table 10–4. The s for the first rural county is 1.36.

• Calculate the mean of the sample means ($\overline{\overline{X}}$).

$$\overline{\overline{X}} = \frac{\overline{X}_1 + \overline{X}_2 + \overline{X}_3 + \ldots \overline{X}_k}{k}$$

where

k = number of subgroups (counties) (20 in this sample)

Thus,

$$\overline{\overline{X}} = \frac{11.5 + 10.7 + 11.0 + 11.4 + \ldots 11.3}{20}$$

$$\overline{\overline{X}} = 11.2$$

• Calculate the mean of the sample standard deviation ($\overline{S}$).

$$\overline{S} = \frac{s_1 + s_2 + s_3 + \ldots s_k}{k}$$

Therefore,

$$\bar{S} = \frac{1.36 + 0.98 + 1.06 + \dots 1.41}{20}$$

$$\bar{S} = 1.1$$

- Calculate the control limits.
  1. $\bar{X}$ chart
     Center line

$$CL_{\bar{x}} = \bar{\bar{X}}$$

$$CL_{\bar{x}} = 11.2$$

Upper control limit

$$UCL_{\bar{x}} = \bar{\bar{X}} + A_3\bar{S}$$

$$UCL_{\bar{x}} = 11.2 + (0.975)(1.1)$$

$$UCL_{\bar{x}} = 11.2 + 1.0725$$

$$UCL_{\bar{x}} = 12.27$$

Lower control limit

$$LCL_{\bar{x}} = \bar{\bar{X}} - A_3\bar{S}$$

$$LCL_{\bar{x}} = 11.2 - (0.975)(1.1)$$

$$LCL_{\bar{x}} = 11.2 - 1.0725$$

$$LCL_{\bar{x}} = 10.13$$

  2. s chart
     Center line

$$CL_s = \bar{S}$$

$$CL_s = 1.1$$

upper control limit

$$UCL_s = B_4 \bar{S}$$

$$UCL_s = (1.716)(1.1)$$

$$UCL_s = 1.89$$

lower control limit

$$LCL_s = B_3 \bar{S}$$

$$LCL_s = (0.284)(1.1)$$

$$LCL_s = 0.31$$

As demonstrated earlier, A_3, B_3, and B_4 are coefficients that are determined by the size of the subgroups (Table 10–3). In this example, the subgroup size is 10.

- Using the CL, UCL, and LCL for the $\bar{X}$ and s, create the control charts by plotting the values (samples) and the limits on the chart (Figure 10–2).

  Therefore

$\bar{X}$ (average)	S (standard deviation)
$CL_{\bar{x}} = 11.2$	$CL_s = 1.1$
$UCL_{\bar{x}} = 12.27$	$UCL_s = 1.89$
$LCL_{\bar{x}} = 10.13$	$LCL_s = 0.31$

- Evaluate the pattern.
  1. no points out of control
- Apply the rules for detecting special causes.

$\tilde{X}$ AND R CHART (MEDIAN AND RANGE)

In situations in which the need is to produce a "quick picture" of a public health program in reference to understanding the process of the information collected or to simplify the manual effort in constructing a control chart, a median ($\tilde{X}$) and range (R) chart is used. Median charts are produced and calculated similarly to mean charts except the standard error of the sample median is used.

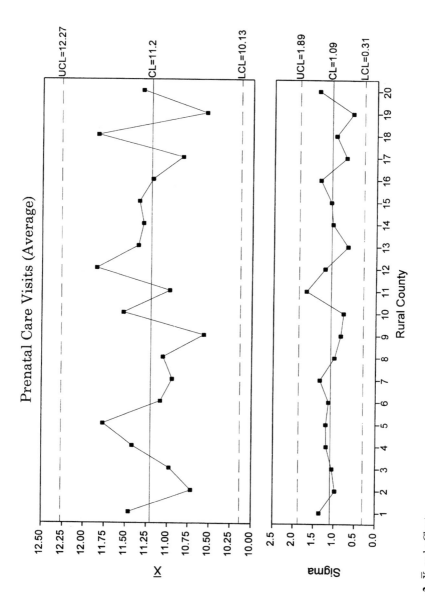

Figure 10-2 $\bar{X}$ and s Chart

Median and range control charts use the median as a measure of central location and the range as a measure of dispersion or process variability. These charts involve very little calculation to produce the normal dimensions of the control chart conditions. The median and range charts should always be replaced by the average and range or standard deviation charts when the skill and expertise are available. In a sense, the median and range charts can be considered a "public health practice screening tool" for early detection and prevention of a program process from getting out of control. In a practical sense the use of these charts requires minimal expertise and can be initially developed at all levels of the public health organization. Clerks, secretaries, administrative personnel, and field representatives can easily monitor their program responsibilities with these types of charts. Also individuals with advanced skills, statisticians, and managers should use this type of chart to evaluate outcomes.

Constructing $\tilde{X}$ and R Charts

The sampling distribution of the medians of the groups analyzed has a mean equal to the average of the median of the groups and a standard error that can be estimated using a coefficient. It may be important to recall that the assumption of normality is not necessary to interpret the standard error of the medians of the groups, and therefore, applying the rules for determining if a process is in control may follow the same assumptions as noted for $\overline{X}$ and R and $\overline{X}$ and s charts. However, to arrive at this point and to make the normality assumption, an Empirical Rule has been developed.[8*]

Basically, the rule states that control charts work well even if the data are not normally distributed.[9] This should address the concern that control charts may be used without the necessity for meeting the assumptions regarding the underlying distribution forms: normal, binomial, Poisson, etc.

The formulas for constructing the median and R charts are as follows:

- based on sample data ($\tilde{X}$)

$$\text{Center line, } CL_{\tilde{x}} = \overline{\overline{X}}$$

$$CL_{\tilde{x}} = \frac{\Sigma \tilde{X}}{k}$$

$$\text{Upper control limit, } UCL_{\tilde{x}} = \overline{\overline{X}} + A_6 \overline{R}$$

$$\text{Lower control limit, } LCL_{\tilde{x}} = \overline{\overline{X}} - A_6 \overline{R}$$

where

$\tilde{X}$ = sample median

$\bar{\tilde{X}}$ = average of the sample medians

k = number of subgroups

Σ = summation

$\bar{R}$ = average of the sample ranges

A_6 = factor used to calculate control limits (UCL, LCL) on a median chart based on the sample range

Thus, to calculate the values and construct a median and range chart, a coefficient (A_6) must be used. A_6 is a factor used to calculate the control limits and is based on the sample size per each subgroup (Table 10–5).

To construct the range part of the chart, the identical formula used in constructing the range (R) portion of the chart in the mean and range chart is used. The generic formula for the range is detailed in the previous section—mean and range chart.

---

[*] In enumerative studies, we often have the opportunity to know something more about the shape of our data. The data points may tend to follow one of a great variety of distributional forms such as the normal, chi square, exponential, uniform, binomial, Poisson, and triangular.

Unfortunately in analytic studies, we usually do not know the distributional form of historical data; there is no guarantee that the form will remain operational in the future. Nevertheless, it is unnecessary to assume that data are normally or otherwise distributed so that control charts work effectively.

W.A. Shewhart demonstrated that the means and standard deviations computed from 25 samples of four observations each drawn from normal, uniform, and triangular distribution all were within three standard errors of their respective means. In Shewhart's words, "In each case all of the points are within the limit as we should expect them to be under the controlled conditions supposed to exist in drawing these samples." (Shewhart, W.A. 1931. *Economic Control of Quality of Manufactured Product*. New York: Van Nostrand. p. 318).

Wheeler and Chambers expand on this point, arguing that "control charts work well even if the data are not normally distributed." (Wheeler, D.J., and D.S. Chambers. 1992. *Understanding Statistical Process Control*. 2d ed. Knoxville: SPC Press. p. 65) They state that when data from a process is stable" no matter how the data 'behave,' virtually all of the data will fall within three sigma units of the average." (Wheeler and Chambers, p. 65) Their Empirical Rule states that for a stable process, "Approximately 99% to 100% of the data will be located with a distance of three sigma units on either side to the average." (Wheeler and Chambers, p. 61) They go on to show that for six widely differing distributions, virtually all the means and ranges computed from samples of sizes 2, 4, and 10 fall within three standard errors of their respective means. Their results indicate that while the distribution of the measurements does affect the percentage falling outside the control limits, the actual effects are quite small. For Subgroup Averages the percentage outside the limits remains about 1% or less. For the Subgroup Ranges the percentage outside the control limits goes above 2% only for the Chi-Square and Exponential Distributions. (Wheeler and Chambers, p. 76)

This provides a very compelling argument for the use of control charts without the necessity for the assumptions regarding any underlying distributional forms.

Table 10–5 Constants for Use in Analyzing a Median Chart Using the Sample Range

Sample Size (n)	Control Factor Limits (A_6)
3	1.187
4	0.796
5	0.691
6	0.548
7	0.508
8	0.433
9	0.412
10	0.362

$\tilde{X}$ and R Chart—Infant Mortality

To understand the trends in infant mortality and assess this outcome measurement for several counties in a state health district over a period of five years or more (up to 10), a median and range control chart may be used. The question to be asked is, Has a special cause of variation caused the central tendency of this process ($\tilde{X}$) to change over the time period observed and has the special cause of variation caused the process distribution (R) to become more or less erratic?

The steps necessary to analyze the problems are

- Collect the data on infant mortality for 10 counties in a health district over a five-year period (1991–1995).

  Usually, for this type of chart, sample sizes are small, less than 10, because size alone is a factor in making the chart simple to construct and understand. Further, the data collected (i.e., the sample size) are generally odd numbers: three, five, seven, or nine. Even numbers require additional calculations to determine the median, not difficult but not really necessary if an odd number is sampled.

- Calculate the median $\tilde{X}$ for each subgroup.

$$\tilde{X} = \text{when } n \text{ is odd, take the middle number}$$

where

  n = sample size (usually fewer than 10)

The calculation for the first county median is

$$\tilde{X} = 15.3, 10.7, 14.2, 12.3, 12.1$$
$$\tilde{X} = 10.7, 12.1, 12.3, 14.2, 15.3$$
$$\tilde{X} = 12.3$$

The median for all the counties is noted in Table 10–6.
• Calculate the range (R) for each subgroup.

$$R = \text{the maximum value} - \text{the minimum value}$$

In our example, for county 1 the range is

$$R = 15.3 - 10.7$$
$$R = 4.6$$

The remainder of the values are noted in Table 10–6.
• Calculate the mean of the sample medians ($\bar{\tilde{X}}$).

$$\bar{\tilde{X}} = \frac{\tilde{X}_1 + \tilde{X}_2 + \tilde{X}_3 + \dots \tilde{X}_k}{k}$$

where

$\tilde{X}$ = the median for each subgroup
k = the number of subgroups (counties) (10 in this example)

Table 10–6 Infant Mortality Rates for a 10-County Area, 1991–1995

| | Years (Measurements) | | | | | Median | Range |
County	1991	1992	1993	1994	1995	($\tilde{X}$)	(R)
1	15.3	10.7	14.2	12.3	12.1	12.3	4.6
2	14.0	11.4	12.8	12.5	11.6	12.5	2.6
3	15.2	13.2	12.6	12.9	13.0	13.0	2.6
4	11.6	13.3	10.0	11.9	10.6	11.6	3.3
5	15.2	15.2	14.7	13.8	12.7	14.7	2.5
6	15.5	14.3	15.0	13.1	12.5	14.3	3.0
7	14.3	15.4	13.7	13.0	12.5	13.7	2.9
8	13.7	14.6	14.3	14.2	12.9	14.2	1.7
9	13.5	7.6	13.1	10.9	10.3	10.9	5.9
10	11.4	8.6	8.8	8.4	7.9	8.6	3.5

$\bar{\tilde{X}} = 12.58$ $\bar{R} = 3.26$

Thus,

$$\bar{\bar{X}} = \frac{12.3 + 12.5 + 13.0 + ...8.6}{10}$$

$$\bar{\bar{X}} = 12.58$$

• Calculate the mean of the sample ranges ($\bar{R}$).

$$\bar{R} = \frac{R_1 + R_2 + R_3 + ...R_k}{k}$$

Thus,

$$\bar{R} = \frac{4.6 + 2.6 + 2.6 + ...3.5}{10}$$

$$\bar{R} = 3.26$$

• Calculate the control limits.
  1. $\tilde{X}$ chart
     Central line

$$CL_{\tilde{x}} = \bar{\bar{X}}$$

$$CL_{\tilde{x}} = 12.58$$

Upper control limit

$$UCL_{\tilde{x}} = \bar{\bar{X}} + A_6\bar{R}$$

$$UCL_{\tilde{x}} = 12.58 + (0.691)(3.26)$$

$$UCL_{\tilde{x}} = 12.58 + 2.25$$

$$UCL_{\tilde{x}} = 14.83$$

Lower control limit

$$LCL_{\tilde{x}} = \bar{\bar{X}} - A_6\bar{R}$$

$$LCL_{\tilde{x}} = 12.58 - (0.691)(3.26)$$

$$\text{LCL}_{\tilde{x}} = 12.58 - 2.25$$

$$\text{LCL}_{\tilde{x}} = 10.33$$

A_6 is the coefficient used for $\tilde{X}$ chart and is determined by the size of the sample (Table 10–5).

2. Calculate the R chart.

Central line

$$\text{CL}_R = \tilde{R}$$

$$\text{CL}_R = 3.26$$

Upper control limit

$$\text{UCL}_R = D_4\bar{R}^*$$

$$\text{UCL}_R = (2.114)(3.26)$$

$$\text{UCL}_R = 6.89$$

Lower control limit

$$\text{LCL}_R = D_3\bar{R}^*$$

$$\text{LCL}_R = (0.0)(3.26)$$

$$\text{LCL}_R = 0 \text{ (zero)}$$

- Using the CL, UCL, and LCL for the $\tilde{X}$ (median) and the R (range), create the control charts by plotting the values (samples) and the limits on the chart (Figure 10–3).

Therefore,

$\tilde{X}$ (median)	R (range)
$\text{CL}_{\tilde{x}} = 12.58$	$\text{CL}_R = 3.26$
$\text{UCL}_{\tilde{x}} = 14.83$	$\text{UCL}_R = 6.89$
$\text{LCL}_{\tilde{x}} = 10.33$	$\text{LCL}_R = 0$

---

*As noted previously, D_4 and D_3 are coefficients that are determined by the size of the subgroups and are shown in Table 10–1.

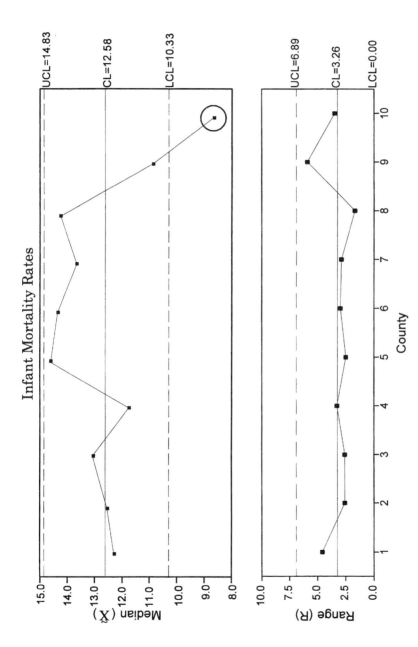

Figure 10–3 $\tilde{X}$ and R Chart

- Evaluate the pattern.
  1. median chart
     – one point outside the control limits
  2. range chart
     – no points out of control
- Apply the rules for detecting special causes.

The rules for detecting special causes were outlined earlier in this chapter, and they also apply to evaluating the pattern of variation for median and range charts. Notably, the five-year trends for the counties sampled are in control for the range chart, but one point outside the $LCL_{\bar{x}}$ suggests that the central tendency variation may be out of control. On closer examination, we see the infant mortality rate of 8.6 per 1,000 live births for county 10 is considered out of control. The public health analyst will realize that this county must be evaluated to determine what has created the unusually low rate, and further the reasons may need to be applied to other counties to bring them to a lower level. As one can see, the control chart may be used for determining low-risk areas that need to be emulated so impact may be made on the remainder of the higher-rate counties over the next period of observation. Also, note the range for this county (10) is in control, indicating that there has not been much change over the past five years in this rate, but yet it is still below the other nine counties.

$\overline{X}$ AND mR CHART (INDIVIDUAL AND MOVING RANGE)

When the data on a process for areas or time periods are obtained for extended periods or intervals and when subgrouping of data are not possible or effective, the data are plotted as individual categories and can be used for a control chart. Because there is only one subgroup, obviously an R (range) cannot be calculated; however, the moving range (mR) of the data may be used to calculate the control limits for X. This allows the analyst to calculate a moving range of up to 10 of the samples or subgroups. These charts are used to evaluate the central tendency of a process over time. Individual charts usually are used when measurements for the variable being investigated are expensive and it is not possible to have multiple samples. In public health practice, there are many situations in which individual measures are appropriate—mortality rates, morbidity rates, and natality rates.

To effectively use these charts, three cautions have been suggested.

1. Charts for individuals are not as sensitive in detecting process changes as $\overline{X}$ and R charts.
2. If process distribution is not symmetrical, care must be taken in interpretation.

3. Charts for individuals obviously do not relate to or isolate the repeatability of a process. For example, several measurements of weight loss in a primary prevention nutrition clinic for 50 women over a period of 6 months represents repeat measurement. If this type of measurement is desired or required, use the $\overline{X}$ and R chart.[10]

Constructing X and mR Charts

The formulas for producing an X and mR chart are as follows:

- Individual (X)

$$\text{Center line, } CL_X = \overline{X}$$

$$CL_X = \frac{\Sigma X}{k}$$

$$\text{Upper control limit, } UCL_X = \overline{X} + E_2 m\overline{R}$$

$$\text{Lower control limit, } LCL_X = \overline{X} - E_2 m\overline{R}$$

where
  X = individual measurement
  k = number of subgroups
  $\overline{X}$ = average of the individual subgroup measurements
  $m\overline{R}$ = average of the subgroups' moving range
  E_2 = a tabulated factor used to calculate the upper and lower control limits on an individual chart based on sample data
  Σ = summation

- moving range (mR)[*]

$$\text{Central line, } CL_{mR} = m\overline{R}$$

$$CL_{mR} = \frac{\Sigma mR}{k-1}$$

$$\text{Upper control limit, } UCL_{mR} = D_4 m\overline{R}$$

$$\text{Lower control limit, } LCL_{mR} = D_3 m\overline{R}$$

---

[*]When the moving range is based on two subgroups when calculating the CL, the denominator is $k-1$, if three subgroups are used the denominator is $k-2$, if four subgroups are used the denominator is $k-3$, and so forth.

where
  mR = moving range
  Σ = summation
  k = number of subgroups
  $m\bar{R}$ = average of the subgroups' moving range
  D_3 = tabulated factor used to calculate the LCL on a range chart based on sample data
  D_4 = tabulated factor used to calculate the UCL on a range chart based on sample data

The constants or coefficients for constructing an X and mR chart are provided in Table 10–7. The coefficients D_3, D_4, and E_2 are defined based on the subgroup size. In the case of the individual coefficient (E_2), it is possible to calculate an average moving range based on two or more subgroups but no more than 10 are recommended. That is, you may have many more subgroups than 10, but in calculating the moving range between the first number and the next number, the calculation should be limited to 10. For example, if you have 20 subgroups (i.e., years in this example), the moving range calculation should be limited to 10 or less. Thus, you could calculate a moving range value based on two-, three-, four-, or five-year intervals up to 10 but no greater.

Table 10–7 Table of Constants and Formulas for Control Charts

| | $\bar{X}$ and mR Charts | | | |
| Subgroup Size | Chart for Individuals (X) Factors for Control Limits | Charts for Ranges (R) Divisors for Estimate of Standard Deviation | Factors for Control Limits | |
n	E_2	d_2	D_3	D_4
2	2.660	1.128	—	3.267
3	1.772	1.693	—	2.574
4	1.457	2.059	—	2.282
5	1.290	2.326	—	2.114
6	1.184	2.534	—	2.004
7	1.109	2.704	0.076	1.924
8	1.054	2.847	0.136	1.864
9	1.010	2.970	0.184	1.816
10	0.975	3.078	0.223	1.777

Source: Copyright ASTM. Reprinted with permission.

X and mR Chart—Prenatal Care Example

In public health, it has been well documented that no or inadequate prenatal care can lead to poor birth outcomes, usually low birth weights. Of particular interest is the trend of no prenatal care over a period of time (i.e., has it improved or worsened and are there any special causes that may be related to the pattern of variation observed?). Thus, to calculate the number of births that occurred that had no prenatal care, an X and mR chart may be used. The data in this instance represent a 17-year period in a health district for the percentage of women who had no prenatal care during pregnancy (Table 10–8). The purpose of this analysis is to evaluate the central tendency over time. More specifically, has there been any change in the pattern that may lead to identifying a special cause? If not, are we satisfied with the pattern we observe or do we need to look at common causes and suggest ways to improve this pattern in our attempts to provide CQI and improve the outcome?

Table 10–8 No Prenatal Care Visits for One County, 1979–1995

Year (k)	No Care (n)	MR
1979	9.0	—
1980	8.0	1.0
1981	8.3	0.3
1982	8.4	0.1
1983	6.0	2.4
1984	5.4	0.6
1985	8.7	3.3
1986	11.2	2.5
1987	11.2	0.0
1988	11.0	0.2
1989	12.0	1.0
1990	13.4	1.4
1991	16.5	3.1
1992	13.8	2.7
1993	12.0	1.8
1994	10.7	1.3
1995	8.7	2.0
TOTAL	174.3	23.7
	$\bar{X} = 10.25$	$m\bar{R} = 1.48$

k = subgroups; n = sample.

The steps necessary to analyze this problem are

- Collect the data on prenatal care for the time period observed (1979–1995) and for the geographic area investigated (i.e., a state, district, county, etc.). Sample size is one, but there may be several subgroups.
- Calculate the moving range (mR).

$$mR = |(\text{measured value}_i) - (\text{measured value}_{i-1})|$$

where
i = observation

The calculation for the first observation is

$$mR = |(8.0) - (9.0)|$$

$$mR = 1$$

The mR value is calculated in the same manner for all observations in the sample (Table 10–8).

- Calculate the ($\overline{X}$) of the sample values.

$$\overline{X} = \frac{X_1 + X_2 + X_3 + \dots X_k}{k}$$

$$\overline{X} = \frac{9.0 + 8.0 + 8.3 + \dots 8.7}{17}$$

$$\overline{X} = 10.25$$

- Calculate the average of the moving range ($\overline{mR}$).

$$\overline{mR} = \frac{\Sigma mR}{k-1}$$

$$\overline{mR} = \frac{R_1 + R_2 + R_3 + \dots R_k}{k-1}$$

$$\overline{mR} = \frac{1 + 0.3 + 0.1 + \dots 2.0}{16}$$

$$\overline{mR} = 1.48$$

- Calculate the control limits.

1. X chart
   Center line

$$CL_X = \bar{X}$$

$$CL_X = 10.25$$

   Upper control limit

$$UCL_X = \bar{X} + E_2 m\bar{R}$$

$$UCL_X = 10.25 + (2.66)(1.48)$$

$$UCL_X = 10.25 + 3.94$$

$$UCL_X = 14.19$$

   Lower control limit

$$LCL_X = \bar{X} - E_2 m\bar{R}$$

$$LCL_X = 10.25 - (2.66)(1.48)$$

$$LCL_X = 10.25 - 3.94$$

$$LCL_X = 6.31$$

E_2 is the coefficient used for the X chart in association with the mR chart and is defined by the size of the sample. In this case, the sample size or subgroup is two, given we use two observations (samples or subgroups) to calculate the moving range (Table 10–7). In this type of control chart, n (sample size) and k (subgroup size) are identical because there is only one sample per one subgroup. This does not mean the values are the same; it means that there is one sample for every one subgroup.

2. mR chart
   Center line

$$CL_{mR} = m\bar{R}$$

$$CL_{mR} = 1.48$$

Upper control limit

$$\text{UCL}_{\text{mR}} = D_4 m\bar{R}$$

$$\text{UCL}_{\text{mR}} = (3.27)(1.48)$$

$$\text{UCL}_{\text{mR}} = 4.84$$

Lower control limit

$$\text{LCL}_{\text{mR}} = D_3 m\bar{R}$$

$$\text{LCL}_{\text{mR}} = (0)(1.48)$$

$$\text{LCL}_{\text{mR}} = 0 \text{ (zero)}$$

As we noted in the last discussion on $\tilde{X}$ and R charts, the constants of D_4 and D_3 were used to determine the control limits. Because this is a form of the R chart, the coefficients for D_4 and D_3 are also used in this situation and are based on the size of the subgroup sample. In this instance, the subgroup size is two because we used two observations to calculate each moving range. If we used three, four, or five observations to calculate the moving range, then the subgroup size would also have been three, four, or five, respectively.

- Using the CL, UCL, and LCL for the X and mR (individual and moving range) chart, create the control charts by plotting the values (samples) and the limits on the chart (Figure 10–4).

    Therefore,

X (individual)	mR (moving range)
$\text{CL}_\text{X} = 10.25$	$\text{CL}_{\text{mR}} = 1.48$
$\text{UCL}_\text{X} = 14.19$	$\text{UCL}_{\text{mR}} = 4.84$
$\text{LCL}_\text{X} = 6.31$	$\text{LCL}_{\text{mR}} = \text{zero}$

- Evaluate the pattern.
    1. X (individual chart)
        −two points outside the LCL
        −one point outside the UCL
    2. mR (moving range chart)
        −no points out of control
- Apply the rules for detecting special causes.

    The same rules apply for detecting special causes as were used for the previous charts discussed in this chapter. However, there are a few issues that

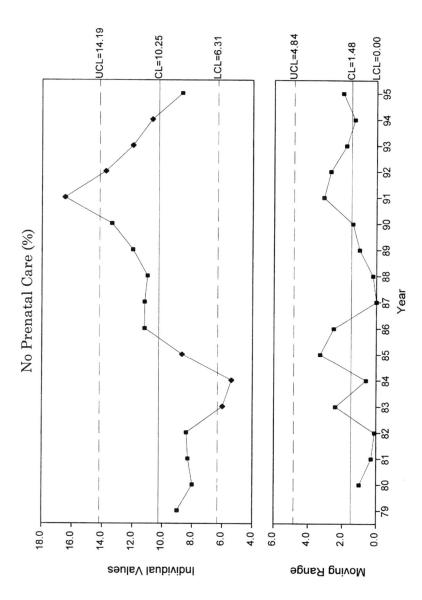

Figure 10-4 X and mR Chart

may have an effect on the interpretation of the pattern of variation. For example, successive moving ranges are correlated, because they have at least one point in common (this would be the minimum number—there could be more). Thus, care must be taken in interpreting trends.

Further, if the process distribution for the sampled data in the individual (X) chart is not symmetrical, then the rules outlined previously may give signals of special causes when none exist. However, the overall effect is almost trivial because, as we noted previously, the Empirical Rule has shown the distribution has little or no effect on the outcome of the control chart interpretation. Remember interpretation is based on values outside standard deviation limits and variation of patterns within the control limits. In our example, it is clear there were two continuous years in which the percentage of no prenatal care was extremely low (special causes), but from 1984 to 1991 there was a steady overall increase to the point where another point is outside the limits (special cause) where the no-prenatal-care rate was beyond the process data limits. This steady increase until 1991 began to turn down during the past five years. The public health analyst now has the option to investigate the two years when low rates of no prenatal care existed for determining improvement variables and obviously to investigate year 1991 for detecting variables that worsened the outcome. Clearly, this use of control charts puts into perspective the pattern of variation in terms of its importance in interpretation by realizing that several points out of control create opportunities on one hand and risks on the other, as opposed to just describing the pattern. What happened in this county during these out-of-control years to produce these results? Now we have a basis for a targeted investigation and hope that we will learn why these patterns occurred so they may be emulated or rejected based on the special causes.

USES OF CONTROL CHARTS

Four variables control charts in this chapter and four attribute control charts in the previous chapter were examined in detail. Clearly, control charts reflect these two broad categories: variables and attributes. In each case, an outcome indicator was investigated (e.g., low birth weight, infant mortality, immunization visit times, and prenatal care) that was measured and then examined. Most important to public health practitioners is to understand why quality improvement methods are used to measure typical health status indicators as defined, to a large degree, by the Year 2000 objectives. In general, control charts are used to

- Evaluate the past.

To evaluate the history of the process for an outcome variable provides some significant insights into public health programs. A retrospective examination of a completed process using control charts answers the question of whether the process for the outcome investigated has been in statistical control. In fact, were decisions based on evidence of statistical control or were the decisions based on the blips in a data set that best support the program position? Certainly, a lack of control (special cause variation) is indicated by applying the tests for detecting special causes. If no special cause is identified, then the retrospective examination could be used for reporting evidence-based results, providing we are content with the trends that the process presented.

• Evaluate the present.

To evaluate the present state of the process for an outcome variable provides some immediate insight into the variation of programs measurement. A cross-sectional examination of a process in progress can be used to generate a signal in the "now" sense of evaluation and whether the program indicator is being measured and/or evaluated as expected. In public health, this real-time evaluation is usually more difficult because many of the outcome indicators are "slow movers" and do not reflect rapid signals of change. However, our definition of present may be adjusted to account for this. The issue is, in any event, that by evaluating the present an intervention may be implemented to retrack the process if indicated. Thus, in this sense, control charts are extremely useful in monitoring the existing state of a process for the outcome characteristic. Further, public health practitioners must expand their "measurement concepts" to include more frequent measurement for many programs and not rely on only two- to five-year measurement horizons. Certainly, in some cases weekly and/or monthly measurements are critical.

• Predict the near future.[11]

To predict the near-future state of a process is a significant responsibility of public health experts. Obviously, to know the past and to maintain the present measurement is important, but to project the future of these outcome characteristics is where public health experts can make the most significant statement. A prospective examination of the program using control charts aids in the ability to predict the near-future condition of an outcome indicator. This is clearly based on statistical evidence of a process's stability and knowledge concerning conditions that could affect the process. The public health practitioner, in this instance, has a tool that is critical to the improvement of public health locally and globally.

For example, if an outcome indicator being evaluated using a control chart shows a stable process and further evaluation by the expert suggests no future source of special cause variations, then the logical conclusion is that the process (outcome indicator) will remain stable in the near future (i.e., no change). Now, curiously what if teenage pregnancy rates are being evaluated (no special cause identified) and there is no movement (no change)? Then unless the common causes are evaluated there will be no change or improvement in the program. Public health, if we want to base our policies and assessments on evidence, now can begin to redirect, provide different interventions, or adapt new policies to pursue future positive change. Of course, if things are progressing forward, then the tools are in place for this conclusion to be expressed also.

Gulezian has suggested additional uses for and/or benefits to the use of quality improvement measurement control charts for program improvement. They are

- to establish what the process is doing
- to determine what the process can do
- to determine whether the process is doing what you want it to do
- to help in deciding whether additional data or charts should be used
- to determine whether to leave a process alone or to make adjustments
- to diagnose a process and decide when to look for special and/or common causes or make adjustments to the process
- to establish the magnitude of inherent or natural variability
- to decide whether to continue using a particular process or whether to change the system or program design
- to become a reference point or basis for continued process improvement.[12]

CONCLUSION

A control chart is a simple graphical device used to observe and monitor the distribution of parameters of outcome measurements to determine change. Specifically, the charts presented in this chapter (variables control charts) are provided to the public health practice field to provide the following:

- for managing the process (i.e., managing the program)
- for analyzing the process using process data (analyzing trends with indicators)
- for detecting if the process is in control based on a standard (Year 2000 objective or other locally defined target) using statistical analysis

The four charts detailed are based on satisfying normal distribution assumptions, but as noted this was not essential to the evaluation based on using the

Empirical Rule. Table 10–9 summarizes the four charts ($\overline{X}$ and R, $\overline{X}$ and s, $\tilde{X}$ and R, and X and mR) in terms of center line, upper control limit, and lower control limit, including sample size requirements and statistical models for evaluation in public health programs. The applications of these charts for public health practice are used to monitor (manage) a process, to analyze a process (in/out of control), and to improve the performance of the outcome indicator over time by studying variation and potentially identifying the cause of this variation. Brassard and Ritter have stated the use and application of these control chart tools. In public health, the application and use of these tools do the following for accomplishing the objectives of the core public health functions of assessment, policy development, and assurance:

- focus attention on detecting and monitoring process variation over time
- distinguish special from common causes of variation, as a guide to local or management action
- serve as a tool for ongoing control of a process
- help improve a process to perform consistently and predictably for higher quality, lower cost, and higher effectiveness
- provide a common language for discussing process performance[13]

Finally, in summary a few "tips" are appropriate for assessing proper use and application of these charts in public health practice. The tips are

- "Control" does not mean that the process of the outcome indicator is what you want it to be—it only means that the process is controlled—could be consistently good or bad. Control is different than targets—do not confuse these two. Targets are the objectives (Year 2000) and are related to customers in our communities, our public, and are not related to the variation of the process.
- Points outside the limits are considered to be out of control—remove the special cause and recalculate the charts (a recalculation example is not provided in this book). Also, look for rules detecting special causes based on the pattern of points within the control limits.
- If a chart is in control (naturally or due to removal of special causes), new data must be put on a new chart. *DO NOT* recalculate the limits. Recalculate only after desired change has occurred.
- Nothing changes just because a chart has been created—you must do something—the chart is the signal to *ACT.*

Most of the charts applied in this chapter have been presented from a temporal point of view; however, in some instances subgroups can be defined as clinics,

Table 10–9 Summary—Variables Control Charts for Public Health Practice

Type	Center Line	Upper Control Limit	Lower Control Limit	Sample Size	Model for Statistical Evaluation
$\bar{X}$ and R chart	$\bar{\bar{X}} = \dfrac{(\bar{X}_1 + \bar{X}_2 + \dots \bar{X}_k)}{k}$ $\bar{R} = \dfrac{(R_1 + R_2 + \dots R_k)}{k}$	$UCL_{\bar{x}} = \bar{\bar{X}} + A_2\bar{R}$ $UCL_R = D_4\bar{R}$	$LCL_{\bar{x}} = \bar{\bar{X}} - A_2\bar{R}$ $LCL_R = D_3\bar{R}$	<10, but usually 3 to 5	Normal
$\bar{X}$ and s chart	$\bar{\bar{X}} = \dfrac{(\bar{X}_1 + \bar{X}_2 + \dots \bar{X}_k)}{k}$ $\bar{S} = \dfrac{(s_1 + s_2 + \dots s_k)}{k}$	$UCL_{\bar{x}} = \bar{\bar{X}} + A_3\bar{S}$ $UCL_s = B_4\bar{S}$	$LCL_{\bar{x}} = \bar{\bar{X}} - A_3\bar{S}$ $LCL_s = B_3\bar{S}$	Usually ≥10	Normal
$\tilde{X}$ and R chart	$\bar{\tilde{X}} = \dfrac{(\tilde{X}_1 + \tilde{X}_2 + \dots \tilde{X}_k)}{k}$ $\bar{R} = \dfrac{(R_1 + R_2 + \dots R_k)}{k}$	$UCL_{\tilde{x}} = \bar{\tilde{X}} + A_6\bar{R}$ $UCL_R = D_4\bar{R}$	$UCL_{\tilde{x}} = \bar{\tilde{X}} - A_6\bar{R}$ $UCL_R = D_3\bar{R}$	<10, but usually 3 or 5	Normal
X and mR chart	$\bar{X} = (X_1 + X_2 + \dots X_k)$ $m\bar{R} = \dfrac{(R_1 + R_2 + \dots R_k)}{k-1}$	$UCL_x = \bar{X} + E_2 m\bar{R}$ $UCL_{mR} = D_4 m\bar{R}$	$UCL_x = \bar{X} - E_2 m\bar{R}$ $UCL_{mR} = D_3 m\bar{R}$	1	Normal

hospitals, counties, etc. The next chapter looks at small area analysis tools and how those methods can be used in understanding the CQI process from a geographic or spatial point of view.

NOTES

1. G.W. Snedecor and W.G. Cochran, *Statistical Methods*, 7th ed. (Ames, IA: Iowa State University Press, 1980), 17.

2. L.S. Nelson, "Control Charts: Rational Subgroups and Effective Applications," *Journal of Quality Technology* 20, 1 (1988): 73–75.

3. The Automotive Division of the American Society for Quality Control Supplier Quality Requirements Task Force (ASQC) and the Automotive Industry Action Group (AIAG), *Fundamental Statistical Process Control: Reference Manual* (Troy, MI: 1991), 18.

4. Ibid.

5. D.J. Wheeler and D.S. Chambers, *Understanding Statistical Process Control*, 2d ed (Knoxville, TN: SPC Press, 1992), 237–249.

6. ASQC/AIAG, *Fundamental Statistical Process Control*, 161–183.

7. H. Gitlow et al., *Quality Management: Tools and Methods for Improvement*, 2d ed. (Burr Ridge, IL: Irwin, 1995), 232–249.

8. Ibid., 255.

9. Ibid., 99.

10. ASQC/AIAG, *Fundamental Statistical Process Control*, 75.

11. Gitlow et al., *Quality Management,* 139–140.

12. R. Gulezian, *Process Control: Statistical Principles and Tools* (New York: QualityAlert Institute, 1991), 165.

13. M. Brassard and D. Ritter, *The Memory Jogger II* (Methuen, MA: GOAL/QPC, 1994), 36.

Chapter 11

Outcome Assessment: Small Area Analysis and Quality Improvement Methods

In public health practice, there is a high demand for assessing—a core public function—the needs of a community from an epidemiologic perspective. Traditionally, there has been a keen interest in using small area analysis, mainly in response to the pressure from federal agencies to monitor the progress of a community toward the Year 2000 objectives. Further, and a more recent development, is the need to develop data systems that will allow effective outcome assessment and quality improvement measurement of a program, community, county, or a customer. Associated with this type of measurement in public health practice is the need to analyze information effectively that represents small areas. To do this public health practitioners need to understand epidemiologic measurement as discussed in Chapter 5 and additionally understand how to analyze communities from a quality improvement perspective using small area analysis (SAA).

A review of the literature reveals two major, almost parallel, uses of small area analysis:

1. small area analysis of epidemiologic data in performing widespread needs assessments
2. small area analysis of community level variations in hospital admissions for various medical and surgical conditions (i.e., variation in hospital utilization statistics)

The *epidemiologic needs assessment approach* using small area analysis dates back to the time of Hippocrates but is probably best recognized with the 1854 analysis of cholera deaths by John Snow in the Soho district of London, England.[1] Of course, this approach of epidemiologic needs assessment is prevalent and very popular in the SAA of health planning, disease investigation, demographic analysis, and indicator profiling providing quality of life reports. All approaches tend to rely heavily on mapping and other geographic methods to display the small area data.

The *hospitalization utilization approach* using small area analysis was reported as early as 1856 by a physician in London (William A. Guy). He noted that annual rates for hospitalization varied from 325 per 1,000 population to 1 per 1,000 population. He hypothesized that the explanation for the variation in use rates between the two areas was related to behavioral characteristics of the populations, specifically to "acts of self indulgence."[2] In the modern era, the study by Coger in 1938 on tonsillectomy is recognized as the landmark report. Of course, now the issues of costs, quality improvement, medical outcomes, and consumer demands have propelled this type of analysis forward.[3]

WHAT IS SMALL AREA ANALYSIS?

Small area analysis is a method of measuring variations and comparing rates of mortality, morbidity, and health care use cost among defined populations.[4] Because considerable variation in mortality, morbidity, and hospital use has been found to exist among small communities, which is often masked when analyzing larger geographic areas, a need to have appropriate statistical/epidemiologic/quality improvement tools is important to proper assessment of public health practices. These tools may be used to address these variations and to determine the significance of the differences and further to monitor these areas over periods of time for variation. Thus, small area analysis identifies variations (differences) in the use (rate) of inpatient hospital services, mortality data, and social, economic, demographic, and psychographic factors, showing those rates in defined small areas (market areas). Each service area (county, city, zip code, census tract, or health market area) rate can be compared with other small areas or the state rate, providing information that could be lost or hidden if only state rates were analyzed.

The data usually have been age and sex adjusted, meaning that any differences cannot be attributed to age or sex. Sometimes such adjustments can obscure age/sex variations when small areas are compared. To use the methods and techniques for small area analysis effectively, there are some simple yet important concepts to know for analyzing small areas.

SIMPLE CONCEPTS IMPORTANT TO KNOW FOR SMALL AREA ANALYSIS

Table 11–1 presents several concepts that must be evaluated by the public health practitioner who takes on the task of quality improvement measurement

Table 11–1 Simple Concepts Important To Know for Quality Improvement Measurement for Small Area Analysis

NUMERATOR	vs.	DENOMINATOR
• Cases (morbidity) • Deaths (mortality) • Visits (utilization)		• Population-at-risk • Service area

NUMBERS	vs.	RATES
• Allocation of resources		• Assessment of health status

SMALL NUMBERS	vs.	LARGE NUMBERS

• Large error, statistically unreliable aggregate:
  ○ Space (geographics)
  ○ Time (years, months, etc.)
  ○ Groups (ages, socioeconomic)
• Identify trends
		• Statistically reliable trends
		• Area comparisons

SIGNIFICANT	vs.	NONSIGNIFICANT
• Clinical vs. statistical • Programmatic vs. statistical		• Sample size too small

SERVICE AREA	vs.	MARKET AREA
• Where *do* patients come from		• Where *should* patients come from

COMMUNITY HEALTH STATUS	vs.	INDIVIDUAL HEALTH STATUS
• Populations in communities • Community diagnosis		• Individuals in clinics • Clinical diagnosis

PROGRAM IMPACT—EVALUATION*	vs.	COMMUNITY IMPACT—EVALUATION*

Must determine the difference between:

1. Program-based evaluation 2. Service-based evaluation	vs.	1. Community-based evaluation 2. Population-based evaluation

*Cannot infer that the program was responsible for improvement in community indicators.

and outcome assessment for small area analysis. Although these concepts are simplistic, they are essential to performing a valid analysis of small areas.

- the numerator/denominator concept

    The numerator/denominator concept is of paramount importance to population-based analysis for small areas. Obviously, the numerator provides counts that may be translated into rates using the appropriate denominator (population-at-risk). Quality improvement measurement in public health practice must understand the nature of a program service-oriented denominator (all patients in the program or clinic) versus a community-based population-oriented denominator (total population in a service area or population-at-risk). When making decisions for improvement in an indicator, public health practitioners must be responsible and report results based on the appropriate target population and use the correct denominator.

- numbers versus rates

The relationships of numbers to rates at first glance seem rather obvious as to their differences in terms of use. However, public health analysts need to be aware that there is a place for both of these values. Specifically, if one is most concerned about resource allocation, then the actual number of events to be addressed must be known because each event would require a certain dollar amount, amount of space, or personnel time. However, if the concern is about the relative health status of one community compared with another, the rates are essential to standardize the comparison for further evaluation. You may recall in the chapter on control charts for attributes that there were occasions for using the counts and occasions for using the rates, depending on the specifics of the chart used.

- small numbers versus large numbers

Small numbers versus large numbers, of course, is the primary issue concerning the analysis of small areas. Notably, small numbers produce large errors and are usually statistically unreliable compared with large numbers, which generally produce statistically reliable trends. The methods described in Chapter 8 based on the binomial and Poisson distributions were presented to deal with the issue of small numbers (counts) in quality improvement. In this chapter, we further make use of the binomial and Poisson distributions to evaluate small areas from a quality improvement perspective. To avoid or compensate for the small number problems, it is customary to aggregate the data by geography (i.e., combining two or more small areas), time (analyzing several time periods or using a three- or five-year moving average), or groups (age, socioeconomic, etc., may be combined to produce a larger number). Further, as proposed in Chapter 7 on the evaluation of runs in a run chart, which is essentially monitoring a trend, the chart becomes an essential tool for public health practitioners whenever small numbers are being evaluated.

- significance versus nonsignificance

A result, if significant or nonsignificant, is usually evaluated by statistical tests. Several tests can determine the significance of numbers for small geographic areas. However, the real issue is the importance of this statistically significant difference in terms of clinical and programmatic policy. The evaluations of all statistical tests must be further evaluated for policy implications—clinically and programmatically. In small area analysis, this is especially true, because small numbers may produce significant results but the confidence limits (control limits as expressed in Chapters 9 and 10) provide the range or interval, which in the case of small numbers may be so wide as to be of no practical value, except to alert the analyst to a potential invalid evaluation.

• service areas versus market areas

The concept of a service area versus a market area is seldom considered as an issue by the public health analyst. In the era of managed care and quality improvement, these terms take on a significant meaning. As public health analysts apply the public health core functions of assessment, policy development, and assurance within their agencies, they must understand that a service area (where do patients come from) and a market area (where should patients come from) is different from a population-based area, which includes both a service area and a market area. In other words, public health is concerned primarily with the population-at-risk for defining needs of a program; however, hospitals have almost always been concerned with service areas and market areas. The future for public health is in the understanding of all these areas because managed care providers are most interested in population-based analysis, and public health agencies at present control many of the data for developing population-based indicators. Managed care providers are desperately seeking to get a handle on this type of information. As a result, public health may be well positioned to meet the needs in the area of managed care and quality improvement.

• individual focus to community (population-based) focus

As discussed in an earlier chapter, there has been a shift away from the individual focus of clients in clinics to the community- or population-based focus of populations in communities. Public health practice has been responsible for assessing the community health status by completing a community diagnosis (population-in-communities) report on the health status of areas. However, as public health shifted into clinical programs (individuals-in-clinics), the health status measurement of individuals was attempted. The result was that very feeble efforts were attempted to evaluate the status of individuals in programs and certainly could be considered as one of the factors contributing to the present disarray of public health. However, public health in the future is well positioned to focus on the population-based assessments and fulfill the core functions of public health.

• program impact versus community impact

Finally, program impact evaluation as opposed to community impact evaluation has been used inappropriately as suggesting impact on both sides of the spectrum—program and community. Traditionally, public health programs have made the inference that if community indicators have improved then the program was responsible. However, there is not always proof available to document this situation. We must, however, begin to evaluate the program that is service-based using proper numerators and denominators to determine if the program has had any influence on improving outcomes. This is not to say the program has not had an effect, but assuming credit for improvement is not based on evidence. Future endeavors, if public health stays in the program business, must be evaluated from the program perspective using program cases (numerators) and program denominators. Of course, public health must continue to evaluate communities and assess change and improvement. The purpose of this book is to bring the appropriate tools to the practice of public health so that quality improvement measurement can become part of the skills advanced and applied by the public health practitioner.

The understanding of the concepts discussed above allows for a more realistic use and application of the statistical tests for small area analysis. In quality improvement, the traditional tools (control charts) are used to understand the variation of a process, and the small area analysis concepts and tools are used to also understand the variation of the characteristic being evaluated but further to determine the significance of the variation based on confidence limits of a count, rate, proportion, ratio, or index. Obviously, the two approaches are almost identical. If one is more concerned with the process over time, the traditional quality improvement tools (control charts) are used, and if one is mostly concerned with process variation in space or geography, then using small area analysis is another tool for quality improvement measurement. No matter the viewpoint, the intent or purpose must be to continuously monitor the situation, hold the gains, and improve the outcomes or process. Using small area analysis as a quality improvement tool must likewise become the skill of the new public health scientist; evaluating small areas (census tracts, ZIP codes, blocks, counties, etc.) is crucial to quality improvement measurement. Obviously, the spatial pattern over time will exhibit characteristics that may be high risk or low risk and, therefore, must be monitored to demonstrate improvement either based on a Year 2000 standard or an objective (such as used in quality assurance) or based on a continuous quality improvement (CQI) model in which no matter if certain geographic areas have met the objective there is always room for continuous improvement in the indicator. A first step toward this process is to know what is expected based on a standard or a predetermined value identified from a specific process (i.e., we know for infant mortality the Year 2000 objective is 7 infant deaths per 1,000 live births—that is a standard; however, an analysis of 15 small areas revealed an infant mortality of 16 infant deaths per 1,000 live births, which is a value based on the process. In both instances, we apply the small area analysis methods to determine the pattern of variation and to see if any of the areas can be determined to be out of control and, thereby, represent a special cause that must be investigated.). Initially, however, the evaluation of small areas must determine the number of expected events (deaths, cases, utilization, etc.) to occur in the area investigated. This concept of determining the number of expected events may also be used in the evaluation of control charts if the process is evaluated against a standard. However, control charts generally evaluate the outcome indicator based on the process and therefore focus on the CQI of the outcome that continues to evaluate levels beyond a standard.

DETERMINING THE NUMBER OF EXPECTED EVENTS

Each of the following two methodologies is statistically valid for small area analysis and should produce the same results. The selection of one methodology over the other, therefore, depends solely on the availability of data and personal preference. The examples provided here are based on determining the number of expected deaths; however, for detecting the number of expected cases for use related to utilization rates, the same methods may apply.

Using the Actual Number of Deaths (Events)

The expected number of deaths can be calculated using the following formula:

$$E = \frac{P_1}{P_2} \times D$$

where
E = expected deaths
P_1 = population being investigated
P_2 = standard population
D = actual deaths in standard population

The ratio, P_1/P_2, should be age-sex-race specific. If the subject is deaths among white men aged 55 to 64, both P_1 and P_2 should refer to the number of white men of these ages; however, if deaths among the overall population are being studied, P_1 and P_2 should refer to the total population.

For example, in a state between 1990 and 1994 there were 52 deaths from fires and flames among men aged 60 to 64. There were 113,128 men of this age in the state; 4,055 were in the city being investigated. Assuming that the risk of dying in a fire was the same in the city as in the state as a whole, the expected number of deaths in the city was calculated as follows:

$$E = \frac{P_1}{P_2} \times D$$

$$E = \frac{4,055}{113,128} \times 52$$

$$E = 1.9 \text{ deaths}$$

Thus, 1.9 (rounded to 2) is the expected number of such deaths in the city among men aged 60 to 64. There were three actual deaths because of fires and flames in the city being investigated, a difference of one death.

Using Death Rates

If, instead of the actual number of deaths (events), death rates are available for the standard population, the expected number of deaths is given by

$$E = P_1 \times M_2$$

where
P_1 = population being investigated
M_2 = specific death rate in the standard population

Because $M_2 = \dfrac{D}{P_2}$, it can be seen that this is algebraically equivalent to the previous method.

Using Death Rates—An Example

Situation: In Burke County, Georgia (small area), the acute myocardial infarction (AMI) rate for 1985–1994 is 147.0 per 100,000 population, representing 306 deaths. The rate in the standard population (Georgia—1985–1994) is 107.9 per 100,000 population.

Solution: $E = P_1 \times M_2$

$$E = 208,224 \times \left(\frac{107.9}{100,000}\right)$$

$$E = 208,224 \times 0.001079$$

$$E = 224.7$$

where E = expected deaths
P_1 = 208,224 (1985–1994 population for Burke County)
M_2 = 107.9 (AMI rate for Georgia)

Thus, we would expect 224.7 deaths in Burke County during 1985–1994 for AMI, and we actually had observed 306 deaths during 1985–1994.

Significance of "Excess Deaths" or "Excess Events"

A problem may also be defined by an excess of morbidity or mortality (i.e., use rate problems or epidemiology/needs assessment problems). In an analysis of "excess deaths," for example, there are two major steps. Initially, it must be determined whether there is a difference between the number of deaths expected and the number that actually occurred (observed). If so, it must be determined whether the excess deaths result merely from chance or are actually significant statistically. This analysis may require the following data on both the population being investigated and the standard population:

- demographic data categorized by age, sex, race, occupation, or other specifics
- mortality data categorized by cause of death, either in actual number observed or in death rates

As we have already noted, if death rates are available for the selected standard population, the expected number of deaths can be derived for the population being investigated.

Testing the Significance of Results (Excess Deaths/Events)

Once the difference between the expected and the observed (actual) deaths has been determined, a statistical test must be applied to determine whether the difference has any significance. If so, a greater than expected number of deaths is not likely to be the result of chance alone; however, there is always a possibility that a certain number of events in 100 could have occurred solely on the basis of chance. The variables control charts discussed in Chapter 10 were based on the same probability by using the normal distribution as the probability model. However, remember that in the use of the control chart, the assumption of normality was not necessary.

The significance of a difference may be tested by means of standardized mortality ratios (SMRs), which are developed and tested using the standard error and confidence intervals, or the chi square "goodness-of-fit" test. Although each of these methods is statistically sound for this purpose, public health analysts with limited statistical backgrounds generally find the SMR easier to use. It requires more subjective judgment in interpreting the results, whereas the chi square test is somewhat more complex and may require some statistical expertise.

Standardized Mortality Ratio

SMR is calculated as follows:

$$\text{SMR} = \frac{\text{Observed deaths}}{\text{Expected deaths}} \times 100$$

A ratio of 100 indicates that the observed number of deaths equals the expected number of deaths. A ratio of 130, for example, indicates that there were 30 percent more deaths than expected; a ratio of 90 indicates 10 percent fewer deaths than expected.

The next step is to calculate the confidence interval of the SMR. The calculation of a 95 percent confidence interval of an SMR is obtained by

$$\text{CI} = \text{SMR} \pm (1.96 \times \text{SE})$$

where

SE = standard error

$$\text{SE} = \frac{\text{SMR}}{\sqrt{d}}$$

d = number of observed deaths

Data on observed and expected deaths in a county, as compared with a state, are presented in Table 11–2. The SMR is 89.97 or rounded to 90 and the SE is 5.58. The resulting confidence interval is 79 to 101. To interpret the confidence interval of an SMR, the following is suggested:

- If the lower confidence limit is below 100 and the upper limit is above 100, there is no significant difference between the number of observed and the number of expected deaths.
- If the lower confidence limit is above 100, then the number of observed deaths is significantly higher than expected, and it is unlikely that the excess is merely a chance occurrence.
- If the upper confidence limit is below 100, the number of observed deaths is significantly fewer than expected.
- If a confidence interval is quite wide, regardless of what the limits are, more data are required or the data should be grouped before any conclusion can be reached. Although no clear-cut rules specify what constitutes a "wide" range, a range of 50 or more is excessive.

In the following example (Table 11–2), it is somewhat difficult to decide whether the result is significant, because the upper confidence limit is barely above 100. It can be concluded that the SMR seems moderately, although not significantly, low at the 95 percent confidence level. A strict interpretation is that it is not significant.

Table 11–2 Observed and Expected Deaths from Heart Disease for County A, by Age Group, 1990–1994

Age Group	Observed Deaths	Expected Deaths
20–29	16	16
30–39	18	20
40–49	22	18
50–59	51	56
60–69	55	72
70–79	62	64
80–89	22	28
90 +	14	15
TOTAL	260	289

$$\text{SMR} = \frac{260}{289} \times 100 = 89.97$$

$$\text{SE} = \frac{\text{SMR}}{\sqrt{d}} = \frac{89.97}{\sqrt{260}} = 5.58$$

95 percent confidence interval,

$$\text{CI}_{95\%} = 89.97 \pm (1.96 \times 5.58)$$

Upper limit $= 89.97 + 10.94 = 100.91$

Lower limit $= 89.97 - 10.94 = 79.03$

$$\text{CI} = 79 \text{ to } 101$$

Chi Square Test

The chi square or "goodness-of-fit" test makes it possible to compare an observed frequency with an expected frequency distribution. The formula for chi square is

$$\chi^2 = \Sigma \frac{(O - E)^2}{E}$$

where

O = observed deaths
E = expected deaths

Table 11–3 presents the calculation of chi square for the data presented in Table 11–2. The computed chi square value of 6.97 is compared with a tabular value of chi square with $(k - r)$ degrees of freedom, where k equals the number of categories that can be calculated for $(O - E)^2/E$ (i.e., the number of age groups in this example), and r equals the number of restrictions (quantities) that were determined from observed data and used in calculating the expected frequencies.

In most cases in which the expected frequencies are determined by using the chi square test (or the SMR), the only observed quantity involved in calculating the expected frequencies is the population (P_1). Under these circumstances, the degree of freedom is $(k - 1)$. However, in the example in Table 11–3 there are no restrictions, as the expected frequencies were not calculated from the observed data but from a standard.

There are eight degrees of freedom (eight age groups). The value of chi square for eight degrees of freedom at the 95 percent level is 15.507.[*] If the calculated value (6.97) is less than the tabular value, as is the case here, then it can be said that there is no significant difference between the observed and the expected deaths. If the calculated value were greater than the tabular value, the difference would be significant. Both methods (i.e., the SMR and the χ^2) provide the same result.

Table 11–3 Calculations of Chi Square for Observed and Expected Deaths from Heart Disease for County A, 1990–1994

Age Group	Observed Deaths	Expected Deaths	$\dfrac{(O - E)^2}{E}$
20–29	16	16	0.00
30–39	18	20	0.20
40–49	22	18	0.89
50–59	51	56	0.45
60–69	55	72	4.01
70–79	62	64	0.06
80–89	22	28	1.29
90+	14	15	0.07
TOTAL	260	289	6.97

$$\chi^2 = 0.00 + 0.20 + 0.89 + 0.45 + 4.01 + 0.06 + 1.29 + 0.07$$
$$\chi^2 = 6.97$$

---

[*]A value obtained by looking at the χ^2 probability distribution.

QUALITY IMPROVEMENT MEASUREMENT AND SMALL AREA ANALYSIS

When analyzing small areas, especially for epidemiology/needs assessment type problems and quality improvement, there are specific methods to be used when the analysis involves:

- counts
- rates
- proportions
- ratios, and
- indexes.

Depending on the assumptions related to the use of the statistical tests and the nature of the data used, it is possible that some of the tests may be appropriate for analyzing hospital utilization statistics (i.e., use rates). If the assumptions are met, then we have a "green light" for analysis.

Small Area Analysis—Hypothesis Testing

To compare one geographic area, time period, or age group with a standard, there are specific tests based on counts, rates, and proportions to use to test the hypotheses of no difference between the two categories. Listed in Table 11–4 is a summary of these statistics for counts, rates, and proportions. Using these tests, we show how they may be applied to the analysis of small areas. Additionally, the use of confidence intervals is demonstrated as a method for assessing the significance of small area variations. The formulas for determining confidence limits for counts, rates, and proportions are also shown in Table 11–4.

Small Area Analysis—Confidence Interval Estimation

Assessing confidence intervals for a single parameter for a small area is an acceptable alternative to significance testing if small proportions or low counts bring into question the approximation model used (i.e., binomial, Poisson, normal), specifically the assumptions concerning the sampling distribution of proportion and counts that are approximated by the binomial and Poisson distributions, respectively. Recall that the binomial and Poisson distributions were the probability models used for the different types of attributes control charts also.

Table 11–4 Small Area Analysis: Area/Standard Comparisons (One-Sample Tests)*

Hypothesis Test On	Test Statistic	Confidence Interval†
One count	$z = \dfrac{x - \mu_0}{\sqrt{\mu_0}}$	$x \pm 1.96\sqrt{x}$
One rate	$z = \dfrac{r - \theta_0}{\sqrt{\theta_0/\text{PYRS}}}$	$r \pm 1.96\sqrt{\dfrac{r}{\text{PYRS}}}$
Alternative rate‡		$\dfrac{1000}{n}(d \pm 1.96\sqrt{d})$
		$SE = \dfrac{r}{\sqrt{d}}$
One proportion	$z = \dfrac{p - \pi_0}{\sqrt{\dfrac{\pi_0(1 - \pi_0)}{n}}}$	$p \pm 1.96\sqrt{\dfrac{p(1-p)}{n}}$
Many proportions§	$\chi^2 = \sum\dfrac{(O - E)^2}{E}$	

*H_0 (Null Hypothesis) = no difference between the observed area (sample) and the expected (population) standard.
†The confidence interval is a range that is expected to contain the population parameter being estimated. The level of probability may be 0.05, 0.01, or 0.001.
‡There are several alternatives to calculating confidence intervals for a rate; each is applicable. The choice to use one over the other is a personal preference.
§The χ^2 may be used for comparing one proportion or many proportions. Because this is the only test presented in this book for measuring variations in many proportions, it is, therefore, included here.

To use these distributions, some facts are essential to an appropriate evaluation of the results. Therefore,

- For *small proportions* or *low counts*, an acceptable alternative is to perform the significant test using the confidence interval approach.
- If the *null value* is included in the confidence interval, the result is equivalent to nonsignificance.
- If the *null value* is not included in the confidence interval, the result is equivalent to significance.

- For *small sample sizes*, the tests for the normal approximation to the binomial or Poisson distribution for proportions and counts, respectively, as outlined in this book may not hold; however, one may use the tables for the binomial and Poisson to determine the exact limits.
- Assessing significance using confidence intervals is a perfectly acceptable procedure and is recommended for small sample sizes (i.e., data representing small areas).

It is always necessary to construct a confidence interval when presenting data derived from a sample of a population or when presenting rates for a population. Such calculations are often based on relatively low numbers of values, and the width of the confidence interval will take this into account. If few values are used, the confidence interval will be quite wide. With a great many values, however, the confidence interval is narrower, indicating that the estimates are more accurate.

The confidence interval can be particularly illuminating for the presentation of nonsignificant results. If the *sample size is too small*, the width of the confidence interval shows clearly the large range of values compatible with the observed result and thus allows one to see the possibly important effects that would be glossed over by giving only the negative result of the significance test. If the sample size is adequate for nonsignificant results, the range covered by the confidence interval should be narrow enough to exclude the possibility of medically important effects.[5]

The probability that the true population rate is contained within the confidence interval is called the degree of confidence. The value most commonly used for the degree of confidence is 0.95, or 95 percent. This indicates that users of the data can be 95 percent confident that the true value lies within the calculated confidence interval. In other words, there is a 95 percent probability that the confidence interval includes the true value and a 5 percent probability that it does not. When a 5 percent chance of error is not acceptable, a 99 percent confidence interval is commonly used.

STATISTICAL GUIDES FOR OUTCOME ASSESSMENT AND QUALITY IMPROVEMENT MEASUREMENT IN ANALYZING SMALL AREAS

This section outlines several statistical guides to be used for evaluating small areas from a quality improvement perspective and assessing outcomes in public health practice. The guides focus on the typical tests of hypotheses and the use of confidence intervals for assessing out-of-control patterns based on defined limits from a spatial perspective. These guides are presented for counts, rates, and proportions.

Statistical Guide 1: Counts (Hypothesis Test)

A Single Count (Comparing a Small Area with a Standard)[*]

- analyzing a single count
- hypothesis test for a count
- problem: Is the number of infant deaths observed in a small area different from an expected number based on a standard (state, region, or national objective—Year 2000 objective may also be used)
- null hypothesis (H_0)

H_0: observed count = standard count (i.e., no difference in the two counts)

- test statistic[†] (normal approximation to the Poisson)
  z test

$$z = \frac{x(\text{observed count}) - x_1(\text{standard count})}{\sqrt{x_1(\text{standard count})}}$$

or

$$z = \frac{x - \mu_0}{\sqrt{\mu_0}}$$

where
  z = normal approximation to the Poisson
  x = observed count in the area
  μ_0 = standard count to be compared (expected count)

- data: infant deaths

Burke County, Georgia (1985–1994) = 62 infant deaths

Georgia (1985–1994) = 12,854 infant deaths

Expected based on standard = 50.9 infant deaths

---

[*]The comparison may be a geographic area, a time period, or an age group.

[†]Assumptions/requirements: that the count is based on independent events and that, for the z test, the count is more than 10. Also the normal approximation can be used when it is reasonable to assume that cases (events) are occurring independently and randomly in time and space. This is less likely to be true for infectious diseases and for diseases in which there is a strong evidence of clustering.

- analysis

$$z = \frac{62 - 50.9}{\sqrt{50.9}}$$

$$z = \frac{11.1}{7.1}$$

$$z = 1.56$$

- determining the expected count (standard)[*]
  1. Infant mortality is based on the number of live births.
  2. Burke County had 3,912 live births; Georgia had 988,147.
  3. Burke County has 0.00396 proportion of the state births.
  4. It would be expected that Burke County would have 0.00396 of the state infant deaths.
  5. The state had 12,854 infant deaths. Therefore,

$$\text{Expected deaths} = 0.00396 \times 12,854 = 50.9$$

- results

  Compare the "*z*" value of 1.56 to the standard normal distribution (critical value) at the 0.05 significance level. The critical value at this level is 1.96.
- interpretation

  Because 1.56 is less than 1.96, there is no significant difference between the number of infant deaths in Burke County compared with the expected number based on the state standard. That is, this one county shows no variation from the standard, so the county is within the limits established by the test using the standard as the expected.

Statistical Guide 2: Counts (Confidence Intervals)

A Single Count (Confidence Intervals for a County Representing a Small Area)

- analyzing a single count using confidence intervals

---

[*]The method used here is "using the actual number of deaths."

$$E = \frac{P_1}{P_2} \times D$$

- confidence intervals for a count draws attention to results actually obtained rather than concentrating on the decision to reject or not to reject. Confidence intervals give a range of values that at a given probability level are likely to contain the true count. Thus, the confidence interval presents the result and conveys the inherent variability in the estimate of that result
- problem: at the 95 percent confidence level, what is the range in the number of infant deaths that we can expect? That is, if the number of infant deaths in an area is assumed to be a sample in time and space, how confident are we that the sample count is reflective of the true count for that area or time period?
- confidence intervals do not require the predetermination or specifications of a null value
- test statistic
  1. For $n \leq 100$, use tables based on Poisson distribution (see Table 11–5—abridged).
  2. For $n > 100$, a normal approximation to the Poisson distribution is used:

$$x \pm 1.96\sqrt{x}$$

  where
$$x = \text{count}$$
  1.96 = critical value at the 95 percent significance level

- data: infant mortality (1985–1994)

$$\text{Burke County} = 62 \text{ infant deaths}$$

- analysis
  1. exact confidence limits per Poisson distribution table (Table 11–5—abridged)

Lower Limit	Actual	Upper Limit
47.5	62	79.5

  2. confidence limits per normal approximation formula:

$$x \pm 1.96\sqrt{x}$$
$$62 \pm 1.96(7.9)$$
$$62 \pm 15.5$$

or

Lower Limit	Actual	Upper Limit
46.5	62	77.5

Table 11–5 Exact Confidence Limits for a Poisson Count*

	95% Confidence Level	
x	x_l	x_u
56	42.302	72.721
57	43.171	73.850
58	44.042	74.978
59	44.914	76.106
60	45.786	77.232
61	46.660	78.357
62	47.535	79.481
63	48.411	80.604
64	49.288	81.727
65	50.166	82.848

*x is an observed Poisson count, x_l and x_u are the lower and upper limits for the population count.

- results

    We are 95 percent confident that the actual number of infant deaths could be as low as 47.5 (46.5) and as high as 79.5 (77.5). Thus, if we sampled another 10-year period from the same small area, we would expect that 95 percent of the time the count of infant deaths would fall between these lower and upper limits. Of course, 5 percent of the time, just by chance, the count could be outside these limits.

- interpretation

    Remembering that the expected count (50.9) calculated from the previous guide on counts was our *null value,* we can then determine if our confidence limits include the value. That is, is 50.9 located between the lower limit (47.5) and the upper limit (79.5)? If they do (and they do in this example), then the result is equivalent to nonsignificance. If the null value was not included, then the result could be considered significant. Our results obtained here verify our earlier results of no significant difference, plus we have a range of possible values the actual count could have been and still be representative of the true count.

Statistical Guide 3: Rates (Hypothesis Test)

*A Single Rate (Comparing a Small Area with a Standard)**

- analyzing a single rate

---

*The comparison may be a geographic area, a time period, or an age group.

- hypothesis test for a rate
- problem: is the infant mortality rate observed in a small area different from an expected rate based on a standard (state, region, or national objective— Year 2000 objective may be used)?
- null hypothesis

    H_0: observed rate = standard rate (i.e., no difference between the two rates)

- test statistic:[*] (normal approximation to the Poisson)
    z test

$$z = \frac{r \text{ (observed rate)} - r_1 \text{ (standard rate)}}{\sqrt{r_1 \text{ (standard rate)/population-at-risk}}}$$

or

$$z = \frac{r - \theta_0}{\sqrt{\theta_0/\text{PYRS}}}$$

where

z = normal approximation to the Poisson
r = observed rate in the area
θ_0 = standard rate to be compared
PYRS = person years-at-risk (population-at-risk), the denominator for the observed rate

- data: infant mortality rate
    1. observed rate

        Burke County, Georgia (1985–1994) = 15.8 per 1,000 live births
        = 62 infant deaths
        = 3,912 live births

    2. standard rate

        Burke County, Georgia (1985–1994) = 13.0 per 1,000 live births
        = 12,854 infant deaths
        = 988,147 live births

---

[*]Assumptions/requirements: that count is based on independent events and that for the z test the count is more than 10. Also the normal approximation can be used when it is reasonable to assume that cases (events) are occurring independently and randomly in time and space. This is less likely to be true for infectious diseases and for diseases in which there is strong evidence of clustering.

- analysis

$$z = \frac{15.8 - 13.0}{\sqrt{13.0/3.912}}$$

$$z = \frac{2.8}{\sqrt{3.323}}$$

$$z = \frac{2.8}{1.82}$$

$$z = 1.54$$

Note: The population at risk must be expressed in 1,000s, because the rate is expressed per 1,000. Thus,

$$3,912/1,000 = 3.912$$

- results

  Compare the *z* value of 1.54 to the standard normal distribution (critical value) at the 0.05 significance level. The critical value at this level is 1.96.
- interpretation

  Since 1.54 is less than 1.96, there is no significant difference between the rate of infant mortality in Burke County compared with the standard rate for the state of Georgia.

  Note: The results obtained here for the rate are similar to that obtained for the counts: no significant difference. Most times, the results will be identical.

Statistical Guide 4: Rates (Confidence Intervals)

A Single Rate (Confidence Intervals for a County Representing a Small Area)

- analyzing a single rate using confidence intervals
- confidence intervals for a rate draws attention to results actually obtained rather than concentrating on the decision to reject or not to reject. Confidence intervals give a range of values that at a given probability level are likely to contain the true rate. Thus, the confidence interval presents the result and conveys the inherent variability in the estimate of that result
- problem: at the 95 percent confidence level, what is the range in the infant mortality rate that we can expect? That is, if the rate in an area is assumed to

be a sample in time and space, how confident are we that the sample rate is reflective of the true rate for that area or time period?

- confidence intervals do not require the predetermination or specification of a null value
- test statistic
  1. For $n \leq 100$ (i.e., if numerator of rate is based on fewer than 100 events), use tables based on Poisson distribution.
  2. For $n \geq 100$, a normal approximation to the Poisson distribution is used.

$$r \pm 1.96 \sqrt{\frac{r}{\text{PYRS}}}$$

where

r = observed rate for the area
1.96 = critical value at the 95 percent significance level
PYRS = person years-at-risk (population-at-risk—the denominator on which the observed rate is based)

- data: infant mortality rate (1985–1994)
  1. observed rate

Burke County, Georgia = 15.8 per 1,000 live births

= 62 infant deaths

= 3,912 live births

  2. standard rate

Georgia = 13.0 per 1,000 live births

= 12,854 infant deaths

= 988,147 live births

- analysis
  1. Exact confidence limits per Poisson distribution table (see abridged Table 11–5):

Lower Limit	Actual	Upper Limit
$47.5 / 15.8 = 3.01$	15.8 (62 deaths)	$79.5 / 15.8 = 5.03$
12.8		20.8

- confidence limits per normal approximation formula[*]

$$r \pm 1.96 \sqrt{\frac{r}{\text{PYRS}}}$$

$$15.8 \pm 1.96 \sqrt{\frac{15.8}{3.912}}$$

$$15.8 \pm 1.96(2.0097)$$

$$15.8 \pm 3.94$$

Lower Limit	Actual	Upper Limit
11.86	15.8	19.74

- results

We are 95 percent confident that the actual rate of infant mortality could be as low as 11.86 (12.8—exact) and as high as 19.74 (20.8—exact). Thus, if we sampled another time period from the same small area, we would expect that 95 percent of the time the rate would fall between these upper and lower limits. Of course, 5 percent of the time, just by chance, the rate could be outside these limits.

- interpretation

Remembering that the expected rate (13.0) noted in the previous guide on rates was or could be our *null value,* we can then determine if our confidence limits include the value. If they do (and they do in this example), then the result is equivalent to nonsignificance. If the *null value* was not included, then the result could be considered significant. The results obtained here verify our earlier results of no significant difference, plus we have a range of possible values that the actual rate could have been and could still be representative of the true rate. *This is an important aspect to the evaluation of variation of events in small area analysis.*

Statistical Guide 5

When Rates Are Not Independent

The two previous guides were based on the fact that the two rates were independent. However, in public health practice there are situations in which the rates

---

[*]*Note:* The population-at-risk (PYRS) must be expressed in 1,000s because the rate is expressed per 1,000. Thus,

$$3{,}912/1{,}000 = 3.912$$

are not independent. Because this is the case, the method for calculating differences in rates when they are not independent must be altered.

- high frequency events (≥ 100)

    When comparing an observed rate with another rate or a standard rate that may not be independent, a slightly modified formula is needed:

$$\mu = (r - s) \sqrt{\frac{n}{s - s^2}}$$

where
    r = the observed rate or rate to be compared
    s = the standard rate (e.g., in the state, region, nation)
    n = the denominator (population on which the rate is based)

The formula is calculated as follows:
1. Square the standard rate s. Change all rates to a per-person basis by dividing by the rate's denominator.
2. Subtract the square of s from s: $s - s^2$.
3. Divide the denominator on which the rate is based, n, by the difference of

    $s - s^2$: $\dfrac{n}{s - s^2}$.

4. Find the square root of the quotient from the last step: $\sqrt{\dfrac{n}{s - s^2}}$.

5. Subtract the standard rate s from the observed rate, r: $r - s$.
6. Multiply the square root in the fourth step by the difference in the fifth

    step: $\mu = (r - s) \sqrt{\dfrac{n}{s - s^2}}$.

If μ exceeds 1.96, it can be concluded that the rate differs significantly at the 95 percent confidence level from the standard rate with which it is compared. If it exceeds 2.58, it is significantly different at the 99 percent level.

If, for example, a county has a population of 16,400 persons and a death rate of 20.9 per 1,000, the objective may be to find out whether the county rate is significantly different from the state rate of 16.8 per 1,000. These rates are not independent since the events that were used to calculate the observed rate are also included in the calculation of the standard rate (i.e., the county is a subset of the state). Thus,

Observed rate: r = 20.9 per 1,000
Standard rate: s = 16.8 per 1,000

Population (denominator n on which the observed rate is based) = 16,400. By applying the above formula

$$\mu = (r - s)\sqrt{\frac{n}{s - s^2}}$$

we set the following six steps:

1. $(0.0168)^2 = 0.0168 \times 0.0168 = 0.000282$
2. $0.0168 - 0.000282 = 0.016518$
3. $\dfrac{16,400}{0.016518} = 992,856.27$
4. $\sqrt{992,856.27} = 996.42173$
5. $0.0209 - 0.0168 = 0.0041$
6. $0.0041 \times 996.42173 = 4.09$ (μ).

Because the value of 4.09 (μ) is greater than 2.58, it can be concluded that the difference between the rates is significant at the 99 percent level. In other words, there is 99 percent confidence that the county death rate is higher than the state death rate.

• low frequency events (at least one rate is based on less than 100 events)

When rates are based on a very low number of events (e.g., births, deaths, cases), the actual number of events is used instead of the rate:

$$\mu = \frac{(o - e)}{\sqrt{e}}$$

where
o = the observed number(s) to be compared
e = the standard number (e.g., state, region, nation)

This formula is calculated as follows:

1. Find the square root of the standard number e: $\sqrt{e}$.
2. Subtract the standard number e from the observed number o: $o - e$.
3. Divide the difference between the observed and standard numbers (step 2) by the square root of e: $\dfrac{(o - e)}{\sqrt{e}}$.

Thus, to determine whether a county infant mortality rate is significantly higher than the state infant mortality rate,

$$\mu = \frac{(o-e)}{\sqrt{e}}$$

where
$o = 20.2$ per 1,000 (65 deaths)
$e = 17.5$ per 1,000 (56 deaths)

Thus,

$$\sqrt{56} = 7.48$$

$$65 - 56 = 9$$

$$\frac{9}{7.48} = 1.20$$

Because the value 1.20 is less than 2.58, it can be concluded that the two rates are not significantly different at the 99 percent confidence level.

Summary—Analyzing Small Areas (One Sample)

A summary of methods for analyzing small areas is provided for (1) counts, (2) rates, and (3) proportions.

Figure 11–1 gives a guide for selecting the appropriate method to use for analyzing one small area or time period or group when counts, rates, or proportions are involved. Further, Figure 11–2 gives the actual formulas used for performing the analysis using counts, rates, and proportions for small areas. Not all methods were discussed in this section; however, in the subsequent section those methods not discussed for one sample are presented for the two or more sample situations.

COMPARING TWO SMALL AREAS

In epidemiologic/needs assessment studies focusing on quality improvement and outcomes measurement, a comparison of two areas is common. A health agency may wish to determine if their geographic area is statistically different from another area. To analyze this type of problem, we usually involve counts (cases), rates, proportions, and the ratio of the two rates. This section provides statistical guides for the purpose of analyzing data from two small areas. Table 11–6 provides an overview of the statistical tests by which we test the null hypothesis that the two areas are not different. Further, Table 11–6 provides the formulas for computing the confidence intervals when data from the two areas are being compared.

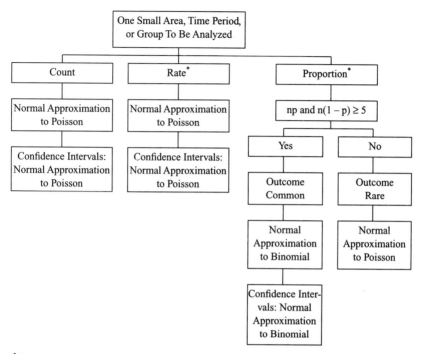

*When rates are not independent, see statistical guide number five for appropriate methods.

Figure 11–1 Selection Guide for Quality Improvement and Small Area Analysis—A Reference Chart for One Sample Situation

---

Statistical Guide 6

Counts: Comparing Two Small Areas*

- analyzing two counts (comparing one group or area with another)
- hypothesis test for the difference between two counts
- problem: is the number of AMI deaths observed in Burke County different from the total cancer deaths observed in Burke County during 1985–1994?

---

*If two counts are to be compared directly, then the counts must be based on the same time period or same underlying distribution in space or time. If this is not the case, then the counts must be converted to rates to correct for the different periods of observation, and it is the rates that must be compared. For the methods presented here, the two counts should be more than 10.

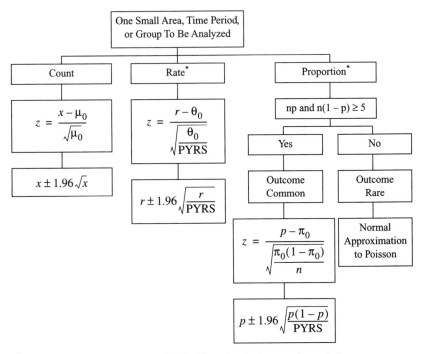

*When rates are not independent, see statistical guide number five for appropriate methods.

Figure 11–2 Selection Guide for Quality Improvement and Small Area Analysis—Formulas for One Sample Situation

- null hypothesis

  H_0: observed number (AMI) = observed number (total cancer) (i.e., no difference in the number of deaths between the two classifications)

- test statistic (normal approximation to Poisson)
  z test

$$z = \frac{x_1 \ (\text{observed count}) - x_2 \ (\text{observed count})}{\sqrt{x_1 \ (\text{observed count}) + x_2 \ (\text{observed count})}}$$

or

$$z = \frac{x_1 - x_2}{\sqrt{x_1 + x_2}}$$

Table 11–6 Small Area Analysis: Comparing Two Small Areas (Two-Sample Tests)

Comparison of:		Hypothesis Test*	Confidence Interval†
Independent counts	(z test)	$z = \dfrac{x_1 - x_2}{\sqrt{x_1 - x_2}}$	$(x_1 - x_2) \pm 1.96 \sqrt{x_1 - x_2}$
Independent rates	(z test)	$z = \dfrac{r_1 - r_2}{\sqrt{\dfrac{r}{\text{PYRS}_1} + \dfrac{r}{\text{PYRS}_2}}}$	$(r_1 - r_2) \pm 1.96 \sqrt{\dfrac{r_1}{\text{PYRS}_1} + \dfrac{r_2}{\text{PYRS}_2}}$
	(z test)	$r = \dfrac{\text{PYRS}_1(r_1) + \text{PYRS}_2(r_2)}{\text{PYRS}_1 + \text{PYRS}_2}$	
Independent proportions		$z = \dfrac{p_1 - p_2}{\sqrt{\dfrac{pq}{n_1} + \dfrac{pq}{n_2}}}$	$(p_1 - p_2) \pm 1.96 \sqrt{\dfrac{p_1 q_1}{n_1} + \dfrac{p_2 q_2}{n_2}}$
		$p = \dfrac{n_1 p_1 + n_2 p_2}{n_1 + n_2}$	
	(χ^2 test)	$\chi^2 = \sum \dfrac{(O - E)^2}{E}$	

*H_0 (null hypothesis): no difference in the two populations from which the samples are selected.
†The confidence interval is a range that is expected to contain a low to high range comparing one sample (region) with another sample (region).

---

where

 z = normal approximation to the Poisson
 x_1 = observed count for area 1 or time period
 x_2 = observed count for area 2 or time period

- data

 AMI: Burke County, Georgia (1985–1994) = 306 deaths (x_1)
 total cancer: Burke County, Georgia (1985–1994) = 344 deaths (x_2)
- analysis

$$z = \frac{306 - 344}{\sqrt{306 + 344}}$$

$$z = \frac{-38}{25.5}$$

$$z = -1.49$$

- results

    Compare the z value of -1.49 to the standard normal distribution (critical value) at the 0.05 significance level. The critical value at this level is ± 1.96.

- interpretation

    Because -1.49 is less than -1.96, there is no significant difference between the AMI deaths (1985–1994) for Burke County and total cancer deaths (1985–1994) for Burke County.

Statistical Guide 7

Rates: Comparing Rates between Two Small Areas

- analyzing two rates (comparing one small area with another)
- hypothesis test for the difference between rates for two areas
- problem: is the infant mortality rate observed in one small area different from the observed mortality rate from another area?
- null hypothesis

    H_0: observed rate (area 1) = observed rate (area 2) (i.e., no difference in the two rates)

- test statistic (normal approximation to Poisson)
    z test

$$z = \frac{\text{rate (area 1)} - \text{rate (area 2)}}{\sqrt{\dfrac{\text{pooled rate}}{\text{population-at-risk (area 1)}} + \dfrac{\text{pooled rate}}{\text{population-at-risk (area 2)}}}}$$

or

$$z = \frac{r_1 - r_2}{\sqrt{\dfrac{r}{\text{PYRS}_1} + \dfrac{r}{\text{PYRS}_2}}}$$

where

z = normal approximation to Poisson
r_1 = rate for area 1
r_2 = rate for area 2

        r = pooled rate (is equivalent to a weighted average of the two observed rates weighted by the person years or population-at-risk [see Exhibit 11–1 for calculating])

    $PYRS_1$ = person-years-at-risk (population-at-risk for area 1)

    $PYRS_2$ = person-years-at-risk (population-at-risk for area 2)

- data: infant mortality rates

  1. area 1

    Burke County, Georgia (1985–1994) = 15.8 per 1,000 live births

                     = 62 infant deaths

                     = 3,912 live births

  2. area 2

    Augusta District, Georgia (1985–1994) = 13.6 per 1,000 live births

                     = 900 infant deaths

                     = 66,067 live births

- analysis

$$z = \frac{15.8 - 13.6}{\sqrt{\dfrac{13.7}{3.912} + \dfrac{13.7}{66.1}}}$$

$$z = \frac{2.2}{\sqrt{3.5 + 0.21}}$$

Exhibit 11–1 How To Calculate the Pooled Rate

Note: The pooled rate is calculated using

$$r = \frac{PYRS_1(r_1) + PYRS_2(r_2)}{PYRS_1 + PYRS_2}$$

$$r = \frac{3,912(15.8) + 66,067(13.6)}{3,912 + 66,067}$$

$$r = 13.7$$

$$z = \frac{2.2}{1.9}$$

$$z = 1.15$$

- results

    Compare the z value of 1.15 to the standard normal distribution (critical value) at the 0.05 significance level. The critical value at this level is 1.96.

- interpretation

    Because 1.15 is less than 1.96, there is no significant difference between the two areas.

- determining confidence intervals for rates in this example

    1. test statistic: normal approximation to Poisson

$$CI = (r_1 - r_2) \pm 1.96 \sqrt{\frac{r_1}{PYRS_1} + \frac{r_2}{PYRS_2}}$$

$$CI = (15.8 - 13.6) \pm 1.96 \sqrt{\frac{15.8}{3.912} + \frac{13.6}{66.067}}$$

$$CI = 2.2 \pm 1.96 \sqrt{4.04 + 0.206}$$

$$CI = 2.2 \pm 1.96(2.06)$$

$$CI = 2.2 \pm 4.04$$

$$CI = -1.84 \text{ to } 6.24$$

2. interpretation

    At the 95 percent level of confidence, Burke County, Georgia, could have an infant mortality rate ranging from a figure of 1.84 per 1,000 lower than Augusta to 6.24 per 1,000 higher.

Statistical Guide 8

Ratio of Two Rates—Using Confidence Intervals To Determine Significance

When comparing an observed rate with an arbitrarily set standard, goal, or target value, the confidence interval for the observed rate provides the significance of the difference. If the standard is included in the confidence interval of the observed rate, there is no significant difference at the level of confidence chosen. The situation is somewhat more complex, however, when comparing rates of two different areas or of two different times for the same area. This requires a direct extension of the concept of a confidence interval. The objective is to determine whether a difference between the rates is significant or whether it is caused solely by random effects. Different methods must be used, depending on whether the rates are independent.

Two rates are independent when they do not include any of the same observations of events (e.g., births, deaths) in their numerator. Thus, rates from overlapping time periods or areas are not independent. For example, rates from a county and the state that the county is in are not independent; rates from two different counties are independent.

To determine whether there is a significant difference between two independent rates, the confidence interval for the ratio between the two rates or the difference between the two independent rates is used.

- ratio of two rates. The ratio is defined as

$$R = \frac{r_1}{r_2}$$

where
R = ratio
r_1 = rate for area 1 or period 1
r_2 = rate for area 2 or period 2

The 95 percent confidence interval for the ratio is defined as

$$R \pm 1.96R \sqrt{\frac{1}{d_1} + \frac{1}{d_2}}$$

where
d_1 = number of events for area 1 or period 1 (i.e., the rate numerator)
d_2 = number of events for area 2 or period 2

To establish a significant difference, it must be determined whether the confidence interval contains the figure 1. If it does not, it can be stated that the two rates are significantly different. If the interval does contain the figure 1, it cannot be concluded that there is a significant difference. Kleinman provided the example in Table 11–7.[6]

$$R = \frac{40}{25} = 1.6$$

- The 95 percent confidence interval is

Table 11–7 Data for Calculating the Ratio of Two Rates

Years	Number of Infant Deaths	Number of Live Births	Infant Mortality Rate per 1,000 Live Births
1961–1965	200	5,000	40
1966–1970	100	4,000	25

Source: Reprinted from J.C. Kleinman, "Infant Mortality," *Statistical Notes for Health Planners*, Vol. 2, 1976, National Center for Health Statistics.

$$\text{CI} = R \pm 1.96R \sqrt{\frac{1}{d_1} + \frac{1}{d_2}}$$

$$\text{CI} = 1.6 \pm 1.96(1.6) \sqrt{\frac{1}{200} + \frac{1}{100}}$$

$$\text{CI} = 1.6 \pm 1.96(1.6) \sqrt{0.015}$$

$$\text{CI} = 1.6 \pm 0.384$$

$$\text{CI} = 1.216 \text{ to } 1.984$$

Thus, the infant mortality rate for 1961–1965 can be said, with 95 percent confidence, to be from 1.22 to 1.98 times the rate for 1966–1970. Because the interval does not contain 1, there is a statistically significant difference in the area's infant mortality rate between the two time periods. If the interval did contain 1, there would not be a statistically significant difference.

A Selection Guide for Analyzing Small Areas (Two Samples)

Test selection to evaluate variation in small areas can be a difficult task. Statistical guides (Figures 11–3 and 11–4) are offered to ease the decision making in selecting appropriate tests when analyzing counts, rates, proportions, or ratios for two or more groups or small areas. The cornerstone of small area analysis is variation. Thus, the significance of the variation must be assessed.

CONCLUSION

The analysis of small areas is of paramount importance in the assessment of outcomes in the quality improvement process. As managed care expands, the

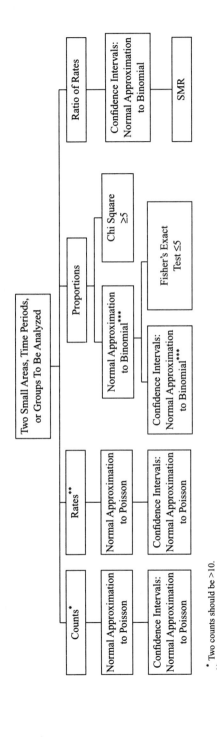

* Two counts should be >10.
** When rates are not independent, see Statistical Guide 8 for appropriate methods.
*** 1. Total sample size >20.
2. n_1p, n_2p, n_1q, n_2q all >5 for sample sizes between 20–40.
3. Valid for total sample size that is in both groups ≥40.

Figure 11–3 Selection Guide for Quality Improvement and Small Area Analysis—A Reference Chart for Two Sample Selections

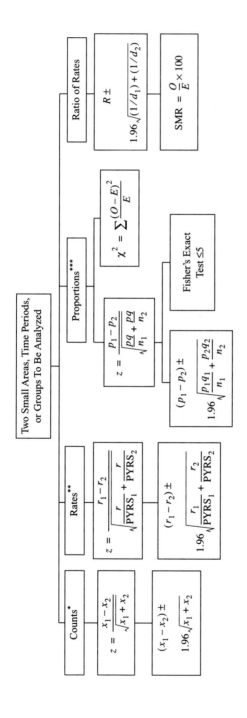

Figure 11–4 Selection Guide for Quality Improvement and Small Area Analysis—Formulas for Two Sample Selections

* Two counts should be >10.

** When rates are not independent, see Statistical Guide 8 for appropriate methods.

*** 1. Total sample size >20.

2. n_1p, n_2p, n_1q, n_2q all >5 for sample sizes between 20–40.

3. Valid for total sample size that is in both groups ≥40.

need for program-based outcome evaluations and the analysis of small areas in the quality improvement environment is critical. This chapter has provided these statistical tools for the public health analyst to provide quality improvement measurement for small areas. Further, public health analysts can use many of the small area analysis techniques and measurements to focus on the core public health functions. The concept of a rate and population-at-risk are central to the analysis of problems related to the management of health services, the understanding of small area variation, and the analysis of communities for monitoring the improvement of outcomes. This chapter has provided the tools and methods for epidemiologic investigation of small areas and the quality improvement measurement for monitoring the effective delivery of health services and improving the process.

The epidemiologic analysis of small areas and the measurement of rates and their significance allow administrators to determine the magnitude of a problem, what warrants further analysis, how to monitor a process to hold the gains, and to identify potential special causes for focusing on improvement. Certainly, a much more practical use for these statistical and epidemiologic methods is to monitor current conditions and establish where improvement can occur in the future. Finally, determining the significance of the results obtained from small area analysis and quality improvement measurement may be more of a practical decision than a statistical one.

NOTES

1. L.D. Stamp, *Some Aspects of Medical Geography* (Oxford University Press, 1964), 16.

2. J.D. Clark, "Variations in Michigan Hospital Use Rates: Do Physician and Hospital Characteristics Provide the Explanation," *Social Science and Medicine* 30, no. 1 (1990): 67–82.

3. Center for the Evaluative Clinical Sciences, Dartmouth Medical School, *The Dartmouth Atlas of Health Care* (Chicago: American Hospital Publishing, 1996).

4. M. Spitzer and P. Caper, "Quality Measurement through Small-Area Analysis Techniques," in *Innovations in Health Care Quality Measurement*, ed. P.L. Spath (Chicago: American Hospital Publishing, 1989), 11–21.

5. L.E. Daly et al., *Interpretation and Uses of Medical Statistics*, 4th ed. (Oxford: Blackwell Scientific Publications, 1991), 136.

6. J.C. Kleinman, "Infant Mortality," *Statistical Notes for Health Planners*. Vol 2 (Washington, DC: National Center for Health Statistics, July 1976), 4.

Index